Waterborne Pathogens

AWWA MANUAL M48

First Edition

FOUNDED 1881

American Water Works Association

Figures

This page intentionally blank.

Tables

This page intentionally blank.

Preface

Waterborne pathogens can cause life-threatening disease in the immunosuppressed populations of the world and illness in the general population. Reports in print and electronic media of recent waterborne outbreaks and emerging pathogens have expanded public awareness of water quality issues. This awareness places greater demands on government agencies and utilities to effectively inform the public about waterborne agents and related health issues. If outbreaks do occur, having accurate information available is a critical need.

The Organisms in Water Committee of the American Water Works Association prepared this manual for water utility management, water quality, and public relations personnel to use as a reference tool. The manual provides scientific information in a concise, readable format that will be helpful to media, city and state government, and water customers who inquire about waterborne pathogenic organisms. Public health and environmental workers will also find it a convenient reference.

This manual includes chapters on waterborne disease outbreaks, water quality in treatment and distribution systems, water quality monitoring, sampling and testing, and sections for organisms classified as parasite, bacteria, or virus. Each organism is described in terms of its taxonomic classification and biology, the disease it causes, its mode of transmission, its occurrence, the effectiveness of water treatment methods in controlling it, and monitoring recommendations. Each chapter has a reference section, and a detailed glossary is included at the end of the manual.

Chapters were selected in consultation with Paul Berger, US Environmental Protection Agency (USEPA) Office of Ground Water and Drinking Water; Barbara Herwaldt, Centers for Disease Control and Prevention; Gary Logsdon, Black & Veatch; Jim Lozier, CH2M Hill; Robert Renner, American Water Works Association; Stuart Smith, Smith-Comeskey, Ltd.; and the Organisms in Water Committee.

Pathogenic organisms reviewed in this manual have been identified in epidemiological investigations of waterborne outbreaks or have the potential to cause such outbreaks. Future editions of this manual will undoubtedly expand this list of waterborne pathogens, as improved detection and identification breakthroughs identify newly emerging or reemerging microbial pathogens.

This is the first edition of the Waterborne Pathogens Manual. The American Water Works Association and the Organisms in Water Committee would appreciate any comments on the manual. Contact the AWWA Water Quality Engineer at (303) 794–7711, 6666 W. Quincy Ave., Denver, CO 80235.

This page intentionally blank.

Acknowledgments

Chapter authors were recruited for their scientific expertise from various fields, including university, state health, and water quality laboratories; drinking water utilities; and federal health and environmental protection agencies. Authors represent North America and the United Kingdom.

Manual Participants

Steering Committee

Marilyn M. Marshall, Manual Chair, University of Arizona, Tucson, Ariz.
Morteza Abbaszadegan, Virus Section Editor, American Water Works Service Company, Belleview, Ill.
Edwin E. Geldreich, Bacteria Section Editor, Cincinnati, Ohio
David Fredericksen, Parasite Section Editor, Upper Mohawk Valley Regional Water Board, Utica, N.Y.

Authors

Section I: Introduction to Water Quality

Waterborne Disease Outbreaks: Gunther F. Craun, Global Consulting for Environmental Health, Staunton, Va., and Rebecca L. Calderon, US Environmental Protection Agency, Research Triangle Park, N.C.
Water Quality in Source Water, Treatment, and Distribution Systems: Kim R. Fox, US Environmental Protection Agency—WSWRD, NRMRL, Cincinnati, Ohio, and Donald J. Reasoner, US Environmental Protection Agency—WSWRD, NRMRL, Cincinnati, Ohio
Water Quality Monitoring, Sampling, and Testing: Jon Bloemker, Michigan Department of Environmental Quality, Lansing, Mich., and Kevin R. Gertig, Fort Collins Water Utility, Fort Collins, Colo.

Section II: Introduction to Bacterial Pathogenic Agents

Acinetobacter: Mic Stewart, Metropolitan Water District of Southern California, LaVerne, Calif.
Aeromonas: Nelson P. Moyer, University of Iowa, Iowa City, Iowa
Campylobacter: Colin R. Fricker, Thames Water Utilities plc, Reading, Berkshire, England
Cyanobacteria: David W. Fredericksen, Upper Mohawk Valley Regional Water Board, Utica, N.Y., and Edwin E. Geldreich, Cincinnati, Ohio
Escherichia coli: Eugene W. Rice, US Environmental Protection Agency, Cincinnati, Ohio
Flavobacterium: Edwin E. Geldreich, Cincinnati, Ohio
Heterotrophic Bacteria: Pierre Payment, Institut Armand Frappier, Laval, Qué.
Klebsiella: Edwin E. Geldreich, Cincinnati, Ohio
Legionella: Nancy H. Hall, University of Iowa, Iowa City, Iowa
Mycobacterium avium Complex: Mark W. LeChevallier, American Water Works Service Company, Voorhees, N.J.
Pseudomonas: Edwin E. Geldreich, Cincinnati, Ohio

Salmonella: Terry C. Covert, US Environmental Protection Agency, Cincinnati, Ohio
Serratia: Edwin E. Geldreich, Cincinnati, Ohio
Shigella: Nelson P. Moyer, University of Iowa, Iowa City, Iowa
Staphylococcus: Edwin E. Geldreich, Cincinnati, Ohio
Vibrio cholerae: Gary A. Toranzos and Alan Toro, Universidad de Puerto Rico, Rio Piedras, Puerto Rico
Yersinia: Colin R. Fricker, Thames Water Utilities plc, Reading, Berkshire, England

Section III: Introduction to Parasitic Pathogenic Agents

Acanthamoeba spp.: Govidina S. Visvesvara and Hercules de Moura, Centers for Disease Control and Prevention, Atlanta, Ga.
Ascaris lumbricoides: Huw Smith, Tony Grimason, SPDL, Stobhill NHS Trust, Glasgow, Scotland, and Celia Holland, Trinity College N. of Dublin, Ireland
Balantidium coli: Lynne S. Garcia, University of California at Los Angeles Medical Center, Los Angeles, Calif.
Blastocystis hominis: Lynne S. Garcia, University of California at Los Angeles Medical Center, Los Angeles, Calif.
Cryptosporidium parvum: Charles R. Sterling and Marilyn M. Marshall, University of Arizona, Tucson, Ariz.
Cyclospora cayetanensis: Ynés Ortega, University of Arizona, Tucson, Ariz.
Dracunculus medinensis: M. Dale Little, Tulane School of Public Health and Tropical Medicine, New Orleans, La.
Entamoeba histolytica: William Keene, Oregon Health Department, Portland, Ore.
Giardia lamblia: Frank W. Schaefer, III, US Environmental Protection Agency, Cincinnati, Ohio
Gnathostoma spinigerum: M. Dale Little, Tulane School of Public Health and Tropical Medicine, New Orleans, La.
Isospora belli: Lynne S. Garcia, University of California at Los Angeles Medical Center, Los Angeles, Calif.
Microsporidia: Ann Cali, Rutgers University, Newark, N.J.
Naegleria fowleri: Govidina S. Visvesvara, Centers for Disease Control, Atlanta, Ga.
Schistosomatidae: Harvey Blankespoor, Utica, N.Y.
Spirometra mansonoides: M. Dale Little, Tulane School of Public Health and Tropical Medicine, New Orleans, La.
Taenia solium: David W. Fredericksen, Upper Mohawk Valley Regional Water Board, Utica, N.Y.
Toxoplasma gondii: J.P. Dubey, US Department of Agriculture—ARS, LPSI, Beltsville, Md.
Trichuris trichiura: Huw Smith and Tony Grimson, SPDL, Stobhill NHS Trust Glasgow, Scotland, and Celia Holland, Trinity College N. of Dublin, Ireland

Section IV: Introduction to Viral Pathogenic Agents

Adenoviruses: Carlos Enriquez, University of Arizona, Tucson, Ariz.
Astroviruses: John E. Hermann, University of Massachusetts, Worcester, Mass.
Caliciviruses: Christon J. Hurst, US Environmental Protection Agency, Cincinnati, Ohio
Enteroviruses: Charles P. Gerba, University of Arizona, Tucson, Ariz.

Hepatitis A: Mark Sobsey, University of North Carolina, Chapel Hill, N.C.

Reoviruses: Syed A. Sattar and V. Susan Springthorpe, University of Ottawa, Ottawa, Ontario, Canada

Rotaviruses: Morteza Abbaszadegan, American Water Works Service Company, Belleville, Ill.

Small, Round, Structured Viruses (Human Caliciviruses): Kellogg Schwab, Baylor College of Medicine, Houston, Texas

Organisms in Water Committee

This manual has been developed under the auspices and support of the American Water Works Association's Organisms in Water Committee:

M. Abbaszadegan, American Water Works Service Company, Belleville, Ill.

J.L. Clancy, Clancy Environmental Consultants, Inc., St. Albans, Vt.

R. DeLeon, Metropolitan Water District of Southern California, La Verne, Calif.

M. Eisenstein, Johnson State College, Johnson, Vt.

D.W. Fredericksen, Upper Mohawk Valley Regional Water Board, Utica, N.Y.

C.R. Fricker, *Chair*, Thames Water Utilities, Berkshire, UK

N.H. Hall, University of Iowa, Iowa City, Iowa

C.M. Hancock, CH Diagnostic and Consulting, Loveland, Colo.

M.M. Marshall, University of Arizona, Tucson, Ariz.

G.A. McFeters, Montana State University, Bozeman, Mont.

D.J. Reasoner, US Environmental Protection Agency—WSWRD, NRMRL, Cincinnati, Ohio

W.J. Robertson, Health Canada, Ottawa, Ontario, Canada

F.W. Schaefer, III, US Environmental Protection Agency, Cincinnati, Ohio

S.A. Schaub, US Environmental Protection Agency, Laurel, Md.

C.D. Smith, Charlotte Smith and Associates, Orinda, Calif.

Special thanks are due to Jennifer Clancy, for the initial momentum for the project, to Marilyn Marshall whose dedication to the project has brought it to completion, and to the section editors Edwin E. Geldreich, David W. Fredericksen, Morteza Abbaszadegan, and Keith Hancock.

This page intentionally blank.

Section I

Introduction to Water Quality

Waterborne Disease Outbreaks: Their Causes, Problems, and Challenges to Treatment Barriers

Water Quality in Source Water, Treatment, and Distribution Systems

Water Quality Monitoring, Sampling, and Testing

The theme used by the Big Thompson Watershed Forum, "The future of water quality is in our hands," is an apt message for our world today.

Water-related stories are commonly reported on national television news—stories such as toxic algal blooms in coastal waters, waterborne disease outbreaks in major cities around the world, and efforts to protect drinking water supplies from feedlot waste. As world economies become increasingly global, waterborne diseases travel independent of national borders. For example, imported agricultural products washed with polluted waters and shipped to the United States have been associated with several waterborne disease outbreaks. These news events have political, economic, and cultural ramifications that either promote or erode water quality and its association with public health.

Although North America has generally pure and safe drinking water, utilities must be active and vigilant to reduce the likelihood of outbreaks of waterborne pathogens. The first step to ensure safe water is to assess current levels of contaminants, both chemical and microbiological, in source waters. Next, a program of protection, education, and improvements to contain these contaminants is begun. Then water treatment plant performance must be enhanced by optimizing treatment processes, and the distribution system must be closely monitored to provide high-quality water to the customer. In-house, private, public health, and university laboratories can help implement and maintain proper sampling techniques and monitoring strategies necessary to meet the goal of providing safe drinking water. Chapters 1 through 3 provide an overview of water quality issues related specifically to waterborne pathogens.

Chapter 1

Waterborne Disease Outbreaks: Their Causes, Problems, and Challenges to Treatment Barriers

Gunther F. Craun and Rebecca L. Calderon

In the United States, state and local public health agencies are responsible for detecting outbreaks, monitoring disease, and performing epidemiological investigations of suspected waterborne outbreaks. When requested, the US Environmental Protection Agency (USEPA) and Centers for Disease Control and Prevention (CDC) help investigate waterborne outbreaks. USEPA and CDC also maintain a national waterborne disease surveillance program, periodically compiling and analyzing statistics for outbreaks that are voluntarily reported.

To be considered a waterborne outbreak, acute illness affecting two or more persons with similar symptoms must be epidemiologically associated with ingesting water (Herwaldt et al. 1992). The exception is a single case of chemical poisoning where the water was found to be chemically contaminated (i.e., infantile methemoglobinemia associated with high nitrate concentrations). During an outbreak investigation, water is usually found to be contaminated with coliform bacteria or a chemical; pathogens have been isolated from water samples in only a few outbreaks.

Most reported outbreaks are associated with water used or intended for drinking or domestic purposes from community, noncommunity, and individual water systems. Outbreaks are also associated with ingesting water not intended for consumption (e.g., the use of contaminated springs and creeks by backpackers and campers, and accidental ingestion of water while swimming). Excluded from this analysis are waterborne outbreaks that occurred on cruise ships operating from US ports.

STATISTICS

Since 1920, 1,884 waterborne outbreaks, 882,144 cases of illness, and 1,169 deaths in the United States have been associated with contaminated drinking and recreational water. Most outbreaks (94 percent), occurred in drinking water systems. Outbreaks caused by the accidental ingestion of water while swimming or other recreation have been systematically reported only since 1971, and these events are not included in the statistics presented (Tables 1-1 to 1-3, and Figures 1-1 to 1-6). During 1971 to 1980, only 15 outbreaks were associated with water recreation; during 1981 to 1990, 45 outbreaks were reported; from 1991 to 1996, 54 outbreaks were reported.

The number of waterborne outbreaks reported in drinking water systems shows somewhat cyclical variations (Figure 1-1). From 1931 to 1950 and 1971 to 1990, the highest number of outbreaks, an annual average of 30, were reported. The fewest outbreaks, 12 per year, were reported from 1951 to 1970. An annual average of 18 outbreaks was reported during the most recent six-year period, 1991 to 1996; the

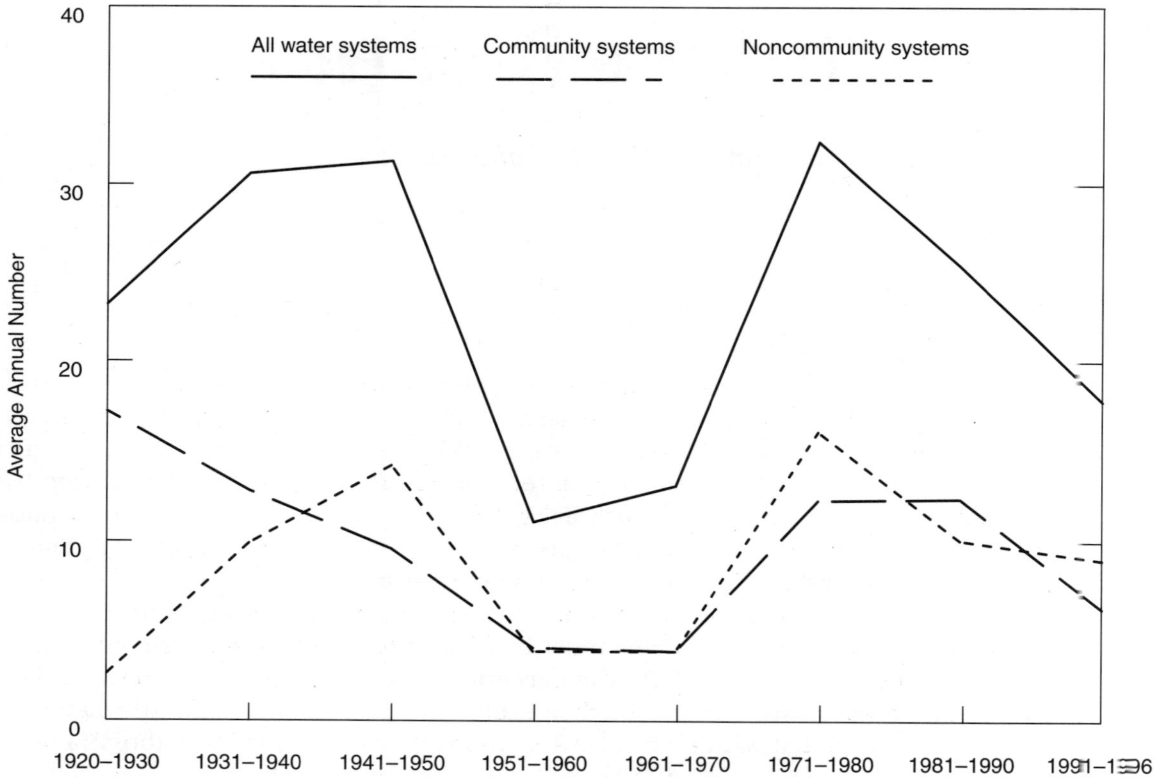

Figure 1-1 Waterborne disease outbreaks, 1920 to 1996

Table 1-1 Illnesses and deaths associated with waterborne outbreaks in the United States, 1920 to 1996

Time Period	Number of Outbreaks	Cases of Illness	Illnesses per Outbreak	Deaths
1920–30	255	102,024	400	669
1931–40	275	93,306	339	320
1941–50	313	53,935	172	61
1951–60	111	12,491	112	10
1961–70	131	46,399	354	20
1971–80	324	78,155	241	5
1981–90	254	63,549	288	6
1991–96	107	426,385	3,985	78
Totals	1,770	876,244	5,891	1,169

number of outbreaks is slightly higher than that reported during 1961 to 1970 (13 per year) and fewer than that reported during 1981 to 1990 (29 per year).

Usually, more outbreaks were reported in noncommunity systems than in community systems (those serving at least 25 year-round residents). Noncommunity water systems also provide water to the public, but they do not give year-round service. These systems serve primarily transient populations such as institutions, industries, camps, parks, hotels, and service stations that have their own water supplies available for use by employees and the public. Individual water systems are used by residents in areas without community systems. After 1931, a similar reporting trend was observed for outbreaks in both noncommunity and community water systems. An annual average of six outbreaks was reported in community water systems from 1991 to 1996, one third the number reported from 1920 to 1930. In noncommunity systems, an annual average of nine outbreaks was reported from 1991 to 1996, more than three times the number reported from 1920 to 1930.

Waterborne outbreaks have caused, on average, 495 cases of illness per outbreak. Case numbers vary considerably, however, depending on the type of water system and time period (Tables 1-1 and 1-2). Outbreaks in community systems usually cause more illness than outbreaks in noncommunity systems. During each decade, cases of illness per outbreak ranged from 247 to 11,052 (median = 268) in community water systems and 51 to 268 cases of illness per outbreak (median = 112) in noncommunity systems. The largest reported waterborne outbreak occurred in the spring of 1993 when contamination of the Milwaukee, Wis., drinking water system

Table 1-2 Waterborne outbreaks and illness by type of water system in the United States, 1920 to 1996

	Community Systems		Noncommunity Systems	
Time Period	Outbreaks per Year	Illnesses per Outbreak	Outbreaks per Year	Illnesses per Outbreak
1920–30	17.2	513	2.6	138
1931–40	12.8	748	8.1	60
1941–50	9.6	467	14.2	57
1951–60	4.1	247	3.9	51
1961–70	3.9	1,023	3.9	111
1971–80	12.3	483	16.1	113
1981–90	12.4	289	10.1	268
1991–96	6.3	11,052	9.3	113

with *Cryptosporidium* caused an estimated 403,000 cases of watery diarrhea (MacKenzie et al. 1994; Kaminski 1994). Because of this single outbreak, the average number of illnesses in community water systems during 1991 to 1994 was 11,052 cases per outbreak, more than 10 times the highest previously reported number of illnesses (Table 1-2). During 1961 to 1970, when two large outbreaks of 16,000 cases each were reported in community systems, an average of 1,023 cases of illness occurred. Excluding the Milwaukee outbreak, 16,960 cases of illness or 443 cases per outbreak occurred in community systems from 1991 to 1996, an illness rate comparable to that observed from 1971 to 1980.

Almost all deaths associated with waterborne outbreaks occurred before 1940 and were caused by typhoid fever (Craun 1986). The deaths reported since 1971 included immunocompromised persons affected during the cryptosporidiosis outbreaks in Milwaukee and in Clark County (including Las Vegas), Nev., in 1993 and 1994. Although accurate statistics are not available for deaths attributed to contaminated water in Milwaukee, it was estimated that 50 to 100 area residents with compromised immune systems died prematurely after being infected with *Cryptosporidium* (Blair 1994; Hoxie et al. 1996). In Clark County, 61 of the 78 laboratory confirmed cases of illness were HIV-infected adults; 32 of these people died within 2 months of the study period, and at least 20 had cryptosporidiosis listed on their death certificates (Goldstein et al. 1996).

Bacterial pathogens caused 13 of the remaining 19 deaths reported since 1971. Seven deaths resulted from community outbreaks of diarrheal illness caused by contamination of water storage tanks with *Salmonella typhimurium*; contamination of water mains with enterohemorrhagic *Escherichia coli* 0157:H7 was responsible for four deaths. Two elderly residents of a nursing home died during an outbreak of shigellosis. Six deaths were caused by chemicals. Two persons died after consuming arsenic-contaminated well water, and single deaths were caused by accidental fluoride contamination of a community water system (two outbreaks), ethylene glycol contamination of drinking water used for hemodialysis, and high nitrate in a farm well.

OUTBREAK REPORTING

These statistics do not reflect the actual incidence of waterborne outbreaks or disease. Rather, the observed trends largely reflect surveillance activities of local and state health agencies during various time periods. Many factors influence the degree to which outbreaks are recognized, investigated, and reported in any single year, including interest in the problem and the capabilities for recognition and investigation at the state and local level (Berkelman et al. 1994). Improved surveillance activities have resulted in increased reporting of waterborne outbreaks (Foster 1990). Waterborne disease surveillance is enhanced by educational outreach programs targeting district public health offices, physicians, and the public. Monitoring programs also benefit from designating one individual to be responsible for disease reporting and outbreak investigations; all water-related complaints and health department inquiries are directed to this person. For example, during a four-year period of intensive waterborne disease surveillance in Colorado from 1980 to 1983, 18 waterborne outbreaks were reported compared to only six during the previous three-year period, when a passive surveillance program was in effect (Hopkins et al. 1985). Several states were found to vary in their reporting. States that reported one third to one half of all outbreaks during certain time periods were found to report much fewer outbreaks in earlier and ensuing time periods.

While it is generally agreed that reporting of waterborne outbreaks is incomplete, the extent of underreporting is difficult to estimate. Rough estimates suggest that only one half to one third, and even as few as 10 percent, of all waterborne outbreaks are detected, investigated, and reported (Craun 1986, 1992). Outbreaks in community water systems are more likely to be recognized and reported than those in noncommunity water systems; problems in individual and recreational water systems are infrequently recognized and reported. Several investigators have attempted to estimate the extent to which epidemic waterborne disease is underreported. Hauschild and Bryan (1980) estimated that 1.4 million to 3.4 million cases of both foodborne and waterborne diseases occurred each year in 1974 and 1975. Carlsten (1993) estimated that 350,000 to 875,000 cases of epidemic waterborne disease may occur each year. Considering both epidemic and endemic waterborne diseases, Morris and Levin (1994) estimated 1.8 million cases and 1,800 deaths annually. Bennett et al. (1987) estimated the annual incidence of waterborne disease to be more than 900,000 cases, accounting for almost 900 deaths. Many believe that Morris and Levin and Bennett et al. have given extreme estimates. One analysis of national morbidity and mortality patterns for selected enteric diseases (Craun 1986) suggests that 230,000 cases of waterborne disease and 50 deaths may occur annually.

CAUSES OF OUTBREAKS

Contaminated groundwater has caused more waterborne outbreaks than contaminated surface water. In each decade since 1920, contaminated, inadequately treated groundwater has caused 44 to 56 percent of all reported outbreaks (Figure 1-2), whereas, inadequately treated surface water has caused 9 to 35 percent of all outbreaks (Figures 1-3 and 1-4). During the last six years, 44 percent of all outbreaks were attributed to contaminated, inadequately treated groundwater; only 9 percent were attributed to inadequately treated surface water.

Since 1971, the incidence of untreated surface water and groundwater as a cause of outbreaks has declined. Contaminated, untreated groundwater was responsible for 25 to 31 percent of all outbreaks during 1971 to 1996. In previous decades, almost half of all outbreaks were reported in untreated groundwater systems (Figure 1-2). Inadequate or interrupted disinfection of groundwater, however, has increasingly caused outbreaks. During the past quarter-century, 19 to 20 percent of all outbreaks were reported in disinfected groundwater systems. In previous decades, only 2 to 6 percent of all outbreaks occurred in these systems. The observed trends in outbreaks occurring in groundwater systems may be due to an increased emphasis on disinfecting groundwater sources with little or no effort to reduce sources of contamination. Also important may be a lack of effective, continuous disinfection, caused perhaps by a perception among some operators that groundwater needs no disinfection. Although most outbreaks in disinfected groundwater systems since 1971 were the result of inadequate chlorination, several occurred in systems using iodine and ultraviolet (UV) light for disinfection.

From 1920 to 1930, almost 20 percent of all outbreaks were reported in untreated surface water systems (Figure 1-3). Surface water is now rarely used without treatment, and only 8 percent and 4 percent of all outbreaks were reported in untreated surface water systems from 1971 to 1980 and 1981 to 1990, respectively. Only one such outbreak was reported from 1991 to 1996. Outbreaks in unfiltered, disinfected surface water systems have also decreased, causing only 4 percent of all outbreaks in 1991 to 1996 (Figure 1-3). During the previous two decades, 13 percent and 15 percent of all outbreaks were reported in unfiltered, disinfected surface water systems. This decrease in reported outbreaks in unfiltered surface water systems is probably largely due to the provisions of the Surface Water Treatment Rule (SWTR) promulgated by USEPA on June 19, 1989 (54 FR 124:27486). The SWTR specifies disinfection criteria for community and noncommunity water systems using surface water sources. The rule also requires filtration for all but exceptionally high-quality surface water sources. Additional requirements to control *Cryptosporidium* are still being considered under the proposed enhanced SWTR (59 FR 145:38832, July 29, 1994).

Outbreaks in filtered surface water systems increased from 1981 to 1990, when 7 percent of all reported outbreaks occurred in these systems. This percentage is about the same for outbreaks reported in filtered systems during 1920 to 1930 (Figure 1-4). Inadequate filtration or pretreatment, or both, was responsible for only 4 percent of all outbreaks reported during 1991 to 1996 and only 1 to 3 percent from 1931 to 1980. Whether or not outbreaks in filtered water systems will remain at these low levels depends largely on the success of current efforts to protect source

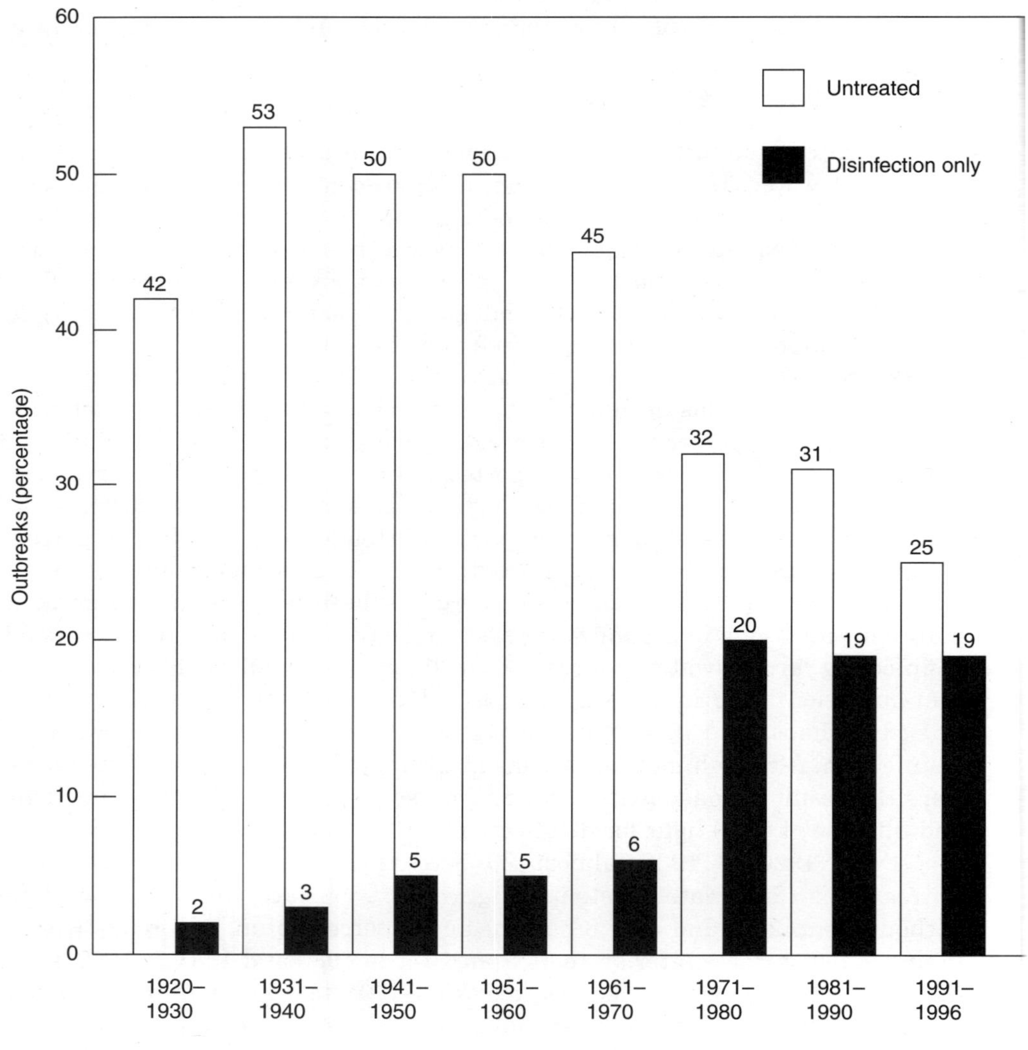

Figure 1-2 Causes of waterborne disease outbreaks from groundwater systems, 1920 to 1996

water quality; optimize filtration facilities to remove particles, turbidity, and pathogens; and provide consistent operation of water treatment plants with effective performance monitoring. Recent programs that identify weaknesses and optimize water treatment have greatly improved performance of surface water treatment plants (Consonery et al. 1997).

In addition to protecting water sources and providing adequate treatment, protecting and maintaining the quality of water during distribution and storage is an important priority. Contamination of water in the distribution system from corrosion products, cross-connections and backsiphonage, inadequately protected storage facilities, and repairs to water mains and plumbing were responsible for 22 percent of the waterborne outbreaks reported from 1991 to 1996. From 1920 to 1990, contamination of distribution systems caused 11 to 18 percent of all outbreaks (Figure 1-5). Additional emphasis is needed on identifying and correcting sources of contamination in distribution systems to reduce the number of these outbreaks.

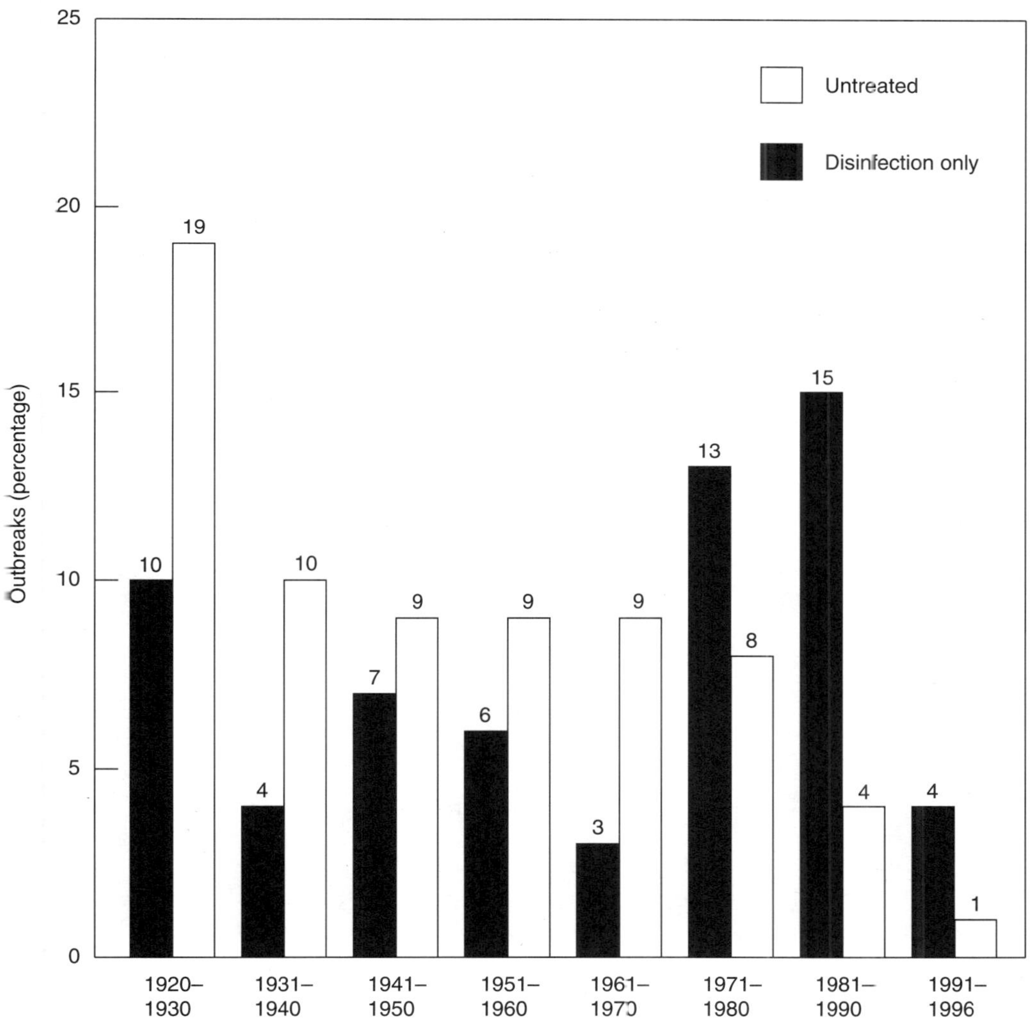

Figure 1-3 Causes of waterborne disease outbreaks from surface water systems, 1920 to 1996

Miscellaneous deficiencies including unknown causes, ingestion of water not intended for drinking, and ingestion of water during recreational activities caused 2[illegible] percent of all outbreaks from 1991 to 1996 (Figure 1-6). In previous time periods miscellaneous deficiencies were responsible for only 4 to 18 percent of outbreaks.

COLIFORM REGULATIONS

Presence of coliform bacteria may indicate the possibility of fecal contamination, a relationship used to assess the microbiological quality of drinking water. USEPA has established a maximum contaminant level (MCL) and routine monitoring requirements for total coliforms in public water systems. The absence of coliform bacteria in a water supply is usually interpreted as evidence of safe drinking water, i.e., water free of pathogens and having a low risk of waterborne infectious disease. However, waterborne outbreaks have occurred even when the MCL for total coliforms has not

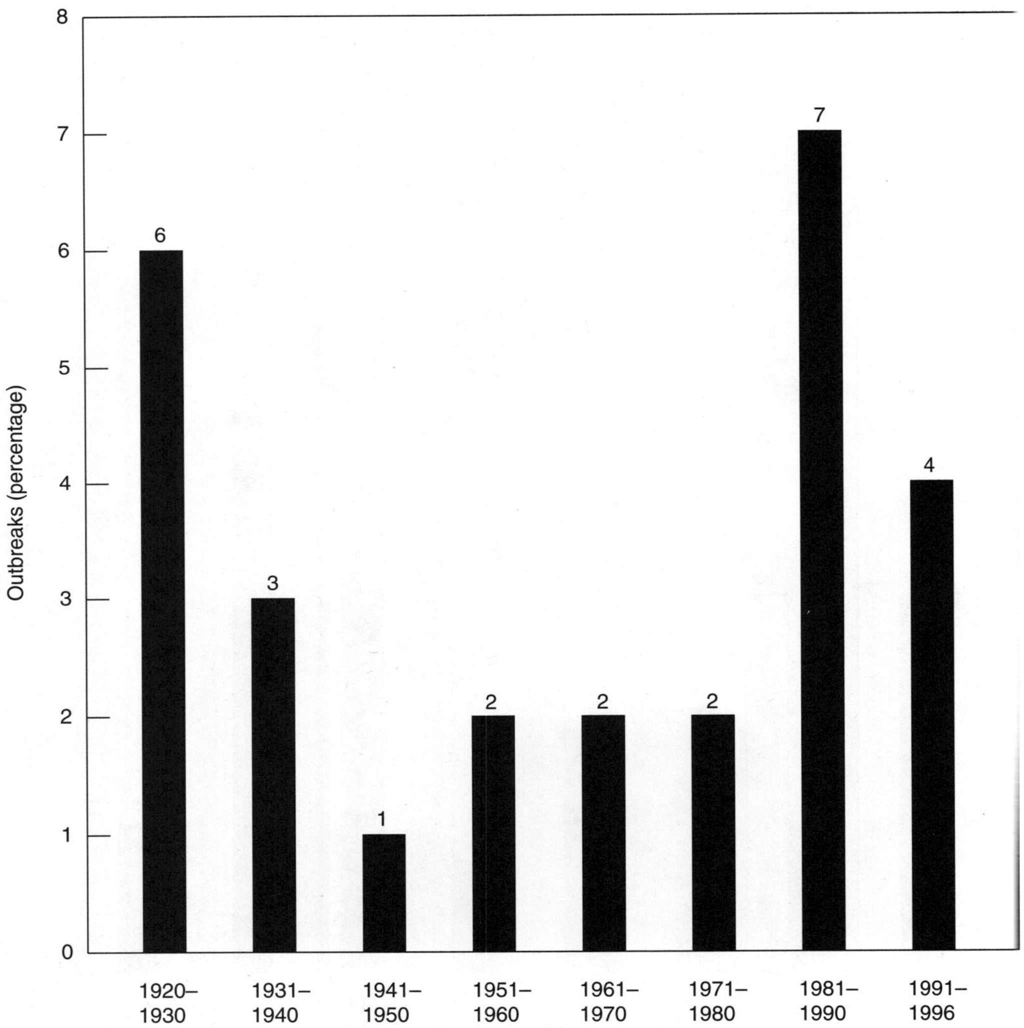

Figure 1-4 Waterborne disease outbreaks from inadequate filtration of surface water, 1920 to 1996

been exceeded. The absence of coliforms, especially in water systems that disinfect, does not exclude the presence of *Cryptosporidium parvum* and *Giardia lamblia*, because these pathogens are more resistant to disinfectants than are coliform organisms (Moore et al. 1994). Water disinfection sufficient to inactivate coliform bacteria may not inactivate *Giardia* or *Cryptosporidium*. An analysis of all protozoan waterborne outbreaks found that the total coliform MCL was not exceeded by any of the community water systems reporting outbreaks of cryptosporidiosis, and few of the systems reporting outbreaks of giardiasis exceeded this level (Craun 1994). From 1993 to 1996, water quality data were available for 35 of 37 waterborne outbreaks with suspected infectious causes of disease. Coliforms were detected in 11 of the 12 outbreaks of bacterial or unknown causes of disease (etiology), but in only 5 of the 9 protozoan outbreaks (Kramer et al. 1996). From 1983 to 1992, coliform bacteria were detected in only half of the outbreaks and caused MCL violations in only one fourth of public water systems in the 3 to 12 months before an outbreak (Craun et al. 1997).

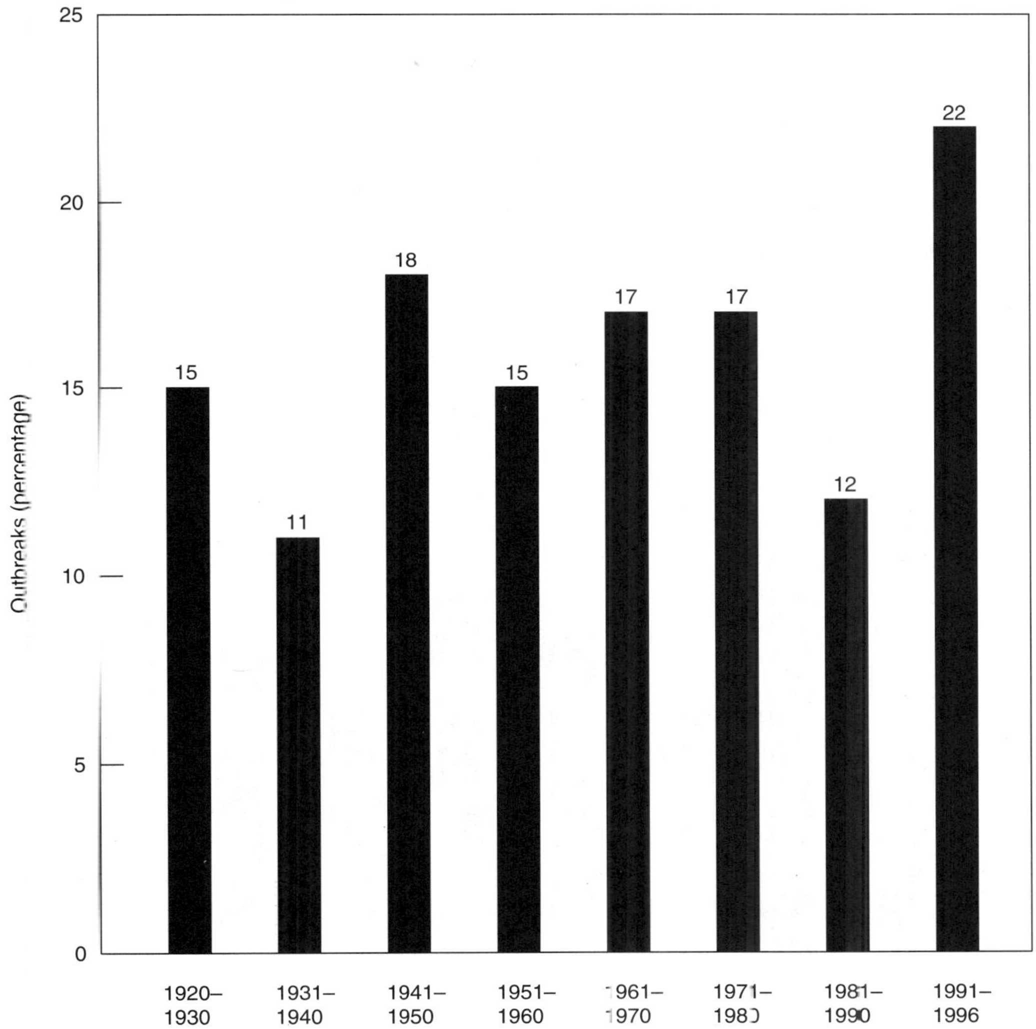

Figure 1-5 Waterborne disease outbreaks from distribution system deficiencies, 1920 to 1996

An analysis of paired communities found that the coliform violation rate was not significantly different between communities that reported and those that did not report waterborne outbreaks; usually both met the MCL.

ETIOLOGIC AGENTS

Waterborne pathogens in which humans are the sole reservoir of infection, such as *V. cholerae*, *Salmonella typhi*, and hepatitis A, are no longer important causes of outbreaks in the United States (Craun 1990). During the late 1800s and at the turn of the century, when water systems were not filtered or chlorinated, waterborne epidemics of cholera and typhoid fever were common in the United States. Filtration and chlorination of drinking water sources were largely responsible for the dramatic reduction of these diseases and decreased importance of water as a mode of transmission. From 1920 to 1960, typhoid fever continued to be transmitted by contaminated water, but no waterborne outbreaks of cholera were reported.

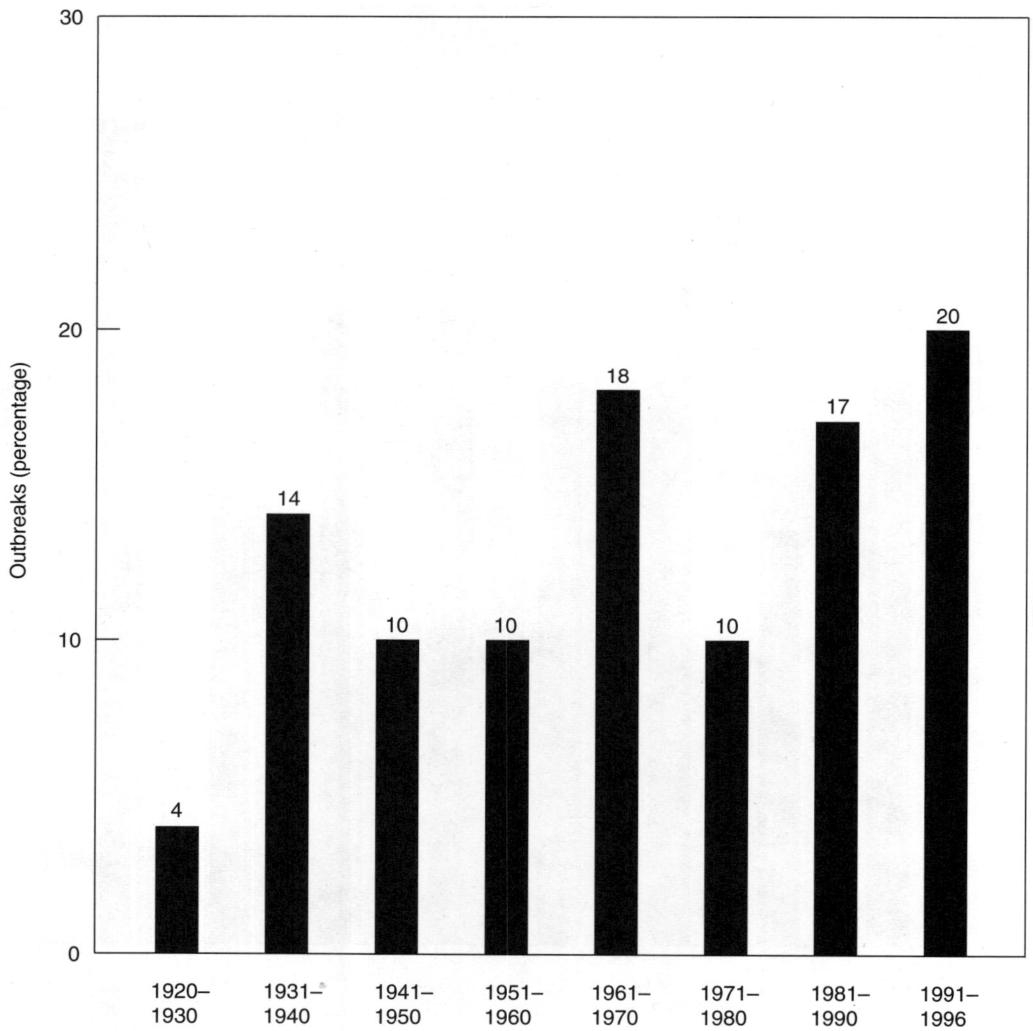

Figure 1-6 Waterborne disease outbreaks from miscellaneous and unknown deficiencies, 1920 to 1996

(Table 1-3). Since 1971, few waterborne outbreaks of typhoid fever have been reported. Hepatitis A virus caused 22 percent of all waterborne outbreaks from 1961 to 1970, but only 4 percent of outbreaks since 1971.

In 1991 and 1992 for the 13th and 14th consecutive years, *G. lamblia* was the most frequently identified etiology of waterborne outbreaks in the United States (Moore et al. 1994). *C. parvum* was the second most commonly identified cause of disease in 1991 and 1992, but in 1993 it was the most frequently identified cause. In 1994, *Giardia* returned to its position as the most frequently identified cause of waterborne outbreaks with *Cryptosporidium* the second most commonly identified cause. From 1995 to 1996, chemical contaminants caused 32 percent of the outbreaks; the most frequently identified infectious agents, *Giardia* and *Shigella*, caused 8 percent of the outbreaks.

Important disease-causing agents in the United States now include protozoa and other pathogens, with wild and domestic animals and humans serving as reservoirs of infection. A number of different animals have been implicated as potential risks for the transmission of giardiasis to humans, including cats, dogs, sheep, pigs, goats, and cattle. Calves are suspected as a major source of water contamination with *Cryptosporidium*, but many other animals are also contaminated with *C. parvum* (Craun 1994). Prevention of waterborne transmission of these pathogens requires protection of water sources from contamination by human sewage and evaluation of the impact of agricultural and urban runoff and other sources of fecal contamination by animals on a water source.

The infective dose for both *Giardia* and *Cryptosporidium* is low. Ten *Giardia* cysts have caused infection (Rendtorff 1954), and recent studies in human volunteers have shown that infection may result from doses of as few as 30 *Cryptosporidium* oocysts (DuPont et al. 1995). Both *Giardia* and *Cryptosporidium* can survive for months in the water environment, especially at low water temperatures, and their occurrence is widespread in US water supplies, including those using relatively pristine sources. High concentrations of water disinfectants and long contact times are required to inactivate *Giardia* and *Cryptosporidium* (Sterling 1990). *C. parvum* has been found to be extremely resistant to water chlorination, but properly designed and operated granular filters with appropriate pretreatment can effectively reduce *Giardia* cysts and *Cryptosporidium* oocysts in drinking water sources (LeChevallier and Norton 1995). Treatment must be optimized for effective removal of cysts and oocysts, however, and frequent monitoring should be conducted to determine the effectiveness of the filtration process (Lytle and Fox 1994). Since granular filters do not provide 100 percent removal of *Giardia* and *Cryptosporidium*, source water must also be protected from sources of contamination. For a water source heavily contaminated with these parasites, filtration may not be able to sufficiently reduce cysts and oocysts below infective dose levels.

WATERBORNE PATHOGENS OF EMERGING CONCERN

Better laboratory methods and quicker, more thorough investigation of outbreaks have helped to identify pathogens responsible for waterborne outbreaks, but an etiologic agent is still not identified in almost half of all reported waterborne outbreaks (Table 1-3). These outbreaks, classified as acute gastroenteritis of undetermined causes, may be caused by familiar waterborne pathogens that are not identified, because investigations were conducted too late to collect clinical specimens or laboratory analysis was inadequate. Outbreaks have also occurred in which an etiologic agent could not be identified, even after extensive laboratory analysis. Newly recognized waterborne pathogens in recent years include *Cryptosporidium*,

Table 1-3 Causes of waterborne disease outbreaks in the United States, 1920 to 1995

Time Period	Disease	Number of Outbreaks	Cases of Illness
1920–40	Typhoid Fever	372	8[illegible],67[illegible]
	AGI, Unidentified	144	10[illegible],81[illegible]
	Shigellosis	10	[illegible],308
	Amebiasis	2	[illegible],41[illegible]
	Hepatitis A	1	28
	Chemical Poisoning	1	[illegible]
1941–60	AGI, Unidentified	265	54,46[illegible]
	Typhoid Fever	94	1,91[illegible]
	Shigellosis	25	8,951
	Hepatitis A	23	930
	Salmonellosis	5	3[illegible]
	Chemical Poisoning	4	4[illegible]
	Para-Typhoid Fever	2	1[illegible]
	Amebiasis	2	[illegible]
	Tularemia	2	3[illegible]
	Leptospirosis	1	[illegible]
	Poliomyelitis	1	1[illegible]
1961–70	AGI, Unidentified	39	26,55[illegible]
	Hepatitis A	29	89[illegible]
	Shigellosis	21	1,73[illegible]
	Typhoid Fever	15	10[illegible]
	Salmonellosis	7	16,651
	Chemical Poisoning	9	4[illegible]
	Toxigenic *E. coli*	4	18[illegible]
	Giardiasis	3	17[illegible]
	Amebiasis	3	3[illegible]
	Para-Typhoid Fever	1	[illegible]
1971–96	AGI, Unidentified	339	82,797
	Giardiasis	115	28,12[illegible]
	Chemical Poisoning	79	4,425
	Shigellosis	42	9,055
	Hepatitis A	28	827
	AGI-Norwalk Agent	21	10,700
	Cryptosporidiosis	11	420,01[illegible]
	Campylobacteriosis	17	5,487
	Salmonellosis	13	2,995
	Typhoid Fever	5	282
	AGI-*E. coli* 0157:H7	4	305
	Yersiniosis	2	102
	Chronic Gastroenteritis	2	94
	Cholera	2	28
	AGI-Rotavirus	1	1,76[illegible]
	AGI-*E. coli* 06:H16	1	1,000
	AGI-Plesiomonas shigelloides	1	60
	AGI-*Cyclospora*	1	2[illegible]
	Amebiasis	1	4

Giardia, Norwalk-like virus, rotavirus, *Yersinia*, *Campylobacter*, and *E. coli* 0157:H7. Also recently identified is a waterborne protozoan pathogen similar to *Cryptosporidium* in some morphologic features. The name *Cyclospora cayetanensis* has been proposed for this pathogen (Ortega et al. 1993). *Cyclospora* has been identified worldwide in stool specimens from patients with diarrhea and in chlorinated drinking water during an outbreak in Nepal (Rabold et al. 1994). *Cyclospora* may be the organism responsible for a waterborne outbreak in a Chicago hospital in 1990, where cyanobacteria-like bodies were identified in ill persons (Herwaldt et al. 1992).

Other unidentified and suspected pathogens may also be important causes of waterborne illness in the United States. For example, no causative agent has yet been identified for a distinctive chronic diarrheal illness characterized by dramatic, urgent watery diarrhea persisting for many months. The first waterborne outbreak of chronic diarrhea was reported in 1987; untreated well water in an Illinois restaurant was implicated as the vehicle of transmission (Parsonnet et al. 1989). Nonbloody diarrhea with a median frequency of 12 stools per day persisted in 87 percent of patients after 6 months. Waterborne transmission is suspected for the atypical *Mycobacteria* (Singh and Yu 1994). Another group of human opportunistic pathogens that might potentially be transmitted by water is the microsporidia (Curry and Canning 1993). A number of other potentially important waterborne pathogens include *Aeromonas* spp., *Helicobacter pylori*, *Toxoplasma*, hepatitis E virus (HEV), enteric adenoviruses, astroviruses, and caliciviruses, which include both the classic calicivirus and small, round, structured viruses, such as Norwalk-like virus (Benenson 1983, 1995). Norwalk-like viruses are an important cause of waterborne outbreaks, and several other pathogens of emerging concern have been associated with the waterborne transmission of disease in other countries. Better assessment of their potential for causing waterborne disease in the United States requires additional information about their occurrence in water sources, their infective doses, and the effectiveness of water treatment processes to remove and inactivate them. Water suppliers should develop their understanding of these waterborne pathogens as more information becomes available in order to assess the vulnerability of their water systems.

SUMMARY

Although waterborne disease has largely been controlled in the United States, outbreaks continue to occur. From 1991 to 1996, 107 waterborne outbreaks and 426,385 cases of illness were reported. As evidenced by the cryptosporidiosis outbreak in Milwaukee, large populations can be affected by outbreaks. The incidence of waterborne disease in the United States is underreported, and even reported outbreaks may not lead to complete epidemiological investigations or documentation of the full extent of the outbreaks. In addition, endemic waterborne disease risks may be important. Sporadic cases are usually never recognized as outbreaks, and specific epidemiological studies must be conducted to estimate these risks of endemic waterborne disease.

Although the severity of disease associated with waterborne outbreaks has decreased in the United States, even outbreaks of mild diarrheal illness can cause time off from work, school, or recreation, resulting in significant economic consequences. The residual number of waterborne outbreaks that still occur in the United States are preventable, but new public health strategies are required for water systems, including increased protection of source water quality; water filtration and continuous disinfection; better monitoring of the effectiveness of water treatment; and increased protection of treated water as it is delivered to the tap.

Waterborne disease outbreaks are caused by many different pathogens, and each require different methods of prevention. For example, typhoid fever and cholera were waterborne diseases in the United States at the turn of the century. Chlorination and protection of water sources from sewage contamination were effective in preventing transmission of these diseases by water, because the pathogens are transmitted exclusively among humans, require large infective doses, and are susceptible to disinfection. *Cryptosporidium* and *Giardia* demand much greater emphasis on water treatment processes, but reliance on water treatment alone may not be effective. Wild and domestic animals are sources of the protozoa, and management practices may be needed to limit sources of contamination. With highly contaminated water sources, infective dose levels may be found in tap water even after filtration. Surface water sources treated only by disinfection may require filtration to ensure against waterborne transmission of *Giardia* and *Cryptosporidium*. Also, outbreaks recently reported in filtered water systems suggest that filtration facilities must be properly designed and operated. Outbreaks of cryptosporidiosis and giardiasis have occurred in groundwater systems with sources subject to contamination by surface water or sewage. Chapter 2 of this manual discusses proper source water protection and treatment. Chapter 3 discusses proper monitoring of source and treated water.

Waterborne outbreaks and endemic waterborne disease can be reduced in the United States by effective water treatment, protection of water sources, and increased surveillance programs that include periodic sanitary surveys. Also needed are improvements in waterborne disease surveillance and the detection of outbreaks. Epidemiological studies should be conducted to better define endemic waterborne disease risks and to assess the effectiveness of improved water quality and more stringent regulations (e.g., filtration of surface water and disinfection of groundwater) in reducing waterborne disease risks.

REFERENCES

Benenson, A.S., ed. 1995. *Control of Communicable Diseases Manual.* Washington, D.C.: American Public Health Association.

Benenson, M.W., E.T. Takafuji, S.M. Lemon, et al. 1983. Oocyst-Transmitted Toxoplasmosis Associated with Ingestion of Contaminated Water. *New England J. Med.,* 307:666–9.

Blair, K. 1994. *Cryptosporidium* and Public Health. *Health and Enviro. Digest,* 8(8):61.

Bennett, J.V., et al. 1987. Infectious and Parasitic Diseases. In *Closing the Gap: The Burden of Unnecessary Illness.* Amler, R.W., and H.B. Dull, eds. Oxford: Oxford University Press.

Berkelman, R.L., R.T. Bryan, M.T. Osterholm, J.W. Leduc, and J.M. Hughes. 1994. Infectious Disease Surveillance: A Crumbling Foundation. *Science,* 264:368.

Carlsten, C. 1993. Water Disinfection By-Products: The Regulatory Negotiation as a Means to Grapple with Uncertainty. Unpublished manuscript.

Consonery, P.J., D.N. Greenfield, and J.[illegible]. Lee. 1997. Pennsylvania's Filtration Evaluation Program. *Jour. AWWA,* 89(8):67.

Craun, G.F., ed. 1986. Statistics on Waterborne Outbreaks in the US (1920–1980). In *Waterborne Disease in the United States.* Boca Raton, Fla.: CRC Press.

Craun, G.F., ed. 1990. *Methods for the Investigation and Prevention of Waterborne Disease Outbreaks.* Cincinnati, Ohio: US Environmental Protection Agency, EPA/600/1-90/005a.

———. 1992. Waterborne Disease Outbreaks in the United States of America: Causes and Prevention. *World Health Statistics Quarterly,* 45:192.

———. 1994. Chairman, Report of New York City's Advisory Panel on Waterborne Disease Assessment. New York: New York City Department of Environmental Protection.

Craun, G.F., P.S. Berger, and R.L. Calderon. 1997. Coliform Bacteria and Waterborne Disease Outbreaks. *Jour. AWWA*, 89(3):16.

Curry, A., and E.U. Canning. 1993. Human Microsporidiosis. *J. Infection*, 27:229–236.

DuPont, H.L., C.L. Chappell, C.R. Sterling, et al. 1995. The Infectivity of *Cryptosporidium parvum* in Healthy Volunteers. *New England J. Med.*, 332:855.

Foster, L.R. 1990. Surveillance for Waterborne Illness and Disease Reporting: State and Local Responsibilities. In *Methods for the Investigation and Prevention of Waterborne Disease Outbreaks*. Craun, G.F, ed. Cincinnati, Ohio: US Environmental Protection Agency.

Goldstein, S.T., D.D. Juranek, O. Ravenholt, et al. 1996. Cryptosporidiosis: an Outbreak Associated with Drinking Water Despite State-of-the Art Treatment. *Annals Intern. Med.*, 124(5):459.

Hauschild, A., and F. Bryan. 1980. Estimate of Cases of Foodborne and Waterborne Illness in Canada and the United States. *J. Food Protection*, 43:435.

Herwaldt, B.L., G.F. Craun, S.L. Stokes, and D.D. Juranek. 1992. Outbreaks of Waterborne-Disease in the United States, 1989–1990. *Jour. AWWA*, 83(4):129.

Hopkins, R.S., P. Shillam, B. Gaspard, L. Eisnach, and R.J. Karlin. 1985. Waterborne Disease in Colorado: Three Years Surveillance and 18 Outbreaks. *Amer. J. Public Health*, 75:254.

Hoxie, N.J., J.P. Davis, and J.M. Vergeront. 1996. Cryptosporidiosis-associated Mortality Following a Massive Waterborne Outbreak in Milwaukee, Wisconsin. Madison, Wis.: Report of Wisconsin Department of Health and Social Services.

Kaminski, J.C. 1994. *Cryptosporidium* and the Public Water Supply. *New England J. Med.*, 331(22):1529.

Kramer, M.H., B.L. Herwaldt, G.F. Craun, et al. 1996. Waterborne Disease: 1993 and 1994. *Jour. AWWA*, 88(3):66.

LeChevallier, M., and W.D. Norton. 1995. *Giardia* and *Cryptosporidium* in Raw and Finished Water. *Jour. AWWA*, 87(9):54.

Levy, D.A., M.S. Bens, G.F. Craun, R.L. Calderon, and B.L. Herwaldt. 1998. Surveillance for Waterborne-disease Outbreaks—United States, 1995–1996. *MMWR* (in press).

Lytle, D.A., and K.R. Fox. 1994. Particle Counting and Zeta Potential Measurements for Optimizing Filtration Treatment Performance. In *Proc. AWWA Water Quality Technology Conference*. pp. 833–856. Denver, Colo.: American Water Works Association.

MacKenzie, W.R., N.J. Hoxie, M.E. Proctor, et al. 1994. A Massive Outbreak in Milwaukee of *Cryptosporidium* Infection Transmitted Through the Public Drinking Water Supply. *New England J. Med.*, 331(3):161.

Moore, A.C., B.L. Herwaldt, G.F. Craun, R.L. Calderon, A.K. Highsmith, and D.D. Juranek. 1994. Waterborne-Disease in the United States, 1991 and 1992. *Jour. AWWA*, 86(2):87.

Morris, R.D., and R. Levin. 1994. Estimating the Incidence of Waterborne Infectious Disease Related to Drinking Water in the United States. Abstract, International Symposium, International Assoc. Hydrological Sciences, Rome, September 13–17.

Ortega, Y.R., C.R. Sterling, R.H. Gilman, V.A. Cama, and F. Diaz. 1993. *Cyclospora* Species—A New Protozoan Pathogen of Humans. *New England J. Med.*, 18:1308.

Parsonnet, J., S.C. Trock, C.A. Bopp, et al. 1989. Chronic Diarrhea Associated with Drinking Untreated Water. *Annals Intern. Med.*, 110:985.

Rabold, J.G., C.W. Hoge, D.R. Shlim, C. Kefford, et al. 1994. *Cyclospora* Outbreak Associated with Chlorinated Drinking Water. *Lancet*, 334 (8933):1360–1361.

Rendtorff, R.C. 1954. The Experimental Transmission of Human Intestinal Protozoan Parasites. II. *Giardia lamblia* Cysts Given in Capsules. *Amer. J. Hygiene*, 59:209–220.

Singh, N., and V.L. Yu. 1994. Potable Water and *Mycobacterium avium* Complex. In HIV Patients: Is Prevention Possible? *Lancet*, 343:1110–1111, May 7.

Sterling, C.R. 1990. Waterborne Cryptosporidiosis. In *Cryptosporidiosis of Man and Animals*. Dubey, J.P., C.A. Speer, and R. Fayer, eds. Boca Raton, Fla.: CRC Press, Inc.

This page intentionally blank.

Chapter 2

Water Quality in Source Water, Treatment, and Distribution Systems

Kim R. Fox and Donald J. Reasoner

Most drinking water utilities practice the multiple-barrier concept as the guiding principle for providing safe water. This chapter discusses multiple barriers as they relate to the basic criteria for selecting and protecting source waters, including known and potential sources of contamination, water treatment and disinfection processes, and educating providers and customers to ensure the highest quality drinking water.

MULTIPLE-BARRIER CONCEPT

The premise behind the multiple-barrier concept is that use of several barriers in a drinking water system is effective in preventing pathogens or other contaminants from reaching the consumer. If one barrier fails, the remaining barriers minimize pathogen presence in the treated water. Although the exact barriers for any single location may differ, essential barriers include

- source water protection
- water treatment plant processes
- disinfection practices
- distribution systems
- education

Source water protection means providing the highest quality source water possible before treatment by controlling use on the watershed, minimizing sewage contamination, protecting the wellhead, and using other strategies that reduce and prevent source water contamination. Finding and developing higher quality source waters also may be necessary or economical.

The water treatment plant barrier encompasses all water treatment processes including (but not limited to) slow sand filters, enhanced coagulation processes, and membrane systems. The treatment plant must be both designed and operated correctly to maintain a contaminant barrier.

Disinfection processes are normally the final barrier to microorganisms. The disinfection barrier consists of a disinfectant residual throughout the distribution system that limits regrowth of microorganisms and possibly prevents subsequent contamination, due to causes like cross-connections.

The distribution system—transmission mains and storage—must be properly maintained to ensure that water quality is not degraded.

Lastly, education of water utility personnel and management, public officials, and water consumers is crucial to maintaining safe drinking water.

SOURCE WATER QUALITY

The quality of surface water and groundwater sources used for drinking water supply varies broadly in the United States, ranging from nearly pristine in some areas to extremely poor in others. Ideally, source water should be free of microbial contamination from human and animal activities, free of toxic natural and synthetic chemical contaminants, and of adequate quantity to meet the needs of the population served. Because of increasing population, pollution from domestic and industrial activities, and, in many cases, lack of alternate water supply sources, many communities must use inferior quality source waters for their water supplies. The poorer the source water quality, the greater the need to provide multiple-step treatment to remove microbial and chemical contaminants.

Source water microbial quality may change drastically in a short time period (perhaps just minutes when related to precipitation events), and vary from day to day because of a variety of activities on the watershed. Natural storm events over the watershed create transient changes in water quality by contributing large amounts of both suspended and dissolved materials to the water. Other relatively constant sources of surface water pollutants include agricultural activities, wastewater treatment plants, septic system drainage, and a variety of industrial and manufacturing operations.

Groundwater Protection

Source water protection minimizes the amount of contamination introduced into water before treatment. A groundwater protection program covers three basic areas:

- protecting the aquifer
- locating wells away from potential sources of pollution
- proper well construction

To protect the aquifer, the extent and type of activities in the recharge zone of that aquifer must be controlled based on aquifer characteristics. A confined aquifer may have a protective barrier between surface contamination and the water. On the other hand, an unconfined aquifer may have porous top layers and contaminated water in the recharge zone surface may percolate quickly into the aquifer. Specific measures to protect a recharge zone include owning and controlling the area, or passing zoning ordinances and regulations that prohibit certain land uses within the recharge area. A formal sanitary inspection can determine how much of a recharge protection program or wellhead protection program is needed.

Wellhead protection prevents surface contamination from entering the well. Installing a well an adequate distance from sources of pollution is a simple means of wellhead protection. Other protective measures include proper design and construction of the well and the wellhead. Decisions must be made concerning the depth of the well, depth of the well casing, depth of the grouting, well pit design, and other factors before construction. Proper design and construction methods are specific to locations and vary with local and state regulations.

Surface Water Protection

When streams, rivers, open ponds, lakes, or open reservoirs must be used as sources of water supply, the danger of contamination is greatly increased. The physical, chemical, and bacteriological contamination of surface water make it necessary to provide greater measures of protection or increased treatment. The three main factors for protecting surface water include

- watershed control
- removing sources of pollution
- properly constructing catchment basins, intakes, and storage facilities

Protecting a surface water source begins with a watershed control program that analyzes watershed hydrology and land ownership, identifies watershed characteristics and activities that could endanger source water quality, and monitors industrial, residential, agricultural, or recreational activities that may adversely impact source water quality. Ownership of the watershed and restricting access is the most stringent control a water utility can have to protect source water quality. When considering operating expenses and capital costs to purchasing costs, it may prove less expensive in the long run to purchase watershed lands. However, control by ownership is less likely as the area of watershed increases. Another way to protect watersheds is to use and enforce zoning restrictions and ordinances. Problems with multiple jurisdictions occur when source watersheds cross political boundaries.

As with groundwater systems, a thorough, periodic sanitary survey to identify specific and potential sources of pollution is necessary to maintain surface source water quality. Ideally, sources of contamination should be identified and corrected before problems occur, but sources can be intermittent and not appear in a cursory sanitary survey. During or after a waterborne disease outbreak, identifying potential sources of the pathogen responsible for the outbreak may prevent future problems or may suggest ways to remove the contaminating source from the watershed or aquifer area. Source waters (both ground and surface) can become contaminated by pathogenic microorganisms from sewage or other waste discharges, septic tank overflows or seepage, urban or agricultural runoff, subsurface movement, recreational usage, or during storage or distribution.

Microbiological Characteristics of Source Water

Source water for a drinking water supply should be the best quality available. The Surface Water Treatment Rule (SWTR) (1989) provides source water quality criteria for water systems wishing to avoid filtration. For such systems, total coliform concentration should be less than 100 per 100 mL, or the fecal coliform concentration less than 20 per 100 mL in 90 percent of samples taken during the previous 6 months. In addition, water turbidity cannot exceed 5 ntu on an ongoing basis, based on grab samples taken every 4 hours (or more frequently) that the system is in operation.

The system must also demonstrate that it maintains disinfection conditions that inactivate 99.9 percent of *Giardia* cysts and 99.99 percent of viruses every day of operation except any one day each month. With some caveats to these requirements, any supply that cannot meet these microbiological quality criteria must install filtration. Any source water that fails to meet these requirements must be treated to render it safe for human consumption. In the future, developing new regulations or tightening current regulations may further limit the number of unfiltered systems by making the requirements to avoid filtration more stringent.

A source water's microbial quality is extremely variable and depends on many factors, including domestic and feral animal activity on the watershed; human activities on the watershed, including recreational, manufacturing and fabrication, and agricultural activities; municipal pollution inputs from raw sewage to primary and secondary wastewater treatment plant effluents; and storm events over the watershed that wash natural and synthetic contaminants into the surface waters or that percolate into the groundwater aquifers. Microbial contaminants associated with these sources include bacteria, viruses, and protozoa, in both pathogenic and nonpathogenic forms.

Densities of bacteria, viruses, and protozoa vary widely because of wastewater effluents from domestic sewage treatment plant processes (e.g., raw wastewater bypass, primary or secondary treatment, and septic effluents) and the frequency and intensity of storm events that both dilute and degrade the receiving water quality by contributing additional contaminants. Heterotrophic bacterial counts may vary from less than 1 to 10 colony-forming units (cfu)/mL in groundwater to more than 1 × 10[illegible] in surface water badly polluted by municipal raw sewage or combined sewage and stormwater overflow effluents. Indicator bacteria (total and fecal coliforms, including *Escherichia coli*) densities in source water can range from less than 1/100 mL in good quality groundwaters to more than 1×10^4/100 mL in surface water badly polluted with municipal raw sewage or combined sewage and stormwater overflow. Few water systems are treating surface water with more than 2×10^4 total coliforms/100 mL or 2×10^3 fecal coliforms/100 mL.

Human viruses found in source waters include enteroviruses (72 types including polio, Coxsackie A and B, and echovirus), reoviruses (six types), hepatitis A, hepatitis E, rotavirus, Norwalk virus, adenovirus (types 1 through 49), parvovirus, corona virus, astrovirus and related viruses not yet classified, epidemic non-A and non-B hepatitis viruses, and caliciviruses. All of these organisms present significant health concerns and, if present in source water, must be removed or inactivated by water treatment processes.

While viruses occur more frequently and in greater abundance in surface source waters, they may also be found in groundwater as a result of septic tank effluents, land application of sewage and sewage sludges, and other sources. Viruses are able to travel long distances as water percolates downward and flows through the soil; the distance of travel depends on the type of soil and the specific geology of a given area. Groundwaters can no longer be considered pristine and safe for consumption. If a groundwater source is directly influenced by surface water intrusions, full conventional treatment may be necessary to ensure that the treated water is safe for consumption.

WATER QUALITY IN TREATMENT SYSTEMS

Water treatment processes that serve as protective barriers against microbial pathogens passing into the distribution system must be operated continuously, optimized for the maximum removal capability, and reliably maintained in order to deal with the most extreme water quality changes anticipated. Microorganisms, including various pathogens, are subject to both physical removal by chemical coagulation–flocculation, sedimentation, and filtration, and to inactivation by chemical oxidizing agents. The SWTR currently requires overall removal and/or inactivation of 99.9 percent (3 logs) of *Giardia* cysts and 99.99 percent (4 logs) of viruses; filtered water turbidities are to be less than 0.5 ntu in 95 percent of measurements taken each month.

Physical removal of microorganisms in water treatment is accomplished by sedimentation during source water storage, coagulation–flocculation, sedimentation, and slow or rapid sand filtration, or by direct filtration with or without filtration aid. Each step results in a reduction of the microbial density in the water, and the cumulative removal ranges from 90 to 99.9 percent, depending on the actual combination of treatment steps. Adding a chemical disinfection step results in further reduction/inactivation of microorganisms to achieve removals of 99.999 to 99.9999 percent (5 to 6 logs) for bacteria, 99.99 percent (4 logs) for viruses, and 99.9 percent (3 logs) for protozoa. Greater removals may occur when all processes are functioning optimally.

Effective rapid sand filtration removal of bacteria and viruses requires the use of chemical coagulants. Without chemical coagulants, only between 1 and 50 percent of influent viruses may be removed at filter rates of 9.8 to 24 m/h. Bacteria removal by filtration without chemical coagulants is in the same range as viruses. Virus removals by water treatment have been reported to range from as little as 10 percent following coagulation–flocculation and sedimentation, to greater than 99.9 percent following full conventional treatment, including disinfection with chlorine. Viruses have been found in fully treated water, indicating the process was not fully effective, possibly because of the association of viruses with particulates that escape the filtration process and also protect the viruses from disinfection.

Heterotrophic bacterial removal by conventional filtration, which includes coagulation, ranges from less than 90 to 99.9 percent (1 to 3 logs) through the filtration process. Final disinfection can achieve an additional 99 to 99.99 percent (2 to 4 logs) removal, yielding a total bacterial reduction of 99.999 to 99.99999 percent (5 to 7 logs). For both bacteria and viruses, the effectiveness of filtration and inactivation by disinfection are adversely impacted by cold water temperatures; therefore, both processes must be continuously monitored and optimized.

Microorganisms are usually inactivated (disinfected) by a chemical oxidant. Specific conditions for maximum inactivation effectiveness of any of these oxidants is beyond the scope of this chapter, but the general order of effectiveness of chemical disinfection is as follows: ozone > chlorine dioxide > hypochlorous acid > hypochlorite ion > chloramines. Time, water pH, and water temperature are significant factors that influence a disinfectant's effectiveness to inactivate microorganisms. The order of relative resistance of microorganisms to inactivation by any chemical disinfectant is as follows: protozoan cysts and oocysts >> animal viruses and bacteriophages > bacteria, including coliforms (except for mycobacteria, which may be more resistant than most of the viruses).

The protozoan pathogens *Giardia lamblia* and *Cryptosporidium parvum* have cysts and oocysts, respectively, that are extremely resistant to chemical disinfectants and other adverse environmental effects. Therefore, the primary means of eliminating cysts and oocysts from water during treatment is by chemical coagulation–flocculation and filtration. This combination of processes in rapid sand filtration treatment is effective for removing cysts and oocysts, providing processes are continuously operated, well run, and closely controlled.

Slow sand filtration is also effective for removing parasite cysts and oocysts because of the filtering action of the schmutzdecke. The schmutzdecke is the top layer (a few centimetres in depth) of sand and particulate materials (fine soil particles, plant debris, microorganisms such as algae, etc.) that have been removed from the water as it percolates downward through the sand filter bed. Diatomaceous earth (DE) filtration can be effective for *Giardia* cyst (10 to 12 µm) removal, but may be less effective for removing the smaller sized *Cryptosporidium* oocysts (4 to 6 µm). Recent studies indicate that *Cryptosporidium* oocysts are effectively removed by these treatment processes only when processes are optimized and continuously operated.

Viruses and bacteriophages are typically only slightly more resistant to inactivation by chemical disinfectants than are bacteria. Both viruses and bacteria, when associated with particulate matter, are more difficult to disinfect than freely suspended viruses and bacteria. Turbidity removal must be maximized during treatment to optimize the effectiveness of the disinfection process for any microorganisms that remain in the water following filtration.

WATER QUALITY IN DISTRIBUTION SYSTEMS

The microbiological quality of treated drinking water as it leaves the treatment plant is the highest it will ever be. As water travels through the distribution pipe system to the consumer, its microbiological quality degrades at a variable rate. The degradation process involves several factors, including loss of disinfectant residual; temperature changes; flow velocity changes; biofilm sloughing and stirred-up pipe sediments caused by rapid changes in flow, or even flow reversals; pipe breaks and replacements, and other maintenance activities; intrusions of contaminants into the pipe network from pressure drops and cross-connections; regrowth of bacteria that survived the treatment processes; and growth of bacteria in biofilms on the pipe walls and surfaces in storage reservoirs and tanks.

Some treatment processes, such as preoxidant treatment (ozone or chlorine) of the source water or coagulated (settled) water before filtration, causes an increase in easily assimilable organic carbon (AOC) that can stimulate bacterial growth or regrowth in the distribution system. Heterotrophic bacterial growth or regrowth usually occurs when the disinfectant residual drops below 0.2 mg/L, the water temperature is greater than 40° F (10° C), and AOC is greater than 50 µg/L. Biological filtration, if practiced, can reduce AOC in filtered, distributed water. This may reduce, but not necessarily eliminate, bacterial regrowth in the distribution system.

Ultimately, the maintenance of an adequate disinfection residual controls bacterial regrowth in the treated distribution water. The SWTR specifies a minimum disinfectant residual of 0.2 mg/L for chlorine or 0.4 mg/L for chloramine in the distribution system to control microbial growth. These disinfectant concentrations may control bacterial growth in the bulk water, but may be inadequate to control biofilm bacterial growth. Thus, the bacterial quality of bulk water leaving the clearwell is usually in the range of less than 1 to 10 cfu/mL measured as heterotrophic plate count (HPC) bacteria. On the other hand, water from other areas of the distribution system (distal areas of the system, dead ends, storage tanks, and reservoirs) may have bacterial densities ranging from 10 cfu/mL to greater than 1×10^5 cfu/mL. Dead-end areas of distribution systems often have high HPC levels along with colored water problems because of corrosion processes, the long residence time of the water, and loss of disinfectant residual.

Elevated storage tanks often have relatively high HPC levels because of loss of disinfectant residual and, during warm weather, high water temperature. Open storage reservoirs may have high HPC levels due to loss of disinfectant residual and contamination from birds, feral and domestic animals, and the surrounding land.

Practical experience indicates that treated water leaving the clearwell must have a disinfectant residual considerably higher than 0.2 to 0.4 mg/L in order to provide the minimum 0.2 to 0.4 mg/L residual at the ends of the system. Just how much disinfectant residual must be applied may vary widely based on a variety of factors, including the total organic carbon (TOC) present in the finished water that will exert a disinfectant demand; water temperature; age and condition of the distribution system piping; extent of biofilm development; residence time of the water; duration of off-line storage in standpipes or reservoirs; type of storage, i.e., covered versus uncovered reservoir; and incidence of posttreatment contamination events that contribute additional disinfectant demand in the form of chemical and microbial contaminants.

Biofilm Effects on Water Quality

Many heterotrophic bacteria that survive or pass through the treatment process are able to adapt to the low nutrient (oligotrophic) conditions of treated drinking water. Once in the distribution system, their ability to associate, temporarily or by colonization (biofilm growth), with surfaces confers survival advantages for the bacteria. Nutrients available to bacteria in the bulk water are usually present at very low levels. This, coupled with the presence of a disinfectant residual, means that bacteria freely suspended in the water are inhibited from growing. However, bacteria associated with surfaces, such as pipe walls and sediments, are exposed to a continuous or even accumulating supply of nutrients from flowing water.

Establishment of a biofilm involves transport of bacteria and nutrients to the pipe wall surface, bacterial adhesion and multiplication, and buildup of microbial growth products. These products include various exopolymeric materials that assist in binding cells to the pipe wall and forming a matrix within which cells are protected from disinfectant. Attachment of bacteria to the pipe wall and other surfaces, or in sediments, provides a 150- to 3,000-fold increase in disinfection resistance, depending on the surface material. Bacteria adapted to growth under low nutrient conditions have been shown to be more resistant to disinfection than bacteria grown under rich nutrient conditions. Effectively disinfecting biofilms in distribution systems is difficult because of the two factors just discussed. Additionally, the transport of the disinfectant into the biofilm is limited by diffusion kinetics. Reactions of the disinfectant with extracellular matrix material, nutrients from the water that diffuse along with disinfectant, and corrosion products from the pipe itself result in a reduced disinfectant residual available to react with the bacterial cell.

The higher the disinfectant residual present in the bulk phase water, the more likely it is that sufficient disinfectant can diffuse into the biofilm to inactivate bacteria found there. There is evidence that a chloramine residual can exert better control of biofilm bacterial growth than does free chlorine. However, once a bacterial biofilm becomes established in a distribution system, it is virtually impossible to get rid of using chlorine or chloramine. Most distribution biofilms appear to be thin and patchy (discontinuous) rather than uniform and continuous. Maintaining an adequate disinfectant residual undoubtedly limits the extent of development of a biofilm, but the disinfectant residual necessary to do so varies with changes in source water quality and with the performance of treatment processes in removing particulates, nutrients, and microorganisms.

Bacterial growth and regrowth in water distribution systems occurs in biofilms, and biofilm bacteria may enter the bulk phase water by release from the biofilm or by sloughing of biofilm particles from hydraulic shearing. Bacterial densities in the biofilm typically range from about 10^5 to 10^8 cfu/cm^2, measured by culture techniques. Maximum biofilm bacterial densities occur when disinfectant residual is low or nonexistent, while lower biofilm densities occur when disinfectant residuals in the bulk water are as high as 1.6 to 1.8 mg/L.

Under some relatively specific conditions, a water utility using a surface water source may experience intermittent or continuous low-level occurrences of coliforms characterized as coliform biofilm, or as growth or regrowth of coliforms in the distribution system. Utilities with such problems are primarily in the northeastern United States, where distribution system age may be part of the problem. Additionally, such coliform biofilm problems have been characterized by

- the inability to maintain a disinfectant residual greater than 0.2 mg/L
- conditioning of the distribution system by exposure to treated water containing relatively high levels of AOC (> 100 µg/L) and TOC (> 2 mg/L)
- warm water temperatures (T ≥ 15° C) occurring from late spring to late fall
- a significant percentage of iron pipe in service for more than 75 years
- lack of a regular flushing program for dead-end areas

Although treatment processes may be producing water that meets microbiological standards, low levels of coliform bacteria do pass through treatment and may survive to colonize the biofilm in some areas of the system. When nutrient levels, disinfectant concentration, and temperature conditions are right, these organisms are able to grow, perhaps to levels sufficient that they are released from the biofilm and appear in the bulk water during sample collection.

SUMMARY

A water utility's ability to produce and maintain high quality drinking water is a major challenge. The pressure to produce ever better quality water, driven by both current and proposed regulations, means that water utilities must evaluate their current ability to meet regulatory goals, forecast and plan for treatment technology changes that may become necessary, and balance the costs and benefits of new technologies against the need to increase costs to consumers.

To maintain or improve the microbial quality of drinking water, utilities must address issues such as watershed management and source water protection; maintain good treatment and disinfection practices, including process optimization; develop a thorough understanding of the hydraulics of their distribution system; be aggressive in managing and operating the distribution system, including active programs for cross-connection control and scheduled hydrant and dead-end flushing; develop a proactive microbial monitoring and data collection program; and make active use of data analysis and information stemming from that analysis to implement better treatment and distribution management practices.

REFERENCES

Block, J.C. 1992. Biofilms in Drinking Water Distribution Systems. In *Biofilms—Science and Technology.* Bott, T.R., L. Melo, M. Fletcher, and B. Capdeville, eds. Dordrechet: Kluwer Publishers.

Bryan, F.L., D. Mason, O.D. Cook, C. Moe, K.R. Fox, R.C. Swanson, J.I. Guzewich, E.C. Todd, and D. Juranek. 1996. *Procedures to Investigate Waterborne Illness.* 2nd International Conf. Association of Milk, Food, and Environmental Sanitarians, Inc., Des Moines, Iowa.

Donlan, R.M., and W.O. Pipes. 1987. Pipewall Biofilm in Drinking Water Mains. In *Proc. AWWA Water Quality Technology Conference.* pp. 637–659. Denver, Colo.: American Water Works Association.

Geldreich, E.E. 1990. Microbiological Quality of Source Waters for Water Supply. In *Drinking Water Microbiology: Progress and Recent Developments.* pp. 3–31. McFeters, G.A., ed. New York: Springer-Verlag.

———. 1993. Microbiological Changes in Source Water Treatment: Reflections in Distribution Water Quality. In *Strategies and Technologies for Meeting SDWA Requirements.* pp. 269–304. Clark, R.M., and R.S. Summers, eds. Lancaster, Pa.: Technomic Publishing Company, Inc.

———. 1996. *Microbial Quality of Water Supply in Distribution Systems.* Boca Raton, Fla.: CRC Press, Inc.

Hurst, C.J. 1991. Presence of Enteric Viruses in Freshwater and Their Removal by the Conventional Drinking Water Treatment Process. *Bull. World Health Org.,* 69(1):113–119.

LeChevallier, M.W., C.D. Cawthon, and R.G. Lee. 1988. Factors Promoting Survival of Bacteria in Chlorinated Water Supplies. *Appl. Environ. Microbiol.,* 54(3):649–654.

LeChevallier, M.W. 1990. Coliform Regrowth in Drinking Water: A Review. *Jour. AWWA,* 82(11):74–86.

Logsdon, G.S. 1990. Microbiology and Drinking Water Filtration. In *Drinking Water Microbiology: Progress and Recent Developments.* pp. 120–146. Brock/Springer Series in Contemporary Bioscience. New York: Springer-Verlag.

McFeters, G.A. 1990. *Drinking Water Microbiology: Progress and Recent Developments.* McFeters, G.A., ed. Brock/Springer Series in Contemporary Bioscience. New York: Springer-Verlag.

Payment, P. 1991. Fate of Human Enteric Viruses, Coliphages and Clostridium perfringens During Drinking-Water Treatment. *Can. J. Microbiol.,* 37:154–157.

Reasoner, D.J., and E.E. Geldreich. 1990. Distribution Systems: Treated Water Quality Versus Coliform Non-Compliance Problems. *In Methods for the Investigation and Prevention of Waterborne Disease Outbreaks.* pp. 207–222. Craun, G., ed. US Environmental Protection Agency, Office of Research and Development. EPA/600/1-90/005a.

Reasoner, D.J., and E.W. Rice. 1993. Bacterial Nutrients and Distribution Drinking Water Quality. In *Strategies and Technologies for Meeting SDWA Requirements.* pp. 305–319. Clark, R.M., and R.S. Summers, eds. Lancaster, Pa.: Technomic Publishing Company, Inc.

Robbins, R.W., R.W. Glicker, D.M. Bloem, and B.M. Niss. 1991. *Effective Watershed Management for Surface Water Supplies.* Denver, Colo.: American Water Works Association Research Foundation and American Water Works Association.

UOP Inc., Johnson Division. 1982. *Ground Water and Wells.* Saint Paul, Minn.: UOP Inc.

US Environmental Protection Agency. 1989. 40 CFR Parts 141 and 142. Drinking Water; National Primary Drinking Water Regulations; Filtration, Disinfection; Turbidity, *Giardia lamblia,* Viruses, *Legionella,* and Heterotrophic Bacteria; Final Rule. *Federal Register,* 54 (No. 124): 27486–27541.

———. 1992. *Basic Need-to-Know on How to Conduct a Sanitary Survey of Small Water Systems.* Cincinnati, Ohio: USEPA.

Van der Wende, E., W.G. Characklis, and D.B. Smith. 1989. Biofilms and Bacterial Drinking Water Quality. *Water Res.,* 23(10):1313–1322.

Viessman, W., and M.J. Hammer. 1985. *Water Supply and Pollution Control.* 4th ed. New York: Harper and Row Publishers.

This page intentionally blank.

Chapter 3

Water Quality Monitoring, Sampling, and Testing

Jon Bloemker and Kevin R. Gertig

Monitoring, sampling, and testing drinking water fulfills two needs—meeting regulatory requirements and anticipating treatment process improvements. The number and types of samples collected and tested to meet regulatory requirements are generally considered the minimum for determining water quality. Increasing the number and types of samples collected and tested provides data more representative of water quality. These data help operators predict changes in water quality, and alter treatment processes or maintenance programs to prevent or reduce the deterioration of finished water quality.

MONITORING

The importance of the timing of sample collection is frequently overlooked and misunderstood. If the timing of sample collection misses the target event, information gained from the program will be deceptive and the best sampling techniques and laboratory quality-control practices will not improve the final results. The only way to avoid this problem is to thoroughly understand the system being sampled. This requires developing an adequate history of water quality changes and identifying indicators that will predict future changes.

Surface Waters and Groundwater Under the Influence of Surface Water

Collecting meaningful samples from public water systems using surface water sources or groundwater under the influence of surface water (subject to the same regulations as surface water) requires several considerations. As discussed in following paragraphs, it is important to clearly define the design and intent of any monitoring program, conduct a program designed to represent average conditions, and use proper timing so samples will not be biased or unrepresentative of true, overall water quality.

As mentioned, a monitoring program must collect far more data than minimum regulatory requirements to effectively represent average conditions. For example, a single, 12-month running average based on samples from four consecutive quarters can be biased from a single atypical result. A more realistic average history requires the monitoring program to be in place for a number of years. Also, increasing the sampling events during periods when water usage is high may be more representative. Another approach is collecting samples at widely spaced intervals during times when water quality is relatively constant and collecting more frequent samples when water quality fluctuates. Average water quality may be better represented by a weighted average based either on the amount of water used or the time between sampling events.

A monitoring program must account for changing activities and conditions within the watershed. Agricultural, recreational, municipal, industrial, and other activities affect downstream water quality. An assessment of the watershed should be performed before a final comprehensive monitoring program is designed and implemented. An inventory of potential point and nonpoint sources of contamination should be performed. If a monitoring program has been established before such an assessment, the results of the data may be more difficult to interpret.

Point source discharges are regulated through National Permit Discharge Elimination System (NPDES) programs in which discharge limits are specified in a permit. Typically, routine point source discharges from these operations will not cause a sudden change in water quality. Most operations meet their limits during routine operations. The assumption that a waste treatment facility operating within its regulatory discharge limits will not be a major source of microbial contaminants appears sound. However, the atypical event may create a problem, such as discharges from combined sewers during periods of heavy precipitation and hydraulically overloaded wastewater treatment plants. Information about point source discharges are usually available through local state primacy agencies.

Nonpoint source discharges from upstream agricultural facilities may degrade water quality. The locations of feed lots, dairy farms, stables, and commercial agricultural businesses, and the waste disposal practices of each operation are factors to consider. Local, county, or state agricultural extension or co-op agents are good starting points for obtaining this information.

The weather may be the most unpredictable influence on water quality. Precipitation, snow melt, wind, drought, and temperature affect water quality. Overland flows of precipitation and snow melt carry contaminants into receiving streams via nonpoint discharges. In addition, precipitation and snow melt are responsible for point source discharges from storm sewers, combined sewers, and treatment plants in urban areas. The direction of the wind may be responsible for the discharge of a stream into a bay or a lake changing course to flow over an intake. Drought conditions result in a reduced dilution factor and may attract wildlife and livestock to the major streams that feed into public water supplies. The influence of discharge from a waste treatment facility is magnified by a reduced dilution factor during droughts. Water temperatures affect the variety and viability of microbiological contaminants, although it may have little bearing on some contaminants' survival in the water environment.

Water providers should be familiar with travel time for the full range of flow conditions in the upstream reaches of their source water. This information may be available for some streams from the US Geological Servey (USGS) or various state agencies. With information on stream flow, a prediction about when an upstream event will affect local water quality can be made and the monitoring schedule and treatment processes adjusted accordingly. Cooperative arrangements with upstream communities and businesses regarding notification of unusual discharges or accidents will aid in short-term changes to monitoring plans.

It may be necessary to develop a monitoring program that includes other potential microbial contaminants besides total coliforms. For source water in the Great Lakes not under the influence of inland streams or shoreline runoff, additional testing beyond total coliforms and heterotrophic bacteria may be unnecessary. At the other extreme, e.g., an inland river location downstream of urban areas or discharge from an overloaded waste treatment facility, routine tracking of microbial contaminants other than total coliforms is crucial to demonstrate the effectiveness of potable water treatment systems. In the majority of situations between these extremes, a baseline understanding of the types of microbial contaminants should be established. Expanded monitoring to include contaminants other than total coliforms, *Escherichia coli*, and fecal coliforms are based on past experiences and overall water quality. Heterotrophic bacteria counts may be useful in clean water conditions. In-house testing programs for *Pseudomonas* sp. or *Klebsiella* sp. may prove useful as indicators of lesser quality source water. Expansion of the monitoring program to *Giardia*, *Cryptosporidium*, or viral testing may yield critical information during nonroutine periods, especially during periods of high runoff.

An example of misleading data is routinely seen in northern US inland streams subject to agricultural runoff. In some such areas, manure is applied to the fields in December and January when the crops are off the fields and the frozen earth supports heavy farm equipment. Immediately following the application, little or no runoff occurs; however, near the end of February or early March, a combination of snow melt and early spring rains carry various contaminants into receiving streams. A monitoring program performed on the first day of each quarter will likely miss the potential problems. Operators responsible for water systems affected by nonpoint discharges should have the flexibility to change monitoring schedules and collect samples that represent periodic and unusual events. During these events, the number and type of samples should be increased.

Monitoring Frequency

Water treatment professionals must maintain consistent finished water quality to protect public health. The Partnership for Safe Water recommends that conventional water plants strive to meet less than 0.1 ntu in finished water at all times. Water treatment can be most challenging during reservoir turnovers, floods, runoff, aquifer changes, and unidentified upstream discharges. Monitoring plans should be site-specific because of the numerous local variables that make monitoring dynamic. After databases are established, certain parameters can be tested less often, while other parameters may need to be added. An example of a weekly matrix is shown in Figure 3-1. Although it is not possible to cover all instances that warrant increased water quality monitoring, the following may be considered for surface waters:

- unusual activity observed in the watershed
- severe weather that affects the source water

Parameter	Process Location	Goal	Minimum Monitoring Winter*	Frequency Other Times	Sampling Location	Method
Turbidity (NTU)	HT Raw	N/A	1/wk	1/wk	Raw Water Sample Station	Nephelometric method using Hach 2100AN Turbidimeter; EPA Approved. †Standard Methods-2130B (*Process Control Lab*)
	PR Raw	N/A	1/wk	1/wk	Raw Water Sample Station	
	PR Raw	N/A	1/month	1/wk	Poudre River Intake	
	T1 Eff.	< 1.0	1/wk	1/wk	T1 Eff. Turbidimeter	
	T2 Eff.	< 1.0	1/wk	1/wk	T2 Eff. Turbidimeter	
	T3 Eff.	< 1.0	1/wk	1/wk	T3 Eff. Turbidimeter	
	T4 Eff.	< 1.0	1/wk	1/wk	T4 Eff. Turbidimeter	
	SS1	< 0.1	1/12 hr	1/12 hr	SS #1 Sample Tap	
	SS2	< 0.1	1/12 hr	1/12 hr	SS #2 Sample Tap	
	Filters 1-23 Effluent	< 0.1	1/2 month	1/2 month	1-23 Filter Eff. Turbidimeters	
	3/4 Mile Michigan Ditch	N/A	N/A	2/wk Apr.–June	Location on upper Poudre River	
	Keal Bridge	N/A	N/A	2/wk Apr.–June	Location on upper Poudre River	
	Narrows Campground	N/A	N/A	2/wk Apr.–June	Location on upper Poudre River	
pH (pH units)	HT Raw	N/A	1/wk	1/wk	Raw Water Sample Station	Electrode method using a two standard calibration; EPA Approved. †Standard Methods-4500 H+ (*Process Control Lab*)
	PR Raw	N/A	1/wk	1/24 hr	Raw Water Sample Station	
	PR Raw	N/A	1/month	1/wk	Poudre River Intake	
	T1 Effluent	> 6.10	1/wk	1/wk	T1 Eff. Turbidimeter	
	T2 Effluent	> 6.10	1/wk	1/wk	T2 Eff. Turbidimeter	
	T3 Effluent	> 6.10	1/wk	1/wk	T3 Eff. Turbidimeter	
	T4 Effluent	> 6.10	1/wk	1/wk	T4 Eff. Turbidimeter	
	T4 Effluent	> 6.10	1/wk	1/wk	T4 Floc Drywell	
	SS1	7.80–8.00	1/12 hr	1/12 hr	SS #1 Sample Tap	
	SS2	7.80–8.00	1/12 hr	1/12 hr	SS #2 Sample Tap	
	Wash Water Return	N/A	1/wk	1/wk	Wash Water Return Overflow	
	3/4 Mile Michigan Ditch	N/A	N/A	2/wk Apr.–June	Location on upper Poudre River	
	Keal Bridge	N/A	N/A	2/wk Apr.–June	Location on upper Poudre River	
	Narrows Campground	N/A	N/A	2/wk Apr.–June	Location on upper Poudre River	

*Is defined as October–March

†*Standard Methods for the Examination of Water and Wastewater*, 19th edition, 1995.

Source. *City of Fort Collins (Colo.) water treatment facility process control laboratory.*

Figure 3-1 Example of a weekly sampling matrix

- deviations in routine chemical, physical, or biological parameters
- accidents involving hazardous materials spilled in the source water
- high pathogen counts in the source water
- elevated heterotrophic plate counts (HPCs)
- elevated coliform counts
- customer complaints regarding quality
- threats to public water supplies
- problems with chemical feed equipment or loss of process
- washwater that must be returned to the head of a plant without pretreatment or disinfection
- algae blooms
- surface water plants not meeting the requirement of less than 0.1 ntu out of individual filters at all times or exceeding 0.3 ntu for 10 minutes after the filter is placed on-line
- cross connections found in the system
- total organic carbon (TOC) levels difficult to reduce in treatment process
- water main breaks or other breaches in the distribution system
- biofilms discovered in the clearwell, storage reservoirs, or distribution system

Reservoir Turnover Monitoring

Another surface water condition that may warrant increased monitoring is reservoir turnover. Facilities that take water from surface water impoundments are subject to annual reservoir turnovers. Although site-specific, turnover typically occurs once in the fall and sometimes in the spring. Turnover is caused by the mixing of a formerly temperature-stratified reservoir. Cold oxygenated water drops to the bottom of the reservoir and replaces warmer water that was anoxic. This turnover can cause quick changes in water quality.

The column of water that exists in most reservoirs has three levels. The upper warmer water is called the epilimnion, the middle level is the metalimnion or thermocline, and the bottom layer is the hypolimnion. Monitoring this column is site-specific and needs to be studied before designing the final monitoring plan. Usually, the more samples that can be taken at various depths, the better the treatment staff will be able to predict water quality changes over time. Depending on the elevation of the intake, the plant may be able to take water at different depths and avert potential problems.

In a stratified reservoir, the three vertical zones (Figure 3-2) of water do not mix and the structure of the water column is determined by the water temperature. Ambient air temperature, influent flow to the reservoir, bacteriological results, algae identification, turbidity, nutrient concentrations, water column dissolved oxygen, and water temperature can all help predict turnover. In some cases, metals such as iron (Fe) and manganese (Mn) may become a problem due to low dissolved oxygen in the hypolimnion layer.

Groundwater Monitoring

Public water supplies using groundwater sources rely on the integrity of the well construction and the natural protection of aquifers. Where well construction is adequate and the aquifer protected, microbiological monitoring programs beyond sampling for total coliforms, *E. coli*, heterotrophic bacteria, and various nuisance environmental bacteria has a limited value. Monitoring programs should be developed to detect changes in water quality that reflect problems with the well itself and natural protective systems. Without adequate well construction or natural protection of the aquifer, expansion of the monitoring program to include other indicator organisms or pathogens may be warranted.

Water quality in wells is not always consistent, for example, water quality in an aquifer can change. Depending on the aquifer, changes in water quality may become evident with an increase in the rate or total volume of water pumped from the well. Fractured limestone and sandstone formations with little protective overburden appear highly susceptible to microbial and chemical contamination. In one epidemiological investigation, clinical evidence indicated that a hepatitis outbreak was due to contamination of a fractured limestone aquifer from septic tank discharges. The same type of fracturing appears to be responsible for high groundwater velocities.

The key to developing a monitoring plan for a groundwater system is obtaining information about the aquifer and the wells in use. Performing a source water assessment or developing a wellhead protection program provides most of the information required to develop a monitoring plan. Information regarding existing well construction practices is invaluable; a poorly constructed well cannot be expected to produce consistent water quality. Typical problem areas with construction include the wellhead, casing, or grouting. Holes, gaps, or other breaches in the systems allow contaminants access to the well.

To determine well construction problems, sampling may be required within the first few minutes or seconds of operating the well. The sample collector may need to determine water volume by measuring the static water level reading to the bottom of the screen or the open bore hole. The primary samples for examining well integrity usually need to be collected within the first two volumes contained in the well. A delay in collecting the sample may risk diluting the contaminants to below detection limits or losing contaminants by flushing the system with fresh water from the surrounding aquifer. A drop in microbiological counts from the initial samples to after the system has been adequately flushed often indicates construction problems. Total coliform or heterotrophic bacteria counts, or both, can be used as indicators

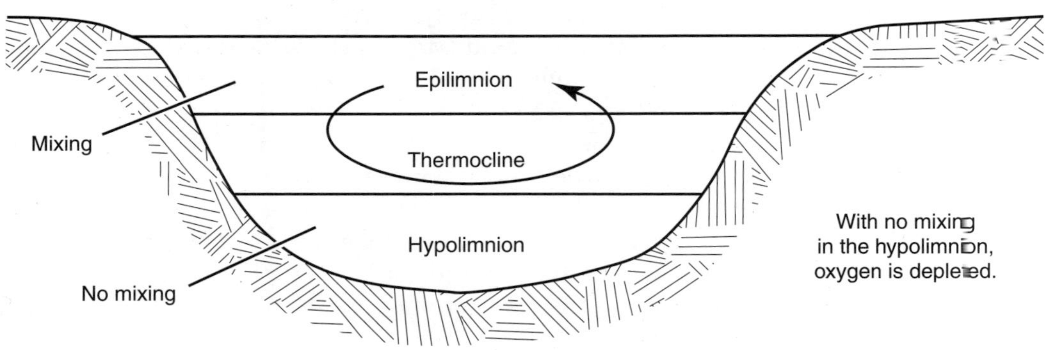

Figure 3-2 Stratification layers of a reservoir

Monitoring aquifer-related problems requires detailed knowledge of existing hydrogeological characteristics. For example, it may be necessary to temporarily seal portions of the well with inflatable bladders to isolate one section of the aquifer from another. Samples may have to be collected at specified intervals throughout a pumping test to detect variations in water quality. In general, an increase in selected indicator counts or values indicates aquifer problems. For example, a correlation between an increase in indicator microbial counts with some surface activities, such as precipitation, indicates direct recharge or groundwater under the influence of surface water. An observed increase in coliform counts over time may justify the expansion of the monitoring program to include other possible microbial contaminants.

Other considerations for increasing the monitoring frequency of well systems are

- increased chlorine demand
- sudden decrease in well production
- high levels of metals, such as manganese (Mn) and iron (Fe)
- biofilm indicators, such as slime observed in the distribution system
- redox potential and pH measurements for biofilms
- temperature changes
- coliforms detected at the source
- increased levels of coliforms in unchlorinated well water
- significant change in total dissolved solids

Monitoring Within Treatment Systems

Since the primary purpose of any treatment system is to improve water quality, a change in microbial quality through the treatment process is expected. The purpose of the monitoring program within treatment systems is to detect those changes. Treatment processes that may change water quality include aeration, coagulation, filtration, softening, and disinfection. Monitoring changes require testing before and after each unit process.

Monitoring changes in groundwater supplies that use simple chemical injection at the discharge piping of a well is straightforward. Sampling is suggested before and following treatment. The untreated or source water tap should be located as close to the wellhead as practical. For wells using vertical turbines, the source water tap should be located far enough from the motor to avoid air currents from the motor. The treated or plant tap should be located downstream from the point of chemical injection at a sufficient distance to permit mixing of the chemical and water. As suggested earlier, the standard indicators of total coliform and heterotrophic bacteria are adequate for most monitoring programs, unless there are problems. Testing for nuisance and fouling bacteria (*Sphaerotilus*, *Leptothrix*, *Crenothrix*, *Gallionella*, and *Clonothrix*) may be performed periodically at the source water tap.

Another way for microbiological contamination to enter the system is a typical iron–manganese removal system with aeration, detention, and filtration. Climatic conditions may assist bacteria in entering the system through the aerator or a poorly sealed detention tank. Inadequate operation and maintenance allows biofilms and slime growths to develop in the various treatment units. Establishing a monitoring program to track coliforms and heterotrophic bacteria in the source, postdetention tank, and filtered water are generally adequate. Monitoring is not as critical in closed or pressure-filtered iron–manganese removal systems using potassium permanganate because of the oxidant's disinfection capabilities.

Developing a monitoring program for a standard coagulation, sedimentation, and filtration treatment plant can become cumbersome. Monitoring lime–soda ash and lime softening plants presents the same dilemma. The main issue to consider when developing a program is how the information will be used. Sampling sites can be set up before and after each unit process. However, most information from the monitoring program may not be used to alter treatment processes. Furthermore, the usefulness of information gained may be questionable. One way to avoid this situation is to focus on optimizing unit processes. Limited information from samples collected at the source and before and after the filters may yield information that will be useful. Consideration should be given to sampling from the effluent of each filter rather than at a point of confluence from all filters.

Routine total coliform monitoring at the water tap, pre- and postfiltration, and finished water effluents should be considered the minimum baseline for complete treatment plants. HPCs after the filters and the reservoir effluent give a better picture of the status of microbial removal efficiencies. Monitoring for other contaminants depends on the source or source water makeup. For filtered water, the total coliform count should be zero colony-forming units per 100 millilitres (0 cfu/100 mL). The HPC for filtered water quality should approach 0 cfu/100 mL. Similarly, for any other microbial indicator counts, filtered water quality before disinfection should approach zero.

Microbial monitoring within the pretreatment or coagulation processes may not produce useful information. Floc particles may interfere with reading and interpreting results. Some test methods are based on color change after a specified incubation period, and iron-based coagulants may discolor the test water. Many analytical techniques are based on the theory that bacteria and other contaminants are uniformly dispersed throughout the entire sample aliquot. Coagulation processes concentrate microbial organisms into the bodies of floc particles, producing artificially low or high results, depending on the sampling technique.

Test results of samples from rapid sand or multimedia filter effluent lines may depend on when the filter was last backwashed or restarted. Filters may produce poor quality water immediately following backwash. Also, filters produce lower quality water for a short duration when returned to service after being off-line. Samples collected in the middle of a filter run may produce microbial counts near a "normal" or "average" condition, whereas samples collected at the beginning or end of a filter run are probably biased.

The possibility of concentrating microbial and other contaminants by recycling filter backwash is a major concern. Depending on regulations and the need to reuse backwash water, a monitoring program may be needed to evaluate the safety of this practice. The monitoring program should compare the quality of the backwash and incoming source water.

The primary sampling locations for any treatment facility should be the effluent point of any on-site reservoir or the point of entry into the distribution system. Daily sampling for total coliforms and HPCs should be the minimum. Sampling for other microbial contaminants should be considered in the event of a treatment system failure. Treatment failures can include sudden increases in filtered water turbidity or an inability to maintain a turbidity of 0.1 ntu or less in the effluent from any single filter. The ultimate treatment failure would be permitting filters to operate to or beyond the point of breakthrough. Additional monitoring at the filter effluent because of treatment failure should include testing for fecal coliforms or *E. coli*, *Pseudomonas* sp., fecal streptococci, *Giardia*, and *Cryptosporidium*. If the filters responsible for the problem are removed from service before sampling, the alternative sampling site should be the plant tap or the point of entry in the distribution system. Natural events warranting expansion of monitoring include turnover in settling basins, heavy precipitation or runoff, or high winds creating unusual conditions in open treatment basins.

The lack of physical system integrity for finished water storage facilities indicates that an expanded monitoring program beyond a total coliform and HPC program is needed. Integrity issues can include open hatches, improperly designed vents, leaky roofs or covers, and open finished water basins. Depending on the severity of the problem, additional monitoring in the distribution system may be needed.

Monitoring Within the Distribution System

Historically, microbial monitoring in the distribution system for many public water supplies has revolved around regulatory requirements for total coliform sampling. Usually, little to no additional information is available about microbiological activity within the distribution system. Additional information, however, may provide a basis for improvements in water treatment operations.

The US Environmental Protection Agency (USEPA) regulations for distribution system total coliform monitoring are designed to reveal catastrophic failures. Strict adherence to the prescribed federal monitoring requirements may not detect the onset of a problem. Additional monitoring beyond the regulatory minimums for the number of samples, frequency, and locations may provide early detection of a problem. It is easier to locate, isolate, and correct problems by sampling additional sites.

The site selection process should address geographical coverage, detention time, and accessibility. Regulatory compliance monitoring and special investigations within the distribution system should occur at representative locations. The entire distribution system should be included in the monitoring program, including pressure districts, isolated areas within the system causing excessive detention times, and materials used for service connections and internal plumbing. Excessive detention times may contribute to undesirable changes in water quality. Usage and storage are two major factors to consider when examining detention time. Limited accessibility to the actual sampling tap may exclude potential sites.

Routine analysis of HPCs is a relatively inexpensive tool for understanding water quality changes occurring within a distribution system. As with all monitoring programs, baseline data for HPCs at various sites must be established. Under ideal conditions, HPC levels should be low. An increase in the cfu/mL may indicate a potential problem. Some authorities have used a 1-log increase in HPC to indicate action is needed. In practice, many utilities start taking action whenever HPC levels for a section of the distribution system increase by a set percentage. When evaluated with other physical, chemical, or microbiological measurements, the potential source or nature of a problem may be identified and corrected.

Microbiological indicator levels not representative of historical background water quality signify additional work is needed. With adequate historical data, HPC can supplement information obtained from standard total coliform testing. HPC levels higher than expected values for a portion of a distribution system may indicate a need to flush water mains or redisinfect.

It may be helpful to use HPC as an indicator in conjunction with the isolation and identification of *Pseudomonas vesicularis* and/or *Flavobacterium* sp. to detect possible biofilm problems. If coliforms are detected, identifying the species of the contaminants (speciation) for *Klebsiella*, *Enterobacter*, *Aerobacter*, and *E. coli* may further help identify a potential biofilm problem. Water distribution system temperatures of 59° F (15° C) or above are normally associated with biofilm activities. The value of pH or TOC as additional potential indicators of biofilm problems typically depends on the specific water system.

Biofilms

Biofilms are patches or masses of living and/or dead microorganisms that accumulate inside water storage reservoirs or pipelines. Because treated water is not sterile, some degree of biofilms exists in all systems. Other types of organisms or material can be "sandwiched" between layers in the biofilm, including nematodes, algae, bacteria, pathogens, fungi, and mineral deposits. See chapter 2 of this manual for more information on biofilms.

New research indicates that biodegradable organic carbon (BDOC) and assimilable organic carbon (AOC) may provide nutrients for many biofilm organisms. Systems with more than 100 µg/L BDOC or AOC tend to have more coliform bacteria than those systems with lower levels. Limiting the amount of BDOC and AOC by optimizing water treatment processes is key to reducing this problem. Temperatures greater than 59° F (15° C) may also increase the growth of some bacteria. Plants using ozone and biologically active filters should monitor the BDOC and AOC levels leaving the treatment plant and throughout the distribution system and establish internal operating goals.

Other monitoring actions for biofilms include

- visually inspect valves and pumps
- use borehole camera inspection
- monitor and record temperature trends
- start and continue a cross-connection control program
- establish sampling methods, such as in-well collectors, filters, and grab samples
- observe and sample during routine systematic flushing
- conduct hydraulic performance tests of the distribution system
- add specific biofilm investigations with analytical methods or presence–absence tests, and direct microscopic analysis, when applicable
- perform basic inorganic chemical tests
- monitor organic carbon (AOC/BDOC) levels in source and finished water, where applicable
- optimize water treatment facilities and strive to meet the Partnership for Safe Drinking Water goal of less than 0.1 ntu at all times
- implement or continue corrosion control programs
- maintain disinfectant residuals throughout the system

- monitor cycling of reservoir levels at various times of the year
- clean and disinfect clearwells and reservoirs on a frequent basis

SAMPLING ISSUES AND TECHNIQUES

The sample collector is responsible for using the correct sample container and sampling technique. If the wrong containers or techniques are used, the validity of the sample results will be questionable. Sampling errors may result in monitoring violations, a loss of laboratory time, and a waste of the public water supply's resources.

The water quality laboratory is usually responsible for providing sample containers for the parameter it intends to analyze. Part of the quality control procedure for any microbiological analytical work requires that the laboratory confirm the sterility of the bottles it uses by testing a portion of the containers it purchases or prepares. For example, the difference between similar sample containers may simply be the preservatives placed in the container before sample collection. Typically, preservatives are dechlorinating agents that must remain in the bottle and not be rinsed out. Laboratories usually do not accept sample containers prepared by or obtained from another laboratory.

Most bacteriological samples have a sample holding time, i.e., the maximum period between the time of sample collection and initiating analysis. The laboratory should supply this information to the sample collector. To meet the holding-time criteria, the sample collector, a courier, or an overnight delivery service may deliver the samples. Whenever practical, samples should be transported iced in a chest or cooler. The laboratory will not accept frozen samples. Samples waiting for delivery should be iced or refrigerated at 4° C. Rapid delivery back to the laboratory is essential to allow sufficient time to perform the analysis.

The sample collector must read and understand the directions for each type of sample. In addition, the sample collector may need to be familiar with field testing for free chlorine or other disinfectant residual monitoring, aseptic sampling procedures, and safe procedures for handling corrosive materials. Either the laboratory or the water supplier should provide this information to the sample collector. Information regarding all sample tap locations and accessibility should be on file.

Example of Directions for Total Coliform or HPC Sampling:

1. Do not open the bottle until ready to collect the sample. Do not touch the inside of the cap or bottle. Retain the cap in your hand. (Do not set it down.)

2. Do not rinse the bottle with the sample. The bottle contains sodium thiosulfate to deactivate chlorine. Go to step 3 if taking a sample from a tap. If collecting a sample from a lake or pool, plunge bottle down and move it in a continuous arc down and back up through the water. Discard the top half-inch (12 mm) of sample. Go to step 4.

3. Select a clean faucet and remove attachments, such as aerators, dishwasher connectors, and so forth. Do not use swivel-arm faucets or faucets at mop sinks. Allow water to run for five min (until cold) at full flow from the sampling tap. Immediately before sample collection, reduce flow to avoid

splashing, and collect the sample directly into the bottle. Do not use an intermediate container. Do not allow water from the outside surface of the faucet to drip into the bottle. Fill the bottle only to the bottom of the neck.

4. Replace the cap. Record the sample time, date, location, disinfectant residual concentration, water temperature, and sampler's initials. It is critical that paperwork or forms submitted to the laboratory with the sample be complete and legible. The laboratory should provide the sampling chain-of-custody forms, which record information needed by the laboratory to ensure all critical quality control elements have been met and to generate valid analytical results.

Tap Selection for Microbiological Samples

A potential problem with any microbial monitoring program is poor sampling tap selection. Failure to select a proper tap produces misleading results. Swing and mixing faucets, and taps with vacuum beakers, aerators, hoses, or filters should not be used. These taps have the potential for bacterial colonies established on surface gaskets and screens to slough off during sample collection. Other potential problems with some taps include the manner in which the flow leaves the faucet. Flow streams that spray or roll up around the end of the faucet are unacceptable.

For microbiological sampling, simplicity in tap design is a key. Manufactured metallic ½-in. (12-mm) faucets with a single shut-off handle and a downturn spout without hose bib threads fulfill this requirement. Sample taps consisting of a petcock or other valve device and approximately 12 in. (300 mm) of ¼-in. (6-mm) tubing formed in a downturned U-shape are ideally suited for sampling. An added advantage of these designs is that the taps can only be used to draw water reducing the likelihood of contamination by other uses. Unintentional contamination by other parties is a major concern for distribution sites or other locations with unrestricted access to taps. Commercially available sampling boxes directly tapped into the water main are another option for distribution systems where freezing and vandalism are not a problem.

Pathogens

One of the greatest challenges water professionals face is selecting an accurate technique to directly quantify the number of enteric pathogens, including *Cryptosporidium parvum* and *Giardia lamblia*. *Giardia* cysts and *Cryptosporidium* oocysts may be required monitoring for certain public water supplies. In some cases, virus monitoring is also necessary, and the search continues for improved techniques for sampling waterborne protozoa (Figure 3-3). Great strides in analytical techniques have been made over the past few years, and research continues for methods that provide quick and accurate results. An overview of the current methods of sampling for pathogens is discussed in following paragraphs.

Field worksheets developed by the laboratory should be filled out completely and checked for errors. They provide key information for the sampler on basic chemistry, physical measurements, and plant statistics at the time of sample. Plant schematics or diagrams are especially helpful when they indicate the exact location of where samples are taken. Information should always be written in waterproof ink on laboratory forms (Figure 3-4). Chain-of-custody forms may be necessary for transport to the laboratory or compliance monitoring situations.

Preparation of the sampling devices as well as carefully planning where and how to take the samples is essential. When using cartridge filter sampling units, recommendations on specific detergents and cleaning techniques should be discussed with the laboratory. Field personnel or staff should be trained on assembly, disassembly, cleaning, and care of cartridge filter units and housing units that can become a problem because of improper set up or poor seals at the top of the housing. Flushing the sample taps, hoses, and housing assembly thoroughly before use is essential. Latex gloves need to be worn when inserting the polypropylene 1-μm filter to limit contamination.

Sampling methods for water containing chlorine residuals require a special procedure involving injecting a flow-proportional dechlorination solution while collecting the sample. The main purpose of the proportional dechlorination system is to eliminate the chlorine residual that may subsequently interfere with identification procedures. Specific attention to flow rate and feed rate of the dechlorination agent is critical. Flowmeters for the 1-μm filter units should be calibrated each year by a meter shop and checked more often with a graduated cylinder to ensure accuracy.

Filter devices such as shown in Figure 3-5 are being developed. This type of unit is self-contained and requires similar sampling protocols to those previously discussed. After sample collection, the inlet and outlet of the unit are simply sealed and delivered to the laboratory for analysis.

Transport and storage of the sample to the laboratory should be expedited by using overnight services. Communication should be already established between the sampler and the laboratory. Coolant materials, such as Blue Ice®, should never be in direct contact with the filters. Coolers need to be cleaned regularly and the coolants sealed to prevent leakage. If care is not taken in sealing the filter before delivery to the laboratory, cross-contamination can occur during transit.

In a critical situation, samples may need to be collected over a short time period, and sampling supplies may be difficult to secure late at night, on weekends, or on holidays. An ample supply of filters and appropriate sampling equipment should always be available for systems known to have the possibility of enteric pathogens in the source or finished water. For smaller systems, the names of several neighboring larger water plants, and after-hours phone numbers for vendors and laboratories should be available. Equipment expense can be overwhelming for the small system, and sharing resources may be the key link in protecting public health.

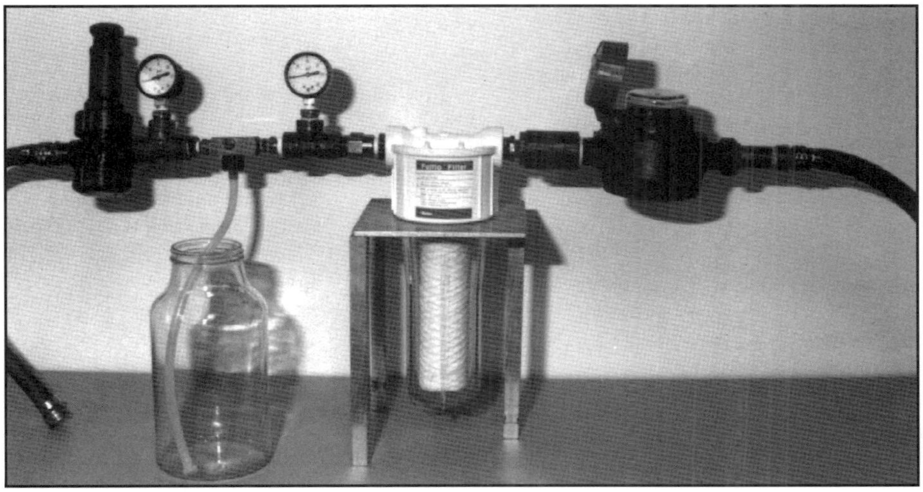

Figure 3-3 Filter housing (1 μm) with appropriate flow-measuring and dechlorinating devices

Analysis Request

Client: ______________________________ Date: __________ PO#: ______________

Person(s) designated to receive results: ______________________________

Address: ______________________________

Phone: ( ) ______________________________ Fax ( ) ______________________________

Address for cooler return: ______________________________

Sample Information: (please print clearly)

Sample Location: ______________________

Sample ID: ______________________

PWSID#: ______________________

Start:

Date: __________ Time: __________

Temperature: ________ pH: ________ NTU: ________

Stop:

Date: __________ Time: __________

NTU: __________

Gallons Sampled: __________ (__________ Litres)

Sample exposed to chlorine? Yes ______ No ________

Sample dechlorinated? Yes ________ No __________

Sampler's Name: ______________________

Please fill in where applicable for this sample:

This sample is a raw surface water _______
finished surface water ________ groundwater ________ or other,
please explain ______________________

Type of Raw Water Source:

_______ Spring
_______ Dug well
_______ Drilled well
_______ Horizontal well
_____ Dug well
_____ Lake/Reservoir
_____ Stream/River
_____ Irrigation canal

If well, depth: ________ ft and distance from
river/stream/lake: ________ ft

Type of Treatment:

______ None
______ Disinfection only
______ Conventional treatment
______ Direct filtration
______ Filter to waste cycle
______ Infiltration gallery

______ Diatomaceous earth
______ Slow sand
______ Pressure filter
______ Other

Filter(s) hydraulic loading ______ gpm/sq.ft.
________ "Clean" filter bed put on line

Type of Disinfection:

_______ Prechlorination
_______ Postchlorination
_______ Postchloramines
_______ Ozone
_______ Other

Courtesy C&H Diagnostics Inc.

Figure 3-4 Example of a laboratory analysis form to be completed in the field

Figure 3-6 shows a pathogen sample kit with various types of hoses, connectors, and dechlorination equipment stored and ready for use. Sampling kits for *Giardia* and *Cryptosporidium* analysis should contain the following items:

- inlet hose with adapters for various sample ports
- backflow preventor
- pressure regulator with pressure gauge
- fluid proportioning injector with pressure gauge
- calibration column for proportioning solution, when applicable
- 1-µm nominal porosity filter and holder
- water meter
- flow control valve–limiting control orifice
- plastic sampling bags
- ice packs with plastic sealed covers
- sample labels
- stopwatch for calculating flow rates
- calculator to determine dechlorination rates, if applicable
- latex gloves
- sodium thiosulfate and reagent-grade water (may be secured through your laboratory)

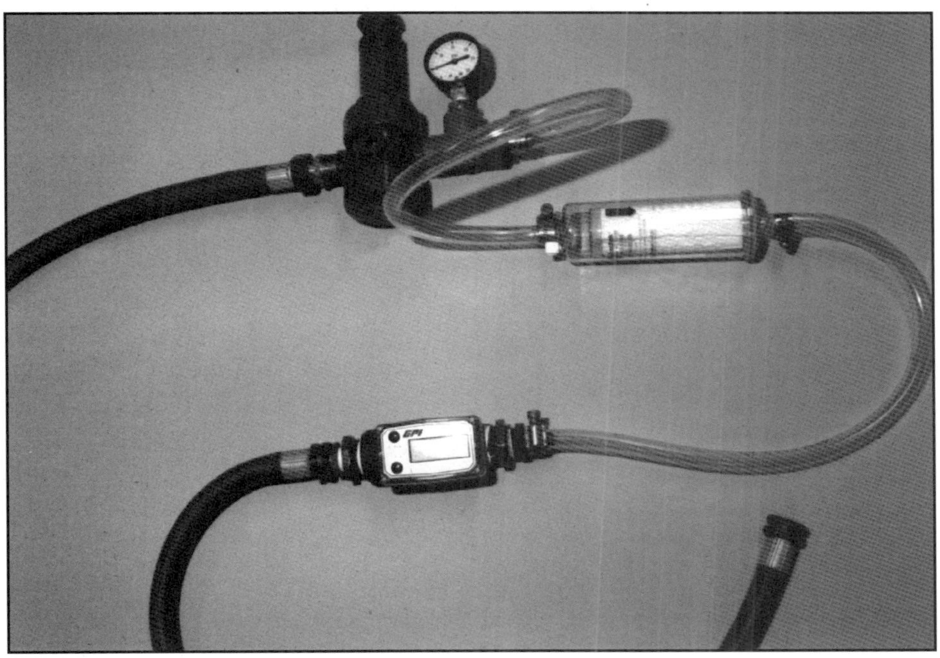

Figure 3-5 Capsule for *Cryptosporidium* and *Giardia* sampling

- graduated cylinders for calibrating sodium thiosulfate additions
- equipment for shipping 10-L samples to the laboratory, if applicable

The following factors should be taken into account when sampling for pathogenic organisms:

Surface water source.

- Confirm the sample point does not have any chemical pretreatment.
- Collect samples after small reservoirs or presedimentation basins, if possible.
- Review the plant process with the laboratory using a plant schematic to describe the sample location. This can help the analyst understand the sample and situation.
- Sample as described by the laboratory using the most recent USEPA-approved method.

Groundwater.

- Sample at the discharge of the pump.
- Flush all lines for a minimum of five min before sampling.
- Discuss with the laboratory all required specific monitoring data.
- Provide a schematic of the system to the laboratory.

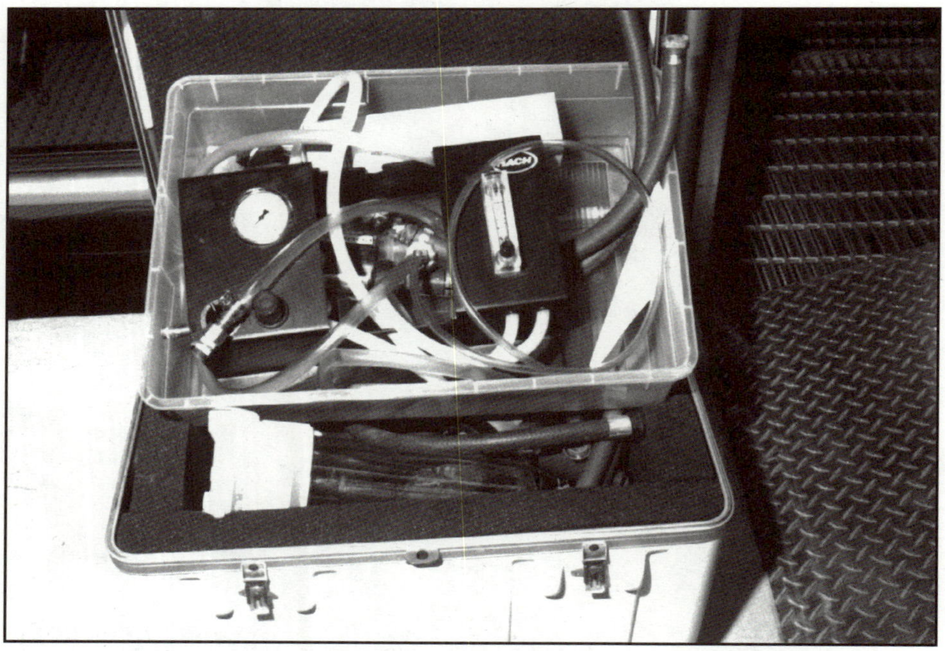

Figure 3-6 Pathogen sampling kit. Various types of hoses, connectors, and dechlorination equipment can be stored and ready for use.

Finished water.

- Sample before chlorination, if possible.
- Dechlorination is required if a sample cannot be taken before chlorination. This procedure requires adding sodium thiosulfate while taking care to maintain proper disinfectant feed rates to the system. Discuss with the laboratory.
- Use the plant schematic to indicate the point of sample for the laboratory.

Sampling Stations or Points

Representative sampling is critical to building a valid database of water quality information. Such a database is valuable because a utility can see seasonal trends, quality improvements, and action plans. Although water quality databases are usually in a computer program, small water suppliers may simply use organized files with specific locations referenced.

Larger systems may prefer establishing sampling station points throughout a water treatment facility and in the water distribution system. One type of sample station is shown in Figure 3-7. If desired, grab samples can be taken at the polyvinyl chloride (PVC) line or pathogen sampling taken at the ¾-in. (19-mm) hose bibs for each filter shown in Figure 3-8. On-line analyzers can be used to monitor filtered water quality. Information from on-line analyzers is then routed through programmable logic controllers and logged onto a computer database for storage. The information can then be archived in database format for retrieval, trending, and establishing control limits for out-of-target results. Because on-line instruments may have different ranges of accuracy, each parameter needs to be evaluated individually. Quality assurance (QA) and quality control (QC) programs to ensure instrument

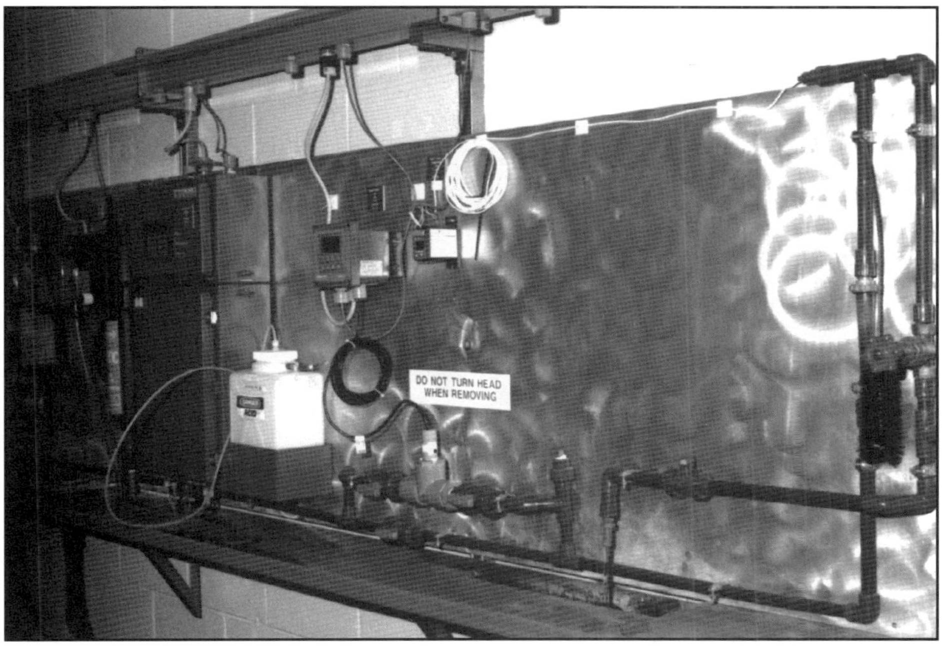

Figure 3-7 Sample station showing on-line analyzers and location for grab samples

calibration or standardization are essential for on-line equipment. One of the major benefits of the sample station concept is that it makes available both real-time data and information on grab samples.

On-line units or running sample taps around the clock may not be justified or practical for smaller systems. Small systems rely on the experience and knowledge of the system operator. Maintaining consistency in the sampling technique and using best judgment to obtain the most representative samples will yield accurate results. The system operator should keep judicious records and ascertain the integrity of the system by sampling the source water and the storage and distribution systems.

Proactive sampling by water systems can be a helpful troubleshooting tool. For example, if a plant or system operates under unusual conditions (e.g., loss of process), sampling with 1-µm units for microscopic particulate analysis (MPA) could provide invaluable information if the units are placed on-line *during* the event. Analysis of the sample filters can provide important information to the water system if used as a proactive tool rather than a reactive test method. Too often, facilities try to piece the puzzle of events together later and not when a problem is taking place.

LABORATORY SELECTION

A certified laboratory must be used to provide analytical data intended to meet the compliance monitoring requirements of the Safe Drinking Water Act (SDWA). However, certification is not a guarantee that the laboratory will always produce valid results. Certification means that the laboratory has successfully met the requirements of the primacy jurisdiction and that certain QC practices are in place.

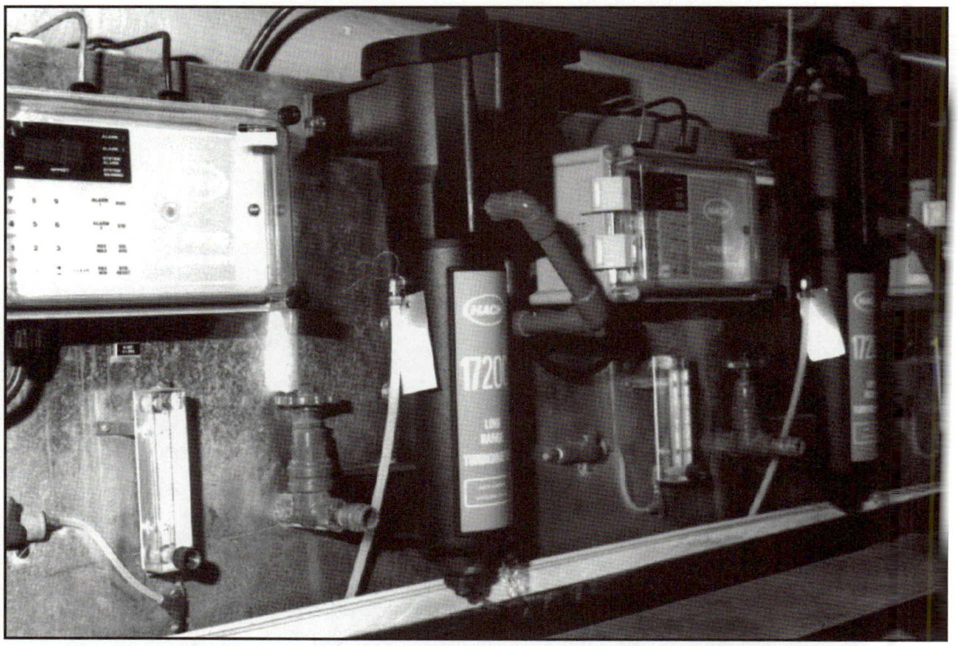

Figure 3-8 On-line turbidimeter sample station with 3/4-in. (19-mm) sample taps for MPA and pathogen monitoring

Most primacy jurisdictions do not require public water supplies to use certified laboratories for testing beyond the monitoring requirements of the SDWA. Also, most primacy agencies do not offer laboratory certification for contaminants for which monitoring has not been specified by the SDWA.

The use of a certified laboratory for optional, nonregulatory testing assures the client that the laboratory is at least aware of certain QC practices that are necessary to produce valid results. One of the certification requirements specifies that laboratories have and maintain an updated QA manual. Depending on contractual arrangements, the laboratory's QA program may be reviewed by the client. A good correlation between the manual and any audit report of the laboratory is an indication of the quality expected from the facility. A review of the QA manual will give the client an idea of the laboratory's capabilities. A failure to fully understand these capabilities and corresponding limitations can become a problem between environmental laboratories and their clients. The capabilities a client should understand include the inherent variabilities in producing microbial data, time required for analysis and reporting of final results, and cost.

Clients of environmental laboratories should understand that different analytical methods may produce different results. Also, there should be an understanding that there is variability in results produced using a single method. Each analytical method has its own recovery rate for a given sample matrix. One method may be capable of recovering 92 percent of the colonies or organisms present, while a different analytical method may have a recovery rate of 87 percent. The difference of 5 percent indicates final results from the two techniques may vary. Microbial techniques report a fixed number of colonies or organisms per a fixed volume or simply as confirming their presence or absence. If the analytical technique was developed to determine the number of colonies per 100 mL and the density is 1 cfu/200 mL, a sample volume of 100 mL will not always yield positive results.

The time needed for an environmental laboratory to return analytical results to its clients depends on a variety of factors, including workload, staffing, equipment, and analytical methods. For bacteriological tests, there may be different incubation periods for two different analytical techniques. In addition, one technique may require subsequent confirmatory testing while another technique may be self-confirmatory. A comparison of two *Standard Methods* procedures, 9221 and 9223, is an excellent example for demonstrating the differences in time required to produce final results. Method 9221, the multiple-tube fermentation technique, requires up to 48 hours for the presumptive stage and possibly an additional 48 hours (for a possible total of 96 hours) for the confirmatory stage of the test. Confirmed and final results are available from Method 9223, Colilert®, within 24 to 48 hours.

Another factor for differences in turnaround times involves how laboratories process sample results. After bench data are produced, time is required to read, interpret, and record the information. Laboratories need to review the QC associated with the sample before the results are released. Lack of staff on weekends or holidays may further slow down reporting time. In some instances, the laboratory may issue verbal or electronic reports as soon as the results are approved as meeting the QC requirements. Under no circumstances should a verbal report be the sole means of reporting the results to the client. Most primacy jurisdictions require either a hard copy or an easily retrievable electronic database report. Forwarding a hard copy of the results requires additional time. Reliance on a mailed hard copy as the only means for reporting results to a client may add potentially unacceptable delays in taking action to correct water quality problems.

USE OF RESULTS

After results are received from the laboratory, the public water utility has legal obligations and several decisions to make regarding the release of the information. The utility must report all monitoring results for contaminants covered by the SDWA to the primacy jurisdiction. Reporting a limited subset of results could be considered an attempt to conceal problems. The public water supply may be required to periodically release information to its consumers in a summarized report. Releasing information provides an opportunity to build support for system improvements and associated costs. In addition, information can prove systems in place are providing high quality water to customers. A utility should avoid releasing information too often, which can result in the message being ignored. Releasing too little or possibly inaccurate information also should be avoided.

Action Plans

Although every water treatment operator strives to produce high quality water, there is a possibility of pathogens passing treatment barriers. Using current methods, simply monitoring for *Giardia* or *Cryptosporidium* cannot assure the water supplier that water is free of pathogens at all times. Therefore, water professionals must develop boil water advisory (BWA) criteria and action plans before there is a problem, not during a crisis.

A course of action should be in place if a test result indicates positive fecal coliform, *Giardia*, or *Cryptosporidium* in finished water. Boil water advisories require a considerable amount of thought if they are to be carried out in timely fashion. One of the most important aspects of BWAs is determining what circumstances will trigger the event, which may involve violation of the total coliform rule, breakdown in treatment, pathogen test result, or an increase in diarrheal disease in the community.

Action plans should be developed by task teams including the operator, local and state health departments, hospitals, nursing homes, physicians, pharmacies, and so forth. A sample flowchart is shown in Figure 3-9. There is no single perfect action plan for all utilities; each must be tailored to the specific area and system. It is essential that plant staff focus on the challenge of fixing the problem that prompted the BWA thus protecting public health. Text of the public notification regulation can be found in the SDWA Reauthorization. Smaller systems might be able to share resources with larger utilities or to network using electronic mail or phone.

Water treatment professionals must regard public health protection as the highest priority. If a test result or condition exists that may breach the public health water quality standard, BWAs must be considered. Boil water advisories should be issued only after carefully evaluating the circumstances. Once the criteria to issue a BWA have been met, prompt action is necessary. Customer confidence may be eroded or elevated depending on the timeliness and accuracy of the information they receive.

Considerations Leading to Boil Water Advisories

The use of analytical results in deciding whether to issue a BWA requires considerable subjective judgment. Professionals at both the public water utility and the primacy jurisdiction making the decision must consider the consequences of issuing a BWA, including its ultimate costs, or delaying its issuance while waiting for additional information.

Boil water advisories erode public confidence if they are not issued in time or issued too often. Financial costs to the public supply can be substantial, but the final

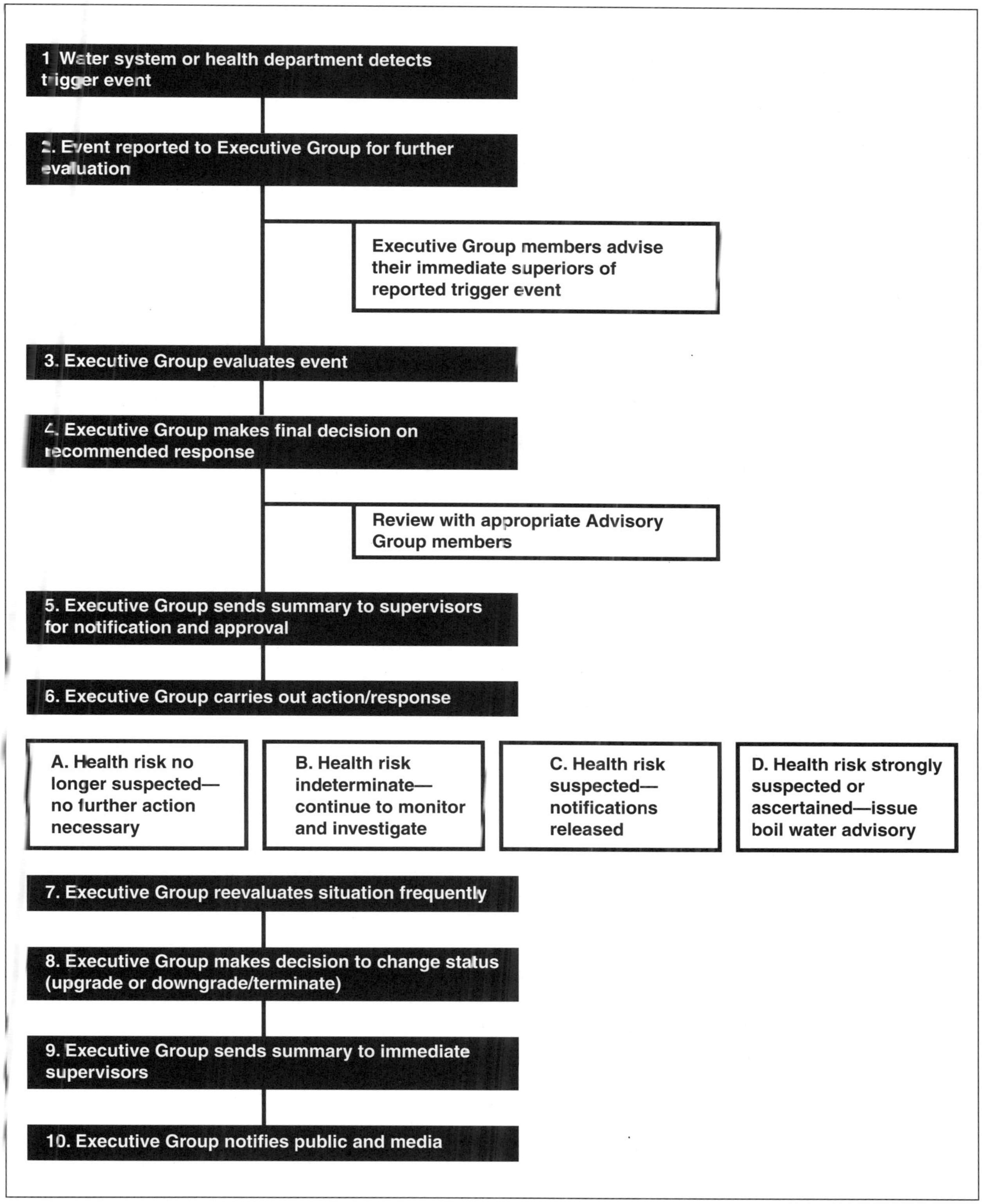

Figure 3-9 Sample flowchart for action–response plan

costs for not issuing an advisory when needed may be devastating. Failure to issue a timely advisory could lead to serious public health, financial, and public relations consequences.

Results from a single sample or set of samples are typically not cause for issuing a BWA. Issuance usually requires additional confirmation, including subsequent sample results, other water quality data, and reports on treatment system operations failure or a breach in the system. Delays in taking action while waiting for additional microbial results may not be prudent.

Public water systems using surface water or groundwater under the influence of surface water are more vulnerable to treatment system breakdowns and may justify immediate issuance of an advisory. Loss of disinfection residuals at the point of entry for these supplies is one reason to take immediate action. Loss of disinfection residuals at the point of entry for protected groundwater supplies in most cases would not be considered cause for the immediate issuance of a BWA without other mitigating circumstances. High filter effluent turbidities should be considered cause for immediate action. If the point-of-entry turbidity levels exceed the regulatory treatment standards or if there are sudden increases in turbidity levels from a single filter, then the water supplier and the primacy agency should determine whether or not an advisory is warranted. Other indicators of treatment system failures needing joint review include sudden changes in water quality or increases in finished water particle counts. Concurrent detection of microbial indicators of fecal contamination and a treatment system failure increases the possible need to issue an advisory.

Professional judgment and discretion are necessary in making decisions on the issuance of an advisory for distribution system failures. Failures include loss of pressure, documented cross-connection backflow, major water main breaks, and breaches in the integrity of water storage facilities. Microbial results supporting the decision to issue a BWA in the event of distribution system problems are not always readily available because of delays associated with analysis. In situations where microbial results are available and system failures are documented, the decision to issue an advisory should be straightforward.

Detection or sudden increase of any microbial indicators in a single sample or set of samples is not sufficient grounds to issue a BWA. However, the change is grounds for other actions such as collecting additional samples. Public water supplies have a regulatory-mandated responsibility to collect additional samples in the event of total coliform detection within the distribution system. Similar, but voluntary, actions regarding sample collection should take place when monitoring for other microbial indicators or pathogens reveals unexpected results. In addition, it may be advisable to consider collecting samples for other indicator organisms in the event of a positive sample, depending on the system and its conditions.

Before the onset of any problems, it is advisable for representatives of a public water supplier to meet with the local primacy jurisdiction agency to discuss the criteria for issuing public notices or BWAs. These discussions should include the actual wording and conditions for issuing the advisory as well as the comfort zones for all parties.

General issues to consider when issuing a BWA include

- reviewing data that may indicate a public health problem and evaluating the integrity of the samples and related quality assurance and control
- repeating the sampling immediately
- involving local and state health departments as soon as possible

- starting with the source water and following analytical results through to the finished water
- trying to identify cause and effect
- determining the identity of the pathogen or organism of concern, identifying and evaluating possible courses of action
- evaluating plant or system performance before, during, and after the sample was taken
- reviewing the last sanitary survey and performing portions again, if warranted
- looking for changes or unusual conditions to see if there is a correlation to sampling results
- reviewing HPC and coliform occurrence data before, during, and after the event
- evaluating the system's capability for contact time (CT) and whether or not the organism can be deactivated

Factors to consider involving the distribution system include

- reviewing water main flushing procedures
- implementing a systematic flushing plan as soon as practical (site-specific or systemwide)
- communicating with restaurants, hospitals, health care, and kidney dialysis centers
- contacting local hospitals, nursing homes, day care centers, and physicians to ascertain recent changes in the public health
- evaluating the area for possible cross-connections
- determining the availability of resources to deal with all of the issues
- establishing additional water quality monitoring sites to determine where other samples will be taken and their frequency
- determining if system line breaks or other unusual situations in the distribution system occurred before the discovery of positive fecal coliform

Considerations When Issuing Boil Water Advisories

Once the decision has been made to issue a BWA, the utility needs to do the following:

- Identify the specific person responsible for communicating with the media.
- Establish one site that will be the command center during the BWA.
- Meet with the task team and identify factors that trigger issuance of a BWA.
- Evaluate criteria for the BWA (e.g., CDC 1997).
- Evaluate the conditions that need to be met to rescind a BWA.
- Include the laboratory in all briefings.

- Increase watershed or well system monitoring and surveillance.
- Acquire extra sterile sample bottles, filters, chlorine-residual test equipment, and other critical supplies.
- Increase monitoring programs for source, treated, and finished water.
- Assign a task team to solve the source water or treatment problem.
- Ask for guidance from local or state health departments, if necessary.
- Maintain close communication with officials at local and state health departments.
- Use technology such as fax machines and electronic mail preprogrammed with contacts for situation updates.
- Identify possible sources of bottled water or mobile tanks for water distribution to customers.
- Have public education materials ready to hand out to all water users.
- Check the CT at the time of the alert and keep time-series logs.
- Sample as frequently as needed, but focus on public health protection.
- Keep one phone line open for internal communications.
- Maintain status boards posted with assignments and updates to ensure communication between staff and town or city leaders.
- Obtain references on action plans from the American Water Works Association (AWWA), the Centers for Disease Control and Prevention (CDC), and USEPA. Correlate these references with what is happening during an event.
- Prepare daily briefing reports understandable to the public. Use care in the spoken and written word; it is easy to say or write something that can be misinterpreted.
- Tailor BWAs to be site-specific for each situation.
- Keep a time-sequenced log of events.

Rescinding the Boil Water Advisory

The following steps should be taken before the BWA is rescinded:

- Determine if treatment is adequate and take immediate action if it is not.
- Check source water and determine if it is acceptable quality.
- Analyze the data that prompted the BWA and determine whether or not it could continue to be an issue due to the sampling as discussed previously.
- Focus on the cause and effect of the BWA.
- Develop a strategy for completion if temporary repairs or remedies are taken.
- Create a document recording all information leading up to, during, and after the incident.
- Work with health departments and the medical community to review epidemiological data.

REFERENCES

American Public Health Association, American Water Works Association, and Water Environment Federation. 1995. *Standard Methods for the Examination of Water and Wastewater*. 19th ed. Eaton, A.D., L.S. Clesceri, and A.E. Greenberg, eds. Washington, D.C.: APHA.

Anon. 1996. *Development of Performance Evaluation (PE) Sample Preparation Protocols for* Giardia *Cysts and* Cryptosporidium *Oocysts*. US Environmental Protection Agency Contract No. 68-C3-0365. Available from the USEPA Water Docket, telephone (202)260-3027.

AWWA. 1993. *So the People May Know.* Denver, Colo.: American Water Works Association.

CDC. 1997. Cryptosporidium *and Water: A Public Health Handbook*. Atlanta, Ga.: Centers for Disease Control.

Craun, G.F. 1993. *Safety of Water Disinfection: Balancing Chemical and Microbial Risks*. ILSI Press.

Frey, M.M., C.M. Hancock, and G.S. Logsdon. 1997. Cryptosporidium*: Answers to the Commonly Asked Questions by Drinking Water Professionals*. Denver, Colo.: American Water Works Association Research Foundation and American Water Works Association.

Geldreich, E.E. 1996. *Microbial Quality of Water Supply in Distribution Systems*. Boca Raton, Fla.: CRC Press.

LeChevallier, M.W., N.J. Shaw, and D.B. Smith. 1996. *Factors Limiting Microbial Growth in the Distribution System, Part II, Full Scale Experiments*. Denver, Colo.: American Water Works Association Research Foundation and American Water Works Association.

LeChevallier, M.W., W.D. Norton, R.G. Lee, and J.B. Rose. 1991. Giardia *and* Cryptosporidium *in Water Supplies*. Denver, Colo.: American Water Works Association Research Foundation and American Water Works Association.

Pontius, F.W. 1994a. Boiling Water Effective for Crypto and Other Microbes. *Opflow*, 20(10):10.

———. 1994b. Surface Water Treatment Rule. In *SDWA Advisor Regulatory Update Service*. Denver, Colo.: American Water Works Association.

Public Law 104-182. Safe Drinking Water Act Amendments of 1996 (Aug. 6, 1996). Section 114. Public Notification.

Renner, R., and R. Hegg. 1997. *Self Assessment Guide for Surface Water Treatment Plant Optimization*. Denver, Colo.: American Water Works Association Research Foundation and American Water Works Association.

Smith, S.A. 1992. *Methods for Monitoring* Iron and Manganese Biofouling in Water Wells. Denver, Colo.: American Water Works Association Research Foundation and American Water Works Association.

USEPA. 1995. *Information Collection Requirements Rule—Protozoa and Enteric Viruses Sample Collection Procedures*. EPA/814-B-95-001. Cincinnati, Ohio: US Environmental Protection Agency.

This page intentionally blank.

Section II

Introduction to Bacterial Pathogenic Agents

Acinetobacter
Aeromonas
Campylobacter
Cyanobacteria
Escherichia coli
Flavobacterium
Heterotrophic Bacteria
Klebsiella
Legionella
Mycobacterium avium Complex
Pseudomonas
Salmonella
Serratia
Shigella
Staphylococcus
Vibrio cholerae
Yersinia

Bacteria are unicellular microorganisms that exist either as free-living organisms or parasites. A number of considerations play a part in establishing a list of recognized waterborne bacterial pathogens. Consequently, some debate exists among professionals as to what should be included in the list. In theory, any organism that can invade the human body and produce a toxic reaction in tissues or organs is a pathogen; in practice, outbreaks of waterborne pathogens must occur in two or more individuals and be spread by water. The major classifications of bacterial pathogens are traditional, new or emerging, opportunistic, and socioeconomic environmental invaders.

TRADITIONAL BACTERIAL PATHOGENS

Major epidemics of typhoid fever and cholera resulting from contaminated water supplies have been documented from ancient civilizations, through the Middle Ages, and in the twentieth century. These disasters led to the development of basic public health measures that reduce contamination of drinking water and food by human waste.

NEW OR EMERGING PATHOGENS

Some organisms reported as new or emerging pathogenic bacteria may be the result of improvements in laboratory methodology or a result of a species mutating into a more aggressive invader of humans. Pathogen *Escherichia coli* 0157:H7 is an example of the latter group.

OPPORTUNISTIC PATHOGENS

This group of bacteria may invade individuals with weakened immune systems, such as the elderly, those with compromised immune systems, and infants with underdeveloped immune barriers. Specific colonization sites may be skin, respiratory system, eyes, ears, nose, or the intestinal tract.

SOCIOECONOMIC ENVIRONMENTAL INVADERS

Differences in socioeconomic environments due to poverty, water scarcity, and political priorities over public health issues can increase the prevalence of certain waterborne pathogens. Some pathogens, such as *Shigella*, are often a threat because of poor sanitation practices and nonexistent water treatment barriers.

Chapter 4

Acinetobacter

Mic Stewart

DESCRIPTION OF THE AGENT

Bacteria of the genus *Acinetobacter* have undergone many taxonomic classifications under at least 15 different generic names. Members of this genus are currently classified in the family Neisseriaceae with one species, *Acinetobacter calcoaceticus*. Further classification of *Acinetobacter* has been based on DNA–DNA homology groups (referred to as *genomic species*). Nineteen DNA–DNA homology groups, including *A. calcoaceticus, A. baumannii, A. haemolyticus, A. johnsonii, A. lwoffii, A. radioresistens,* and 12 unnamed genomic species are currently recognized. *Acinetobacter* may eventually be classified under the family Moraxellaceae, which includes *Moraxella*, *Acinetobacter*, *Psychrobacter*, and other related organisms.

Acinetobacters are rod-shaped, 0.9 to 1.6 µm in diameter and 1.5 to 2.5 µm in length, but become more spherical in shape during stationary growth. These organisms are aerobic, do not form spores, and are gram-negative, but may be gram-variable in pure culture. Cells exhibit “twitching motility” due to the presence of polar fimbriae. Many strains are encapsulated and can demonstrate considerable aggregation depending on growth conditions. Strains grow between 20 and 30° C with a temperature optima of 33 to 35° C. Acinetobacters are catalase-positive, oxidase-negative, and nonfermentative. Most strains grow in defined media containing a single carbon and energy source. The DNA G+C content is 38 to 47 mol percent.

DESCRIPTION OF THE DISEASE

A. baumannii is the genomic species of *Acinetobacter* of greatest clinical significance; however, definitive identification of many acinetobacters associated with infections is commonly incomplete. Acinetobacters, generally considered to be of low virulence, have been increasingly associated with nosocomial (hospital-acquired) infections, including septicemia, meningitis, endocarditis, brain abscesses, lung abscesses, pneumonia, empyema, urinary tract infections, eye infections, and skin and wound infections. A survey of nosocomial infections indicated that this organism was responsible for 0.3 percent of endemic nosocomial infections in critically ill patients and 1 percent of hospitalwide bacterial nosocomial infections. Studies have indicated that 3 to 24 percent of pneumonia patients using mechanical ventilation devices were infected with at least one *Acinetobacter* sp., which suggests this organism is an emerging pathogen under these conditions. Importantly, with the exception of *Pseudomonas aeruginosa*, mortality rates associated with nosocomial *Acinetobacter* infections were higher than those for other bacterial species. Acinetobacters associated with bacteremia may act as a single pathogen or be associated with other microbes. Factors enhancing the virulence of acinetobacters include (1) presence of a capsule, (2) adhesion to human epithelial cells due to fimbriae, capsular polysaccharide, or both, (3) production of enzymes that may damage tissue lipids, and (4) production of an endotoxin. Factors that predispose persons to infection by *Acinetobacter* include advanced age, chronic lung disease, immunosuppression, neonates, surgery, use of antimicrobial agents, presence of invasive devices (e.g., endotracheal tubes), and use of respiratory equipment. Antibiotic treatment for *Acinetobacter* infections includes amikacin, imipenem, ceftazidime, pefloxacin, or ciprofloxacin.

RESERVOIRS FOR THE AGENT

Acinetobacters can be isolated from soil, seawater, fresh water, estuaries, sewage, contaminated food, and mucosal and outer surfaces of animals (including fish) and humans. Acinetobacters may be part of the normal bacterial flora in over 25 percent of healthy humans and have been isolated from moist areas of the body, including the axillae, groin, oral cavity, respiratory tract, between the toes, and, to a lesser extent, the digestive tract. In hospital patients, 7 to 45 percent were found to harbor this organism. *Acinetobacter* spp. have been found in 27 percent of hospital sink traps, 20 percent of hospital floor swab cultures, and in 12 percent of air samples in wards containing patients infected by this organism. Studies documenting the prevalence of *Acinetobacter* in soil, surface water, estuaries, thermal springs, and groundwater found 93, 96, 50, 42, and 38 percent, respectively, of the samples tested from these environments contained this organism.

MODE OF TRANSMISSION

The ubiquitous nature and environmental persistence of acinetobacters aid in the transmission of these organisms in hospitals. High colonization rates of the skin, throat, respiratory system, and digestive tract of hospital patients together with the occurrence of acinetobacters as part of the normal bacterial flora in humans provide a significant source of this organism. Consequently, transmission of this organism through person-to-person contact or contact with medical instrumentation, equipment, or surfaces throughout the hospital ensures the continual persistence of acinetobacters. Studies documenting acinetobacters in air samples collected in the vicinity of infected patients indicate that aerosolization may also be an important transmission method. Water supply may be another important mode of transmission because these organisms are often part of the profile of heterotrophic bacteria found on granular activated carbon (GAC) and sand filters, in pipe biofilm, and point-of-use devices.

METHODS FOR DETECTING THE AGENT

Acinetobacters can be isolated and cultivated on ordinary laboratory media. Organic Medium 79, Mineral Medium with Crude Oil, Peptone Yeast Extract Medium, Trypticase Soy Agar with Glycerol, and Trypticase Phytone Medium may all be used to cultivate the organism. Selective and differential media, such as Sellers Agar, Herella Agar, and MacConkey Agar, may also be used. Eosin-Methylene Blue Agar and mAC agar may be used to differentiate *Acinetobacter* species isolated from potable water environments. Optimum growth temperatures for most strains is 33 to 35° C; however, growth at lower temperatures also occurs. Acinetobacters from soil and water can be enriched by inoculation of 20 mL of an acetate–mineral medium with 5 mL of a water sample or a filtered 10 percent soil suspension followed by vigorous aeration at 30° C or at room temperature. Acinetobacters favor a slightly acidic (pH 5.5 to 6.0) growth environment. Biotyping, serotyping, phage typing, bacteriocin typing, protein profiles, multilocus enzyme electrophoretic typing, plasmid profiles, pulsed-field gel electrophoresis, ribotyping, and other molecular-based methods help discriminate among acinetobacters.

OCCURRENCE OF THE AGENT IN PEOPLE, ANIMALS, AND THE ENVIRONMENT

In one study, *Acinetobacter* was detected in 38 percent of groundwater samples with an arithmetic mean of 8 colony-forming units (cfu)/100 mL (range, <1–178), but represented less than 0.1 percent of the heterotrophic plate count (HPC) population. Other studies, however, have reported that 54 percent of HPC isolates obtained from a groundwater site were acinetobacters. Acinetobacters were isolated in 16 percent of the samples not containing coliforms, which suggests the inadequacy of coliforms as an indicator of these organisms. Preliminary testing also established that groundwater isolates of *Acinetobacter* contained at least one virulence factor similar to clinical isolates. In addition, some of the groundwater isolates of *Acinetobacter* were found to interfere with the detection of total coliforms when using standard selective media. In a study of a chlorinated distribution system, *Acinetobacter* was found to be the most commonly isolated organism and comprised 5.5 percent of the total organisms identified. Sampling conducted during a chlorine failure of the same system indicated that *Acinetobacter* comprised the second highest portion of the HPC population. In similar studies conducted in Canada, approximately 1 to 2 percent of organisms isolated from the distribution system were identified as *Acinetobacter*.

SURVIVAL OF THE AGENT IN THE ENVIRONMENT

The occurrence of acinetobacters in water environments, contaminated food, and as flora of humans and animals provide evidence of the ubiquitous and adaptive nature of these organisms. Studies of *Acinetobacter*-infected patients indicated that this organism could be recovered from articles contained in the room for up to 13 days after discharge of the patient. Acinetobacters have also been isolated from contaminated mattresses, feather pillows, telephone handles, door pushplates, patient charts, tabletops, and from various equipment and surfaces in the hospital environment. A strain of *Acinetobacter* spp. was shown to survive for up to six days after inoculation on dry filter paper. That period is comparable to *Staphylococcus aureus*, but considerably longer than *Escherichia coli* and *Pseudomonas* spp. Survival on hospital floors and washcloths have also been documented.

DOCUMENTED WATERBORNE OUTBREAKS

Acinetobacters have been associated with outbreaks in hospital settings but not in treated public drinking water supplies.

EFFECTIVENESS OF WATER TREATMENT PROCESSES

Conventional treatment by coagulation and filtration removes between 75 and 99 percent (0.6 to 2 logs) and 50 and 99.5 percent (0.3 to 2.3 logs), respectively of bacteria. Disinfection results during the treatment process can vary appreciably depending on the disinfectant used and the relative resistance of the organism; however, typical removals range from 99 to 99.99 percent (2 to 4 logs). The use of a disinfectant residual in the distribution system provides additional microbial inactivation. Naturally-occurring *Acinetobacter* spp. were observed to have inactivation rates similar to other heterotrophic bacteria, such as *Moraxella*, *Aeromonas*, *Pseudomonas*, and *Alcaligenes*, when exposed to chloramines. Other studies, however, have indicated that acinetobacters can develop increased resistance to chlorine, chloramines, and chlorine dioxide when grown under conditions favoring cell aggregation.

NATIONAL OR INTERNATIONAL GUIDELINES AND MONITORING RECOMMENDATIONS

No regulatory guidelines for acinetobacters in drinking water have been established in the United States. Treatment of drinking water and effective distribution maintenance programs are important in controlling acinetobacters in drinking water. Control of antibiotic usage to minimize development of resistant strains, and good housekeeping practices, including equipment decontamination, strict attention to hand washing, and effective isolation procedures of infected patients, are important control factors for acinetobacters in hospitals.

INFORMATION SOURCES

Atlas, R.M. 1997. *Handbook of Microbiological Media*. Parks, L.C., ed. Boca Raton, Fla.: CRC Press, Inc.

Baumann, P. 1968. Isolation of *Acinetobacter* from Soil and Water. *J. Bacteriol.*, 96(1):39–42.

Bergogne-Berezin, E., and K.J. Towner. 1996. *Acinetobacter* spp. as Nosocomial Pathogens: Microbiological, Clinical, and Epidemiological Features. *Clinical Microbiol. Reviews*, 9(2):148–165.

Bifulco, J.H., J.J. Shirey, and G.K. Bissonnette. 1989. Detection of *Acinetobacter* spp. in Rural Drinking Water Supplies. *Appl. Environ. Microbiol.*, 55(9):2214–2219.

Grimes, D.J. 1991. Ecology of Estuarine Bacteria Capable of Causing Human Disease: A Review. *Estuaries*, 14(4):345–360.

J.M. Montgomery Consulting Engineers, Inc. 1985. *Water Treatment Principles and Design*. New York: John Wiley & Sons, Inc.

LeChevallier, M.W., R.J. Seidler, and T.M. Evans. 1980. Enumeration and Characterization of Standard Plate Count Bacteria in Chlorinated and Raw Water Supplies. *Appl. Environ. Microbiol.*, 40(5):922–930.

Mosso, M.A., M.C. Rosa, C. Vivar, and M.R. Medina. 1994. Heterotrophic Bacterial Populations in the Mineral Waters of Thermal Springs in Spain. *J. Appl. Bacteriol.*, 77:370–381.

Olson, B.H., and M.H. Stewart. 1990. Factors that Change Bacterial Resistance to Disinfection. In *Water Chlorination Chemistry, Environmental Impact and Health Effects*. Jolley, R.L., L.W. Condie, J.D. Johnson, S. Katz, R.A. Minear, J.S. Mattice, and V.A. Jacobs, eds. Chelsea, Mich.: Lewis Publishers.

Payment, P., F. Gamache, and G. Paquette. 1988. Microbiological and Virological Analysis from Two Water Filtration Plants and their Distribution Systems. *Can. J. Microbiol.*, 34:1304–1309.

Spino, D.G., and E.E. Geldreich. 1981. *Acinetobacter* spp.: Distinct Morphology on Eosin Methylene Blue Agar as an Aid to Identification in Drinking Water. *Appl. Environ. Microbiol.*, 41(4):1063–1064.

Starr, M.P., H. Stolp, H.G. Truper, A. Balows, and H.G. Schegel, eds. 1981. *The Prokaryotes: A Handbook on Habits, Isolation, and Identification of Bacteria*. New York: Springer-Verlag.

Stetzenbach, L.O., L.M. Kelley, and N.A. Sinclair. 1986. Isolation, Identification and Growth of Well-water Bacteria. *Ground Water*, 24:6–10.

Wolfe, R.L., N.R. Ward, and B.H. Olson. 1985. Inactivation of Heterotrophic Bacterial Populations in Finished Drinking Water by Chlorine and Chloramines. *Water Res.*, 19(11):1393–1403.

This page intentionally blank.

Chapter 5

Aeromonas

Nelson P. Moyer

DESCRIPTION OF THE AGENT

The genus *Aeromonas* of the family Aeromonadaceae consists of 19 recognized DNA hybridization groups, comprising 17 genospecies and 14 phenospecies (3 genospecies remain unnamed). Aeromonads are facultatively anaerobic, chemoorganotrophic, nonsporulating, oxidase positive, gram-negative rods or coccobacilli, 0.3 to 1.0 µm in diameter and 1.0 to 3.5 µm in length, motile by a monotrichous polar flagellum, and appearing singly or in short chains. The psychrophilic aeromonads pathogenic for fish are nonmotile. The mesophilic aeromonads important to environmental microbiologists and the water industry are *A. hydrophila*, *A. sobria*, and *A. caviae*. These grow in a temperature range between 15 and 38°C on a variety of eugonic media. When grown at 35°C for 18 hours on sheep blood agar plates, colonies are round, convex, measuring 2 to 3 mm in diameter, creamy to mucoid in consistency, translucent gray in appearance, with or without hemolysin production. They are strongly hydrolytic, producing a number of proteolytic, saccharolytic, hemolytic, and lipolytic extracellular enzymes. They are differentiated from similar oxidase positive bacteria, such as *Plesiomonas*, by gelatin hydrolysis and failure to ferment inositol, and from the *Vibrio* by their resistance to O/129 (150 µg) and inability to grow in the presence of 6 percent sodium chloride.

DESCRIPTION OF THE DISEASE

Aeromonads are pathogenic for fish and aquatic animals, and they represent an economic threat to the aquaculture industry. Human disease is characterized by a broad range of pathology, from self-limiting gastrointestinal illness to septicemia and death. Soft-tissue infections occur within hours following penetrating injuries in aquatic environments, or wound contamination with surface water. Local suppurative infections are characterized by pain, swelling, erythema, and edema. Fever accompanies septicemia and disseminated infections. Complications of soft-tissue infections include cellulitis, necrotizing fasciitis, myositis, sepsis, meningitis, pneumonia, peritonitis, osteomylitis, and endocarditis, among others. Gastrointestinal disease develops within a few days following ingestion of contaminated food or water, and may be an acute, cholera-like illness characterized by profuse watery diarrhea, or a less-severe diarrhea, with fever and abdominal cramping.

A chronic form of the disease with multiple soft to loose stools per day, but without marked dehydration, is characteristically associated with children under the age of five years, who have a history of therapy with antibiotics to which aeromonads are resistant. Repeated or prolonged antibiotic therapy disrupts normal intestinal flora and provides a competitive environment for aeromonads in which they can opportunistically colonize. Untreated water from wells that contain aeromonads places infants and children at risk of chronic *Aeromonas* gastroenteritis. Adults diagnosed with "irritable bowel" syndrome may be suffering from undiagnosed chronic *Aeromonas* gastroenteritis. Rapid diagnosis by bacterial culture and performance of antimicrobial susceptibility tests is necessary for successful treatment of extra-intestinal *Aeromonas* infections. Shock-chlorinating wells and distribution systems may be necessary to suppress aeromonads.

RESERVOIRS FOR THE AGENT

Aeromonads are found in fresh water, estuarine and marine environments, sediments, sludge, and sewage. They have been recovered from chlorinated and nonchlorinated drinking water supplies worldwide, where they contribute to regrowth and biofilm problems in distribution systems. They are readily isolated from surface waters, flocs, and sediments in nature, and from the surfaces and intestinal contents of aquatic animals. Aeromonads have been cultured from domestic and hospital water systems, bottled drinking water, renal dialysis units, and home aquaria. Their presence in groundwater indicates surface water or aquatic animal contamination. Aeromonads have been isolated from produce, meats, and shellfish. Water may be the major source of contamination of foods.

MODE OF TRANSMISSION

Soft-tissue infections occur following traumatic exposure to contaminated water, as do wound and eye infections. Persons with underlying disease or immunosuppression are at increased risk of dissemination following infection. Gastrointestinal infections result from ingestion of contaminated food or water. Aeromonads have been reported as a cause of travelers' diarrhea. Person-to-person transmission occurs through the fecal–oral route, typically from substandard personal hygiene or diapering infected infants. Aeromonads enter water supplies from incomplete treatment, new construction, and maintenance and repair activities.

METHODS FOR DETECTING THE AGENT

Direct plating methods are recommended for culturing aeromonads from polymicrobic sources, such as surface water, sewage, sediments, and sludge, when they are present in sufficient number (≥1 colony-forming unit [cfu]/mL). Spread plates or pour plates of diluted samples are required to isolate aeromonads present in high numbers. Membrane filtration and multiple tube fermentation techniques have been used to enumerate aeromonads with differential and selective media. Recovery of aeromonads from groundwater or treated drinking water may require resuscitation or enrichment when present in low numbers (≤10 cfu/100 mL). Alkaline peptone water, pH 8.6, may be used directly, with Moore swabs or Spira bottles, or with membrane filtration for enrichment of aeromonads at very low levels or when aeromonads are heavily outnumbered in a sample by competitive bacteria. Aeromonads are presumptively identified by their colony morphology and hemolytic reaction on blood agar plates, the oxidase test, and growth characteristics in either TSI/LIA/MIO (see glossary) or Kaper's Multi-test medium. Complete identification of phenospecies depends on biochemical tests.

OCCURRENCE OF THE AGENT IN PEOPLE, ANIMALS, AND THE ENVIRONMENT

Aeromonads grow to high numbers in surface waters containing organic material (total organic carbon [TOC], assimilable organic carbon [AOC], biochemical oxygen demand [BOD], or biodegradable organic matter [BDOM]) and they have been proposed as indicators of water pollution and the trophic state of water. Populations of aeromonads exhibit marked seasonal variation, with the highest counts occurring in the summer. The incidence of gastroenteritis cases in humans parallels the seasonal peak in natural *Aeromonas* populations. *A. caviae* is the predominant species in fecally contaminated waters. While aeromonads have been isolated from up to 27 percent of chlorinated drinking water supplies, their numbers do not correlate with the presence of coliform bacteria, which suggests regrowth or biofilm colonization in the distribution system. The percentage of humans found to have aeromonads in their intestines and show no symptoms of disease ranges from a low of 0.1 percent in developed countries to a high of 30 to 50 percent in countries without effective water and sewage sanitation. Swine, sheep, cattle, and poultry harbor aeromonads in their intestinal tracts at low levels without evidence of disease.

SURVIVAL OF THE AGENT IN THE ENVIRONMENT

Aeromonads survive in the environment at temperatures between 2 and 42° C, and association with sediments and aquatic animals ensures their survival at ambient temperature extremes. They tolerate a range between pH 5.2 and 9.8. Population densities in sewage sludge (>10^8 cfu/mL), wastewater (10^2–10^7 cfu/mL), rivers (10–10^4 cfu/mL), and lakes and reservoirs (1–10^2 cfu/mL) illustrate the ubiquitous nature of aeromonads in the environment. Counts of 10^{-2}–10 cfu/mL and 10^{-2}–10^3 cfu/mL have been recorded in finished water and distribution water, respectively. Uncontaminated groundwater will have *Aeromonas* counts of <1 cfu/mL.

DOCUMENTED WATERBORNE OUTBREAKS

Recently, aeromonads have been recognized as the cause of waterborne and foodborne outbreaks of disease; however, no outbreaks of *Aeromonas* gastroenteritis have been documented in association with treated public drinking water supplies. Counts of aeromonads in contaminated well water associated with cases of gastroenteritis range between 0.7 and 460 cfu/mL. The potential for outbreaks is likely to occur only in susceptible individuals, e.g., infants, children on ampicillin, persons with underlying disease, or the immunosuppressed.

Because significant contamination is unlikely in a municipal system, the probability of a large identifiable outbreak is remote. Recognition of increased numbers of sporadic cases in a community is equally unlikely, because sporadic cases are below the detection threshold of current epidemiological surveillance systems. *Aeromonas* gastroenteritis is not a reportable disease in most states, and clinical laboratories rarely include a search for aeromonads in their routine stool culture procedures, except by physician request. Colonization of treatment plants and distribution systems has been documented, and anecdotal information suggests that susceptible persons may be at risk of developing *Aeromonas* gastroenteritis as the result of continuous exposure to low levels of aeromonads in treated drinking water.

EFFECTIVENESS OF WATER TREATMENT PROCESSES

Chlorination is sufficient to control aeromonads in public drinking water supplies with properly maintained distribution systems, provided the free chlorine residual remains above 0.5 ppm at the distal ends of the system. Free chlorine residuals below 0.5 ppm are associated with an increased number of positive water samples, and growth in filter beds, softeners, and flocculation and sedimentation basins. Aeromonads colonize pipes and plumbing fixtures at the distal ends of distribution systems in biofilms. Granular activated carbon (GAC) sequesters nutrients that promote growth of aeromonads. Regular removal of sludge from sedimentation basins, and proper chlorination, filter maintenance, backwashing procedures, and hydrant flushing are required to control *Aeromonas* colonization of public water supplies.

NATIONAL OR INTERNATIONAL GUIDELINES AND MONITORING RECOMMENDATIONS

While no regulatory standards for the permissible number of aeromonads in drinking water have been established in the United States, operators can assume that their systems are functioning properly when the heterotrophic plate counts (HPCs) remain below 10 cfu/100 mL in distribution water. The European Community has established a drinking water standard of no more than 20 cfu/100 mL for aeromonads in water leaving the treatment plant, and no more than 200 cfu/100 mL in distribution system water. Use of biologically activated filters, and aging distribution systems with established biofilm, make it difficult to completely eradicate aeromonads from drinking water supplies. Aeromonads have been reported as a cause of heterotrophic interference in coliform tests. Using the MTF method, lightly turbid lauryl tryptose broth (LTB) tubes that are clear at 44.5°C usually contain aeromonads. Canada recently established an *Aeromonas* maximum contaminant level (MCL) of 0 cfu/100 mL for bottled drinking water.

INFORMATION SOURCES

Austin, B., M. Altwegg, P.J. Gosling, and S.W. Joseph. 1996. *The Genus* Aeromonas. Chichester, UK: John Wiley & Sons.

Farmer, J.J., III, M.J. Arduino, and F.W. Hickman-Brenner. 1992. The Genera *Aeromonas* and *Plesiomonas*. In *The Prokaryotes, Second Edition, Vol. 3*. pp. 3012–3045. Balows, A., H.G. Trüper, M. Dworkin, W. Harder, and K.-H. Schleifer, eds. New York: Springer-Verlag.

Janda, J.M., A.L. Abbott, and A.M. Carnahan. 1995. *Aeromonas* and *Plesiomonas*. In *Manual of Clinical Microbiology, Sixth Edition*. pp. 477–482. Murray P.R., E.J. Baron, M.A. Pfaller, F.C Tenover, and R.H. Yolken, eds. Washington, D.C.: ASM Press.

Chapter 6

Campylobacter

Colin R. Fricker

DESCRIPTION OF THE AGENT

The genus *Campylobacter* belongs to the family Vibrioaceae and contains 14 species including several that may be pathogenic to both humans or animals. Campylobacters are microaerophilic, oxidase positive, gram-negative, slender, curved rods that are motile by means of a single polar flagellum. Healthy cells are spiral or curved, 0.2 to 0.5 µm wide and 0.5 to 5.0 µm long. Older or damaged cells may form coccal bodies. The campylobacters of concern to the water industry are the "thermophilic" group. Of greatest concern to human infection are *C. jejuni*, *C. coli*, and *C. upsaliensis*.

DESCRIPTION OF THE DISEASE

The campylobacters cause a variety of diseases in a wide range of animals and in humans. In humans, the principal symptom is acute diarrhea that clinically cannot be distinguished from most other acute bacterial infections of the gut. While the incubation period may range from 1 to 8 days, 2 to 3 days is more common. The onset of diarrhea is usually sudden and may be preceded by a prodromal flu-like illness, acute abdominal pain, or both, which may mimic the symptoms of appendicitis. The diarrhea may be profuse and watery, probably due to the production of a cholera-like enterotoxin, or may be dysenteric and contain blood and mucus. The disease is usually self-limiting and patients stools are normally culture negative after three weeks, although occasionally excretion persists in excess of three months. Complications of *Campylobacter* enteritis are relatively uncommon; 1 to 2 percent of patients may suffer from a reactive arthritis and infection has also been linked with Guillain-Barré syndrome. In human volunteer studies, the infectious dose has been shown to vary considerably, although infection has been caused by ingestion of a few hundred organisms.

RESERVOIRS FOR THE AGENT

Campylobacter enteritis is principally a zoonotic disease and the organisms are harbored in the intestines of a wide variety of domestic and wild animals, particularly birds. Campylobacters have been found in almost all bird species that have been examined. They are particularly prevalent in poultry, likely a major source of human infection. Water probably has a major role in disseminating infection in flocks of poultry. Campylobacters can be found in most natural fresh and marine waters, even in remote areas, and their occurrence tends to be higher during autumn and winter. They are also found in high numbers in domestic sewage and undisinfected treated sewage effluents.

MODE OF TRANSMISSION

Campylobacters are transmitted by the fecal–oral route. Person-to-person transmission is relatively uncommon and is usually restricted to young children. Direct transmission from animals to humans is relatively common, either through occupational exposure to infected animals or from household pets. Indirect transmission, through consumption of contaminated food or water, is by far the most common route of infection, despite the fact that campylobacters are easily killed by normal cooking temperatures. Poorly prepared or undercooked chicken is probably the major cause of human infection. Outbreaks associated with consumption of unpasteurized milk or contaminated water have frequently been reported.

METHODS FOR DETECTING THE AGENT

Most strains of campylobacters are sensitive to oxygen and require CO_2 for adequate growth. Both *C. jejuni* and *C. coli* can use hydrogen as a major energy source. While most strains will grow on relatively simple media, either complex or defined, they prefer the addition of blood, serum, or powdered carbon. *C. jejuni* and *C. coli* grow optimally at 42 to 43° C but will not grow below 30° C. Biochemically the campylobacters are relatively inactive and do not use sugars. Several biotyping schemes have been developed based on tests such as H_2S production, hippurate hydrolysis, and DNA hydrolysis.

Since the first successful isolation of campylobacters from human feces in the early 1970s, a wide spectrum of media have been formulated, although most have been designed with detection from food or feces rather than water. In the 1980s most work on the detection of campylobacters in water and the environment used Preston broth (a nutrient broth base containing lysed blood, trimethoprim, rifampicin, polymyxin B, and amphotericin B) together with a supplement known as FBP (containing ferrous sulfate, sodium metabisulfite, and sodium pyruvate) followed by plating on Preston agar. Further work, aimed at eliminating the need for inclusion of blood, demonstrated that the use of ceferaperazone in a charcoal-containing medium worked well. For optimal recovery of campylobacters from water, a preenrichment culture should be used lasting for two to four hours, followed by enrichment and plating on to selective media. However, procedures have not been optimized and some degree of experimentation may be required.

As a general procedure for the detection of *C. jejuni* and *C. coli*, water samples should be concentrated by filtration through a 0.22-µm filter. Then the filter is placed in nonselective broth containing FBP supplement, incubated at 42° C for 4 hours, after which antibiotics are added. Incubation is continued for 24 hours, then the broth plated onto Preston agar and incubated for 48 hours in a microaerobic environment before examination. Isolates should then be examined by gram stain and oxidase and catalase reactions and then further identified where required using the limited number of biochemical tests available. Serotyping schemes are available based on either heat labile or heat stable antigens; the procedure based on heat stable (lipopolysaccharide) antigens is preferred for routine use. Several procedures based on a combination of enrichment culture and the polymerase chain reaction (PCR) have been described, but there are few situations, if any, where their use can be justified.

OCCURRENCE OF THE AGENT IN PEOPLE, ANIMALS, AND THE ENVIRONMENT

The campylobacters that cause infection in humans are unable to grow in water, but they may still be present in relatively high numbers. Marked seasonal variation occurs in naturally contaminated waters, with higher numbers being found during the cooler months of the year. *C. jejuni* appears to be the predominant species in aquatic environments, the source of which is often sewage or wildlife, particularly birds. Experiments have suggested that *C. jejuni* may survive better in water than *C. coli* or *C. lari*, although this has not been extensively researched. The number of individuals without symptoms carrying campylobacters is low in developed countries, but may be significant in developing areas where poor standards of hygiene exist. Campylobacters are rarely found in chlorinated drinking water, and when present are usually the result of posttreatment contamination and are always found together with *Escherichia coli*.

SURVIVAL OF THE AGENT IN THE ENVIRONMENT

Campylobacters survive well in aquatic environments, particularly at temperatures below 5° C. Their survival appears to be enhanced by the presence of organic material and low dissolved oxygen. The numbers present in surface waters are usually low (< 100/mL), although in wastewater numbers as high as 10^4/mL have occasionally been detected. Groundwater contains no campylobacters unless contaminated with surface water. Fully treated water subject to adequate disinfection will be free from *Campylobacter*.

DOCUMENTED WATERBORNE OUTBREAKS

A large number of waterborne outbreaks of *Campylobacter* have been reported in the literature, often affecting hundreds or even thousands of individuals. Despite these large outbreaks, the organism causing the outbreaks has seldom been isolated from the drinking water supply. The lack of isolation may be due to sporadic occurrence, poor detection techniques, or the presence of viable but nonculturable organisms. Sources of these waterborne outbreaks have included surface water, unchlorinated water storage tanks contaminated with bird feces, groundwater contaminated by surface runoff, and mains contaminated by cross-connection. While drinking water may be a major risk factor, there is no evidence that campylobacters can colonize or even survive in water distribution systems, thus, consumption of properly treated water is unlikely to result in infection.

EFFECTIVENESS OF WATER TREATMENT PROCESSES

Normal disinfection procedures using chlorine are sufficient to kill campylobacters in drinking water supplies and the organisms appear to be somewhat more susceptible to chlorine than *E. coli*. In laboratory experiments, *E. coli* survived better than campylobacters and is likely a good indicator for the potential presence of campylobacters. Campylobacters are not found in water in the absence of *E. coli*. Water systems that are maintained free of *E. coli* will be free of campylobacters.

NATIONAL OR INTERNATIONAL GUIDELINES AND MONITORING RECOMMENDATIONS

While there are no specific standards for the presence of campylobacters in drinking water, their potential presence is covered by the *E. coli* standard.

INFORMATION SOURCES

Melby, K., B. Gondrosen, S. Gregusson, H. Ribe, and O.P. Dahl. 1991. Waterborne Campylobacteriosis in Northern Norway. *International Journal of Food Microbiology*, 12:151–156.

Sacks, J.J., S. Liele, L.M. Baldy, S. Berta, C.M. Patton, M.C. White, W.J. Bigler, and J.J. White. 1986. Epidemic Campylobacteriosis Associated with a Community Water Supply. *Amer. J. Pub. Health*, 76:424–428.

Skirrow, M.B. 1990. *Campylobacter* and *Helicobacter* Infections of Man and Animals. *Topley and Wilson's Principles of Bacteriology, Virology and Immunity. Volume 3. Bacterial Diseases*. Smith, G.R., and C.S.F. Easmon, eds. London: Edward Arnold.

Stern, N.J. 1992. Reservoirs for *Campylobacter jejuni* and Approaches for Intervention in Poultry. In Campylobacter jejuni: *Current Status and Future Trends*. pp. 49–60. Nachamkin, I., M. Blamer, and L. Tompkins, eds. Washington, D.C.: Amer. Soc. Microbiol.

Vogt, R.L., H.E. Sours, T. Barett, R.A. Feldman, R.J. Dickinson, and L. Witherell. 1982. Campylobacter Enteritis Associated with Contaminated Water. *Amer. Intern. Med.*, 96:292–296.

Chapter 7

Cyanobacteria

David W. Fredericksen and Edwin E. Geldreich

DESCRIPTION OF THE AGENT

Cyanobacteria (blue–green algae) are best known for the unsightly scum they produce during summer blooms in eutrophic freshwater lakes, reservoirs, and in the sluggish backwaters of rivers. These organisms are more closely related to bacteria than to types of algae. Worldwide, six genera, at least 13 species, and several strains have been identified. In North America, five genera have been identified as toxin producers, including two strains of *Anabaena flos aquae*, *Aphanizomenon flos-aquae*, *Microcystis aeruginosa*, and *Nodularia* sp. Illustrations of these organisms may be found in an appendix to the current edition of *Standard Methods for the Examination of Water and Wastewater.*

In size, cyanobacteria range from 1 µm for unicellular types to over 30 µm for multicellular species. The group is gram-negative and has a metabolic pathway that can fix nitrogen in the dark. They also carry out oxygenic photosynthesis, like higher plants, by splitting water to free oxygen in aerobic sunlight environments. Some produce gas vacuoles that allow them to float, and all have a gliding mechanism that is poorly understood. There are also two different types of differentiated cells in their structure—heterocysts and akinetes (spores). These characteristics suggest that the cyanobacteria are truly an intermediate group of organism that are neither algae or bacteria.

DESCRIPTION OF THE DISEASE

Some cyanobacteria can produce toxins that, if ingested in sufficient concentration, may cause gastrointestinal upsets. Body contact exposure through water recreation may induce skin irritations that lead to a rash. The most convincing case history reported is that of a physician who fell into a lake containing a heavy bloom of cyanobacteria and swallowed an estimated 250 mL of water. A few hours later, he suffered stomach pains, nausea, vomiting, painful diarrhea, fever, headache, and pains in limb muscles and joints that lasted for 2 days. Samples of slimy green stool from the patient were subjected to laboratory analysis for pathogens (including virus) and revealed no *Salmonella* or *Entamoeba*, but many cells of *Anabaena* and *Microcystis*.

Two categories of toxins are produced by cyanobacteria—neurotoxins and hepatotoxins. Observations of poisoning of domestic animals show that when mucous membranes are exposed to cyanobacterial neurotoxins, symptoms develop in 4 to 10 minutes and death within 30 minutes. The effects of hepatotoxins can cause symptoms in exposed animals within 30 minutes and death within 24 hours. Using cobra venom as a point of reference, the alkaloid neurotoxins produced by species of *Anabaena flos-aquae* and *Nodularia spumigena* range from equally potent with 20 µg per kilogram body weight as the lethal dose (LD_{50} of 200 µg/kg). The hepatotoxins produced by *Microcystis aeruginosa* and some strains of *Aphanizomenon flos-aquae* are over twice as potent as cobra venom with 9 µg/kg being the LD_{50}.

Some of these toxins have been found to be tumor promoters and oncogenic in laboratory animals. One of the toxins isolated from *Anabaena* is an alkaloid that can cause neuromuscular blocking activity. Another toxin, isolated from *Microcystis aeruginosa*, affects the cardiovascular systems and produces lesions on the livers of a variety of laboratory animals when administered orally or by intraperitoneal injection. Fortunately, because large doses of toxins are necessary to produce these symptoms in animals, any residual toxins that might pass through a drinking water supply after conventional treatment would be further diluted by vast volumes of water. This safety factor places the concentration far below any known human toxicity level.

RESERVOIRS FOR THE AGENT

Stagnant water, sediments, and soil appear to be significant reservoirs for these organisms. While high densities of cyanobacteria may appear in the feces of infected animals, there is no evidence to support their common presence in the normal intestinal flora of healthy warm-blooded individuals.

MODE OF TRANSMISSION

The most frequent mode of transmission is by water ingestion, however, body contact water sports in areas of massive blooms of cyanobacteria is also of serious concern.

METHODS FOR DETECTING THE AGENT

To detect cyanobacteria, water samples are first blended with glass beads or treated by ultrasound to break filamentous forms prior to streaking on agar plates. There are a variety of selected mineral media available (D-medium, ASM-1, BG-11, and WC) with incubation at 25°C under cool white fluorescent light. Some recalcitrant cyanobacteria may not be freed easily of contaminants, thus, physical and chemical separation schemes may be necessary. Success in achieving pure cultures depends on persistence and patience. Microscopic examination using simple wet-mount staining techniques with India ink and methylene blue are used to identify morphological characteristics.

OCCURRENCE OF THE AGENT IN PEOPLE, ANIMALS, AND THE ENVIRONMENT

Since cyanobacteria are not dependent on a fixed source of carbon, they are widely distributed throughout aquatic environments. Cyanobacteria are to be found in the early stages of soil formation, whether it is converting bare rock or decomposing debris. They are also naturally occurring in stream sediments, overlying surfaces of slow-moving streams, receiving waters for a variety of waste discharges and treated effluents, rural storm runoff, marshes, drainage canals, rice fields, and marine waters. Massive growths of these bacteria often occur during the summer in surface waters at densities of 500 cells or more per millilitre.

SURVIVAL OF THE AGENT IN THE ENVIRONMENT

Polluted surface waters that become stagnant due to slow flows under summertime drought conditions often support persisting populations of cyanobacteria. These organisms, like many algae, are stimulated by water temperature and high concentrations of inorganic nitrogen (N) and phosphorus (P). Most of these growths occur when nitrogen and phosphorus concentrations reach 0.8 and 0.4 mg/L, respectively. Their capability to be a source of biological nitrogen fixation in soils and water is also a significant contributor to long-term survival and an important role in the ecological succession of microorganisms in the environment.

DOCUMENTED WATERBORNE OUTBREAKS

There have been numerous reports of poisonings of livestock, pets, and wildlife by waters laden with cyanobacteria. Outbreaks of human gastroenteritis from ingestion of toxic cyanobacteria in public water supply occurred in Charleston, W. Va., and the area served by the Anacostia Reservoir near Washington, D.C., during the drought years of 1930 and 1931. More recently (1981), an outbreak of human poisoning occurred in northeastern Pennsylvania where 12 children and one adult were affected by an *Anabaena* sp. bloom. In another case study (1990), a localized outbreak of diarrhea occurred among residents of a Chicago apartment building. This incidence was traced to cyanobacteria toxins in the open water supply storage tank. Apparently, the cover to the tank had been inadvertently left ajar so that light and airborne cyanobacteria in dust particles gained access, grew, and in time, released toxic by-products throughout the plumbing system.

EFFECTIVENESS OF WATER TREATMENT PROCESSES

For utilities using surface water supplies, cyanobacteria are well known for their association with taste-and-odor problems, often regarded as a matter of aesthetics. Many utilities with seasonal taste-and-odor occurrences spend millions of dollars on powdered activated carbon (PAC) to remove the offending compounds. In light of recent information on cyanobacteria, PAC and granular activated carbon (GAC) may be very important to toxin removal. Furthermore, for those water systems using disinfection as the only surface water treatment, there is always the threat of a seasonal passage of cyanobacteria and deposition of their dead cells in the distribution pipe network. Such an occurrence provides a source of assimilable organic carbon (AOC), which is a potential nutrient for bacterial regrowth.

NATIONAL OR INTERNATIONAL GUIDELINES AND MONITORING RECOMMENDATIONS

Neither cyanobacteria nor their obnoxious metabolites are regulated by the US Environmental Protection Agency (USEPA) or by states, except under guidelines stating that drinking water must be potable. As defined, potable water must not only be safe, but clear and free from any objectionable tastes and odors, regardless of origin.

INFORMATION SOURCES

American Public Health Association, American Water Works Association, and Water Environment Federation. 1995. *Standard Methods for the Examination of Water and Wastewater.* 19th ed. Eaton, A.D., L.S. Clesceri, and A.E. Greenberg, eds. Washington, D.C.: APHA.

Billings, W.A. 1981. Water-Associated Human Illness in Northeast Pennsylvania and Its Suspected Association with Blue-Green Algae Blooms. In *Water Environment Algal Toxins and Health.* p. 243. Carmichael, W.W., ed. New York: Plenum Press.

Carmichael, W.W. 1991. Blue-Green Algae: An Overlooked Health Threat. *Health and Enviro. Digest*, 5(6):1.

Committee on the Challenges of Modern Society (NATO/CCMS). 1987. *Drinking Water Microbiology.* Cliver, D.O., and R.A. Newman, eds. *J. Environ. Path. Toxicol. Oncol.,* 7(5/6)1.

Epidemiologic Notes and Reports. 1990. Outbreaks of Diarrheal Illness Associated with Cyanobacteria (Blue-Green Algae)-Like Bodies—Chicago and Nepal, 1989 and 1990. *MMWR*, 40:325.

Francis, G. 1878. Poisonous Australian Lake. *Nature*, 18:11.

Kotak, B.G., S.L. Kenefick, D.L. Fritz, C.G. Rosseaux, E.E. Prepas, and S.E. Hrudey. 1992. Occurrence and Toxicological Evaluation of Cyanobacterial Toxins in Alberta Lakes and Farm Dugouts. *Water Res.,* 27(3):495.

Olson, T.A. 1949. History of Toxic Plankton Associated Phenomena. Algae-Laden Water Causes of Death in Domestic Animals. *Sewage Works Eng.*, 20(2):71.

———. 1952. Toxic Plankton. *Water Sewage Works*, 99:75.

———. 1955. Studies of Algae Poisoning: With Special Reference to the Relationship of This Phenomena to Losses of Wildfowl and Other Birds. *Flicker*, 27:105

———. 1960. Water Poisoning—a Study of Poisonous Algal Blooms in Minnesota. *Amer. J. Public Health*, 50:883.

Repavich, W.M., W.L. Sonzogni, J.H. Standridge, R.E. Wedgpohl, and L.F. Meisner. 1990. Cyanobacteria in Wisconsin Waters: Acute and Chronic Toxicity. *Water Res.,* 24:225.

Runnegar, M.T., A.R. Jackson, and I.R. Falconer. 1988. Toxicity to Mice and Sheep of a Bloom of the Cyanobacterium (Blue-Green Algae) *Anabaena circinalis. Toxicon*, 26:599.

Society for Applied Bacteriology, Symposium Series No. 6. Aquatic Microbiology. 1997. Skinner, F.A., and J.M. Shewan, eds. New York: Academic Press.

Carmichael, W.W., ed. 1981. *The Water Environment: Algal Toxins and Health.* New York: Plenum.

Chapter 8

Escherichia coli

Eugene W. Rice

DESCRIPTION OF THE AGENT

Escherichia coli is a bacterial species that is a major constituent of the normal intestinal flora of man and warm-blooded animals. *E. coli* is the predominant species comprising the fecal coliform group of bacteria. The organism is a gram-negative, facultatively anaerobic, rod-shaped bacterium about 0.5 to 2.0 µm in size. While most members of this species are considered harmless commensal organisms, some strains are responsible for gastrointestinal illness. Pathogenic *E. coli* causes diarrheal illness, especially among children in developing countries and in travelers to these locales. Pathogenic strains have been categorized into six groups, based on serological and virulence characteristics. These groups include enteropathogenic *E. coli* (EPEC), enterotoxigenic *E. coli* (ETEC), enteroinvasive *E. coli* (EIEC), enterohemorrhagic *E. coli* (EHEC), enteroaggregative *E. coli* (EAggEC), and diffuse adherent *E. coli* (DAEC). Because there is little information about the mode of transmission for the last two groups they will not be discussed.

DESCRIPTION OF THE DISEASE

Symptoms and pathology vary among the groups of pathogenic *E. coli*. Infectious dose studies have shown that, with the exception of the EHEC group, in which the infectious dose is considered quite low, 10^8 to 10^{10} organisms are required to produce infection. The infectious dose may be about 10^6 organisms when stomach acids are neutralized before ingestion.

Infections caused by EPEC have most commonly been associated with diarrhea in infants, with some reports of high mortality rates. Acquisition of immunity is thought to be the primary reason for the low occurrence rate in adults. Typical symptoms include watery diarrhea, fever, and dehydration. The incubation period in infants is not known. The duration of illness is generally 1 to 3 days, however, persistent diarrhea for more than 14 days has been reported. Adherence to intestinal mucosa with eventual destruction of microvilli is the primary mode of pathogenesis. Adhesion has been linked to a specific plasmid encoded adherence factor.

ETEC is a common cause of travelers' diarrhea and pediatric diarrhea in developing countries. Symptoms include watery diarrhea, abdominal pain, and vomiting. Fever, if present, is generally low-grade. The incubation time is approximately one to two days. The illness may last from three days to several weeks. ETEC strains produce enterotoxins, which may be either heat-labile, heat-stable, or both. The heat-stable toxin is very similar to the toxin produced by *Vibrio cholerae*.

Strains of EIEC produce a disease similar to that caused by *Shigella*. Watery diarrhea accompanied by abdominal cramps, fever, and muscle pain characterize this illness. In most cases, blood is not present in the stool. The incubation period is relatively short, with symptoms usually occurring in less than 24 hours after exposure. The ability to invade and multiply within epithelial cells is associated with a plasmid carried by these bacteria.

Diarrhea caused by EHEC may vary from extremely bloody to nonbloody stools. Abdominal pain accompanies the diarrhea, but usually the infected individual does not have a fever. The average incubation time is three to four days. The duration of the illness is generally about one week, but may persist for longer periods. The development of hemolytic uremic syndrome is a major risk factor for young children. EHEC organisms produce potent phage-mediated toxins referred to as Shiga-like or Vero toxins types I and II. A plasmid-dependent adherence factor has also been associated with these organisms.

RESERVOIRS FOR THE AGENT

Humans serve as the principal reservoir for all pathogenic *E. coli* groups, with the exception of EHEC. Cattle are thought to be a primary reservoir for EHEC organisms. Nonpathogenic *E. coli* are derived from all warm-blooded animals and may represent 95 to 99 percent of all coliforms found in feces of these animals.

MODE OF TRANSMISSION

Pathogenic *E. coli* groups are spread by the fecal–oral route. Fecally contaminated food or water as well as direct contact are primary modes of transmission. Water contaminated with sewage has been implicated in both recreational and drinking water disease outbreaks.

METHODS FOR DETECTING THE AGENT

Typical biochemical reactions used for identification of *E. coli* include fermentation of lactose, production of indole from tryptophane, a positive methyl red test, a negative Voges-Proskauer test, inability to use citrate as a sole carbon source, and presence of the enzyme ß-glucuronidase. In most instances, with the possible exception of suspected outbreak situations, standard methods for detecting fecal coliforms or *E. coli* should be sufficient for determining the sanitary quality of water. During outbreaks, standard procedures for *E. coli* may be used to analyze for the presence of EPEC and ETEC groups.

Members of the EIEC group are negative or slow lactose fermenting organisms. Thus lactose-based media, commonly used for coliform analyses, would not be appropriate for isolating EIEC. The EHEC group, specifically *E. coli* serotype 0157:H7, grows poorly at 44.5°C and is routinely negative in tests for ß-glucuronidase. Fecal coliform and *E. coli* methods that rely on these characteristics would not detect this pathogen. Total coliform assays, however, incubated at 35°C, may be used to screen for this serotype. Additional tests, such as sorbitol fermentation and assays for glutamate decarboxylase, may be used in differentiating this group.

When analyzing for specific pathogens it is always advisable to assay large volumes of water (1 L or more). Samples may be concentrated by membrane filtration or centrifugation and assayed using appropriate media. The use of enrichment broths facilitates the recovery of stressed organisms. Definitive identifications must be based on both biochemical and serological characterizations.

OCCURRENCE OF THE AGENT IN PEOPLE, ANIMALS, AND THE ENVIRONMENT

All four of the major pathogenic *E. coli* groups have been associated with water. Human sewage is the major source for EPEC, EIEC, and ETEC in contaminated water. Fecal pollution from bovine species appears to be the primary source for EHEC organisms. In any fecal contamination event, nonpathogenic *E. coli* should always occur in numbers exceeding pathogenic strains. Thus, wild type *E. coli* may be used as an indicator for the presence of these pathogens.

SURVIVAL OF THE AGENT IN THE ENVIRONMENT

Numerous reports have shown that *E. coli* is capable of surviving in the aquatic environment. Factors such as water type (i.e., surface or ground), water temperature, and nutrient levels directly affect survival mechanisms. Research studies have usually found that survival times for pathogenic *E. coli* do not vary widely from survival times for normal wild type *E. coli* strains under similar conditions in the aquatic environment.

DOCUMENTED WATERBORNE OUTBREAKS

Waterborne transmission is an important factor in the epidemiology of diarrheogenic *E. coli*. EPEC infections, while being most common in children, can also occur in adults. A major EPEC outbreak affecting more than 100 individuals attending a conference center occurred in 1971 near Washington, D.C. The pathogen (serotype 0111) was isolated from drinking water and fecal specimens. An unchlorinated groundwater source contaminated by sewage was the source of the outbreak. A similar waterborne outbreak of EPEC had been previously reported from Sweden in 1965.

One of the largest waterborne pathogenic *E. coli* outbreaks in the United States occurred in 1975 at Crater Lake National Park in southwestern Oregon. More than 2,000 individuals experienced gastrointestinal disease. The causative organism was an ETEC strain (serotype 06) that produced both heat-labile and heat-stable toxins. This serotype was found in both the water and fecal samples. A shallow spring supplying the park's drinking water supply was found to be contaminated by sewage. Although chlorination was used, areas of the distribution system were found to contain no detectable chlorine residual. Two ETEC (serotype 0159) outbreaks reported from Japan were also linked to contaminated drinking water.

A waterborne outbreak caused by EIEC (serotype 0124) was reported from a children's camp in Hungary. A leaking sewer was implicated in contaminating the drinking water. The causative organism was isolated from patients' stools and a reservoir supplied by a spring water source.

While considered primarily a foodborne pathogen, the EHEC group has also emerged as an agent of waterborne disease. Both drinking water and recreational water exposure have served as vehicles of transmission for EHEC (serotype 0157). An outbreak of EHEC (serotype 0157:H7) in Cabool, Mo., was epidemiologically linked to an unchlorinated drinking water supply. The source of contamination was attributed to disturbances through line breaks in the distribution system.

EFFECTIVENESS OF WATER TREATMENT PROCESSES

Proper disinfection of drinking water should control pathogenic strains of *E. coli*. Various studies have shown that *E. coli* is readily inactivated by chlorination, with $C \times T_{99}$ values reported at 0.2 mg-min/L or less. In the United States, current disinfection guidelines targeting protozoan and viral pathogens in surface water supplies are sufficient for controlling *E. coli*. An adequate disinfectant residual must be maintained in all areas of the water distribution system.

NATIONAL OR INTERNATIONAL GUIDELINES AND MONITORING RECOMMENDATIONS

Adherence to national standards for coliform bacteria in drinking water provides the best protection from waterborne disease outbreaks caused by pathogenic *E. coli*. Suspected outbreaks should be reported to local and national public health authorities. International measures should be instituted if an epidemic involves the populations of more than one country. The World Health Organization established International Collaborating Centres to assist in disease management on the global level. Diarrheal illness caused by *E. coli* is one of the diseases covered by these centers.

INFORMATION SOURCES

American Public Health Association, American Water Works Association, and Water Environment Federation. 1995. *Standard Methods for the Examination of Water and Wastewater.* 19th ed. Washington, D.C.: APHA.

Benenson, A.S. 1995. *Control of Communicable Diseases Manual*. Washington, D.C.: APHA.

Doyle, M.P., and V.V. Padhye. 1989. Escherichia coli. In *Foodborne Bacterial Pathogens*. Doyle, M.P. ed. New York: Marcel Dekker.

Geldreich, E.E., K.R. Fox, J.A. Goodrich, E.W. Rice, R.M. Clark, and D.L. Swerdlow. 1992. Searching for a Water supply Connection in the Cabool, Missouri Outbreak of *Escherichia coli* 0157:H7. *Water Res.*, 26(8):1127–1137.

Chapter 9

Flavobacterium

Edwin E. Geldreich

DESCRIPTION OF THE AGENT

The genus *Flavobacterium* contains aerobic, gram-negative, asporogenous bacilli that are nonmotile, oxidase-positive, nonfermentative, nonglucose oxidizers. They produce pigmented colonies (when grown at incubation temperature below 35° C) that may be yellow, orange, and red to brown. These pigments are nonsoluble in media. The exact taxonomy of some of these organisms is still in debate because they usually do not demonstrate typical reactions (or any at all unless incubated for an extended time) in most biochemical identification media used to speciate gram-negative bacteria. As a consequence, estimates of the number of species vary from 30 to 70.

DESCRIPTION OF THE DISEASE

Clinically, the most important species of *Flavobacterium* are *F. meningosepticum*, *F. breve*, and *F. odoratum*. *F. meningosepticum* is the species most frequently involved as an opportunistic pathogen in nosocomial infections, including meningitis (particularly in infants), pneumonia, endocarditis, and septicemia.

RESERVOIRS FOR THE AGENT

Soil and water appear to be significant reservoirs for *Flavobacterium*. Detecting these chlorine-resistant organisms to some degree in any water supply is not unusual. Stagnation of building plumbing systems can provide opportunities for *Flavobacterium* colonization and they can be found in hospitals. *Flavobacterium* may also be introduced through microbial growth on devices connected to the water supply.

MODE OF TRANSMISSION

The route of exposure may be by ingestion, body contact with water supply, or by person-to-person contact in hospitals.

METHODS FOR DETECTING THE AGENT

The most successful recovery of *Flavobacterium* in water supply is with R2A spread plates or as microfiltrated (MF) medium with incubation at 28° C for 5 to 7 days. Pigmented colonies that develop need to be purified and tested for reactions to various biochemicals. While some success may be achieved using commercially prepared multitest kits, more definitive results may be achieved by placing the biochemical agent in a diluted R2A formulation and incubated for extended time at 28° C.

OCCURRENCE OF THE AGENT IN PEOPLE, ANIMALS, AND THE ENVIRONMENT

Normally, flavobacteria are not part of the resident microflora of humans. In the aquatic environment, flavobacteria are ubiquitous, being found in soil, water, sewage, vegetation, and dairy products.

SURVIVAL OF THE AGENT IN THE ENVIRONMENT

Little is known about the environmental conditions in the distribution system that favor the colonization of these heterotrophic bacteria, but the available organic concentration needed may be less than 1 µg of carbon per litre. Current evidence suggests that conditions contributing to *Flavobacterium* regrowth include absence of free chlorine residual, water temperatures above 15° C, accumulations of bacterial nutrients (assimilable organic carbon [AOC] and specific inorganics) in pipe sediments, and static water conditions.

DOCUMENTED WATERBORNE OUTBREAKS

Waterborne outbreaks are thought to be caused by *Flavobacterium* colonization in stagnant plumbing systems. Six office workers complained about intense abdominal cramping six to eight hours after drinking water from fountains demonstrated to contain high counts of *Flavobacterium*. A sufficient quantity of *Flavobacterium* was likely ingested through water consumption to cause endotoxin gastroenteritis. Further investigation of the plumbing pipe network suggested that the bacterial colonization occurred in ½-in. copper lines leading to drinking fountains. *Flavobacterium* was not isolated from the tubing or reservoirs within the refrigerated fountains. No stagnation was evident in the public water supply lines entering the modular office buildings.

EFFECTIVENESS OF WATER TREATMENT PROCESSES

Flavobacterium species appear to be chlorine-resistant. One strain was shown to survive a 10-minute exposure to 10 mg of chlorine per litre. During a five-month study of a New England metropolitan water supply, *Flavobacterium* species were detected in the disinfected water from five of nine finished water reservoirs. In another study of the seasonal occurrence of various pigmented bacteria (including *Flavobacterium*) in a treated municipal water system in the Midwest, these organisms were detected not only in the raw water supply but thought to enter from soil in line breaks and subsequent repairs to the distribution system. The predominant pigmented bacteria at most locations in the treatment basins or from distribution sites were yellow and orange strains. A small number of pink organisms also occurred in water collected at selected distribution sites.

NATIONAL OR INTERNATIONAL GUIDELINES AND MONITORING RECOMMENDATIONS

There are no national or international guidelines for this opportunistic pathogen in water supply, recreational waters, and sewage effluents.

INFORMATION SOURCES

Geldreich, E.E. 1996. *Microbial Quality of Water Supply in Distribution Systems.* Boca Raton, Fla.: CRC Press.

Reasoner, D.J., and E.E. Geldreich. 1985. A New Medium for the Enumeration and Subculture of Bacteria from Potable Water. *Appl. Environ. Microbiol.,* 49:1–7.

Rubin, S.J., P.A. Granato, and B.L. Wasilauskas. 1985. Glucose-Nonfermenting Gram-Negative Bacteria. In *Manual of Clinical Microbiology*, 4th ed. pp. 330–349. Lennette, E.H., A. Balows, W.J. Hausler, Jr., and H.J. Shadomy, eds. Washington, D.C.: ASM Press.

Chapter 10

Heterotrophic Bacteria

Pierre Payment

DESCRIPTION OF THE AGENT

The heterotrophic plate count (HPC) enumerates aerobic and facultative aerobic bacteria found in water. The bacteria must be capable of growing on simple organic compounds (primarily carbohydrates, amino acids, and peptides) found in the culture medium, and under specified incubation time and temperature. HPC bacteria can be any bacteria that meet this definition-by-method; they can be different species at different geographic locations and at different times. Populations detected also differ according to the culture medium used, incubation conditions, and temperature.

The number of HPC bacteria in drinking water can be as high as 10,000/mL in the absence of a free chlorine residual, high turbidity, and the warm water temperatures of summer. HPC bacteria indicate a deterioration in drinking water quality.

The predominant HPC bacterial genera are *Alcaligenes*, *Acinetobacter*, *Flavobacterium*, and *Pseudomonas*. The types of bacteria present on pipe surfaces are similar to those reported in drinking water. Pigmented bacteria can be found in water and form a significant percentage of the HPC population of treated water. Other bacteria of potential medical importance, such as *Staphylococcus*, *Mycobacterium*, and *Serratia*, have been found in water. HPC bacteria are also found in large numbers in point-of-use and point-of-entry devices; they grow readily in the carbon filter of these devices unless a bacteriostatic agent has been added to prevent regrowth. However, some bacteria grow even in the presence of a bacteriostatic agent.

DESCRIPTION OF THE DISEASE

HPC bacteria are not normally used as an indicator of disease, and bacteria in this group are usually not directly associated with a specific illness or disease. However, bacteria *within* the HPC can cause disease, both as primary pathogens and as opportunistic pathogens, including pathogenic *Escherichia coli* (gastrointestinal illnesses), and the opportunistic *Pseudomonas* (skin or lung infections) and *Aeromonas* (possibly gastrointestinal illnesses). Because the media used for HPC are not designed to be selective and do not include differential indicators for specific bacterial groups, all these bacteria remain as unspecified bacterial species.

The relationship of HPC to gastrointestinal disease has been reported as part of an epidemiological study of the gastrointestinal health effects of drinking water. An apparent relationship between the HPC counts on medium R2A at 35°C and gastrointestinal illness was reported for consumers of water produced by reverse osmosis units. Very high bacterial counts were observed in the reservoir containing the treated water, and bacteria with virulence characteristics could have been responsible for this observation. Immunologically compromised people (due to microbial infections, age, cancer treatments, etc.) are generally considered to be susceptible to any infections, and opportunistic pathogens could play a role in such infections. In a second epidemiological study, fully treated tap water bottled immediately after production was found to also support high HPC numbers but to have no health effect.

RESERVOIRS FOR THE AGENT

Heterotrophic bacteria are ubiquitous in the environment. Distinct reservoirs for large numbers of these organisms occur wherever there are readily decomposable sources of bacterial nutrients, such as decaying biological entities, polluted water, and wastewater discharges.

MODE OF TRANSMISSION

Because heterotrophic bacteria are ubiquitous, transmission in the water environment may come from ingestion, bathing or body contact, and inhalation.

METHODS FOR DETECTING THE AGENT

The first plate count procedures used nutrient gelatin at 20°C for 48 hours. Plate count on nutrient agar at 37°C for 24 hours was later added. Incubation at 20°C was not recommended for several years. The terminology was changed to heterotrophic plate count (HPC) bacteria in the 16th edition (1985) of *Standard Methods for the Analysis of Water and Wastewater*. This edition introduced several new procedures, such as the membrane filtration (MF), spread plate, low-nutrient medium (R2A), different incubation temperatures (20, 28, and 35°C), and incubation times. The pour plate technique with incubation at 35°C for 48 hours has gradually been replaced by the R2A medium in a spread plate or MF procedure, the latter permitting analysis of larger sample volumes. The R2A low-nutrient agar medium was developed to maximize bacterial recoveries. It yields higher counts when incubated for 5 to 7 days at 20 or 28°C. The m-HPC medium also may be used to examine larger sample volumes, but the limited inclusion of fewer nutrients at higher concentration causes the medium to detect fewer different species of the diverse heterotrophic bacterial population.

Bacteria in low-nutrient aquatic environments are stressed, and culture conditions in the pour plate and spread plate are often unfavorable. The MF method allows analysis of larger sample volumes and enumeration of low concentrations of bacteria, provided the water is relatively low in turbidity. The 37°C plate count could be related to pathogenic bacterial types, while the 20°C plate count replicates the normal flora of water.

HPC bacteria at levels higher than 500 colony-forming units (cfu)/mL at 35°C have been reported to interfere with fecal coliforms detection by MF. The current use of chromagenic substrate media to detect coliforms by presence–absence tests apparently does not suffer from this interference.

OCCURRENCE OF THE AGENT IN PEOPLE, ANIMALS, AND THE ENVIRONMENT

Heterotrophic bacteria constitute part of the normal flora encountered on the body and in the fecal discharges of all animals, on the surfaces of plants, in soil, water, and the dust nuclei of rain drops.

SURVIVAL OF THE AGENT IN THE ENVIRONMENT

Survival of heterotrophic bacteria is influenced by nutrients, substrate, desiccation, algae and bacterial predators, sunlight exposure, pH, temperature, aerobic and anaerobic conditions, and the presence of heavy metals and disinfectants. Studies of the effect of nutrients in treated water in relationship to their growth in distribution systems has been extensive. Bacteriological quality changes due to heterotrophic bacteria in distribution systems may cause aesthetic problems involving taste and odor, discolored water, and slime growths, and economic problems, including corrosion of pipes and biodeterioration of materials such as gaskets and lubricants.

DOCUMENTED WATERBORNE OUTBREAKS

No waterborne outbreaks or illnesses resulting from high heterotrophic bacterial densities in public water supplies have been documented. There is, however, some concern for the health of subpopulations with deficient or suppressed immune systems.

EFFECTIVENESS OF WATER TREATMENT PROCESSES

HPC bacteria in drinking water are being used to gain better information on the effects of water treatment processes and the bacteriological quality of distributed drinking water. HPC monitoring provides water quality information and bacterial quality changes in water during treatment, storage, and distribution.

Because of the large number of these bacteria, especially at 20° C, HPC has been used to monitor the efficiency of water treatment processes, changes in water quality during distribution and storage, microbial growth on materials, and bacterial regrowth or aftergrowth potential. Conventional water treatment, including final disinfection with chlorine, reduces HPC bacteria to almost undetectable levels. However, culturable bacteria constitute only a minor part of the total bacterial counts and they are able to grow in low-nutrient environments. Thus, they will rapidly regrow in the absence of residual disinfectant or in treated water that contains enough nutrients for their growth. Biologically stable treated drinking water (i.e., after biological filtration) significantly reduces the potential for regrowth.

Bacteriological quality changes may cause aesthetic problems involving tastes and odors, discolored water, and slime growths, and treatment plant problems, including pipe corrosion and biodeterioration of materials. Bacterial numbers tend to increase during distribution. The density reached is influenced by a number of factors, including the bacterial quality of the finished water entering the distribution system, temperature, residence time, presence or absence of disinfectant residual, construction materials, and availability of nutrients for growth.

Attached bacteria (biofilm organisms) are more difficult to inactivate than those freely suspended in the water. Extensive literature, mostly work done in Europe, is available on the growth of microorganisms on materials in contact with drinking water. Maintaining adequate disinfection residuals throughout the distribution system, reducing available nutrients in treated waters, and routine maintenance (i.e., regular flushing programs) are effective means of controlling HPC. See chapter 2 of this manual for further information.

NATIONAL OR INTERNATIONAL GUIDELINES AND MONITORING RECOMMENDATIONS

Various guidelines, both national and international, set allowable levels of HPC bacteria in drinking water. These guidelines must be carefully interpreted because the methods used for enumeration can be different in methodology (plate count versus membrane filtration), medium used (nutrient agar, m-HPC, or m-R2A), incubation temperature (20, 28, 35, or 37°C), and incubation period (2 to 7 days). In general, the maximum recommended counts are on the order of 500 cfu/mL but some countries have suggested lower levels, e.g., not more than 100 cfu/mL. Because the scientific basis for these numbers has been seriously questioned, most countries use the values to suggest that increases in HPC bacteria indicate inefficient disinfection or water degradation that should be investigated and corrective measures taken, if required.

INFORMATION SOURCES

American Public Health Association, American Water Works Association, and Water Environment Federation. 1995. *Standard Methods for the Examination of Water and Wastewater.* 18th ed. Washington, D.C.: APHA.

Colbourne, J.S. 1985. Materials Usage and Their Effects on the Microbiological Quality of Water Supplies. *J. Appl. Micro.,* 59:47S–59S. Symposium Supplement.

Geldreich, E.E., H.D. Nash, D.J. Reasoner, and R.H. Taylor. 1972. The Necessity of Controlling Bacterial Populations in Potable Water: Community Water Supply. *Jour. AWWA*, 64:596–602.

Health Canada. 1996. *Guidelines for Canadian Drinking Water Quality.* 6th ed. Publication H48-10/1996E. Ottawa, Ont.: Health Canada.

LeChevallier, M.W., C.D. Cawthon, and R.G. Lee. 1988. Inactivation of Biofilm Bacteria. *Appl. Environ. Microbiol.,* 54:2492–2499.

Olson, B.H., and L.A. Nagy. 1984. Microbiology of Potable Water. *Advances in Applied Microbiology,* 30:73–132.

Payment, P. 1995. Health Significance of Bacterial Regrowth in Drinking Water. *J. Water Sci.,* 8:301–305.

———. 1996. Should We Regulate the Bacterial Heterotrophic Plate Count (HPC) in Drinking Water. In *Proc. AWWA Annual Conference*. pp. 19–24. Denver, Colo.: American Water Works Association.

Payment, P., E. Franco, L. Richardson, and J. Siemiatycki. 1991. Gastrointestinal Health Effects Associated with the Consumption of Drinking Water Produced by Point-of-Use Domestic Reverse-Osmosis Filtration Units. *Appl. Environ. Microbiol.,* 57: 945–948.

Payment, P., J. Siemiatycki, L. Richardson, G. Renaud, E. Franco, and M. Prévost. 1997. A Prospective Epidemiological Study of Gastro-Intestinal Health Effects Due to the Consumption of Drinking Water. *Intern. J. Environ. Health Res.,* 7:5–31.

Reasoner, D.J. 1990. Monitoring Heterotrophic Bacteria in Potable Water. In *Drinking Water Microbiology.* McFeters, G.A., ed. New York: Springer-Verlag.

US Environmental Protection Agency. 1989. National Primary Drinking Water Rules and Regulations, USEPA Surface Water Rule. Filtration, Disinfection, Turbidity, *Giardia lamblia*, Viruses,

Legionella, Heterotrophic Bacteria. *Federal Register*, 54(124):27486–27541.

World Health Organization. 1996. *Guidelines for Drinking Water Quality.* 2nd ed., Vol. 2: Health Criteria and Other Supporting Information. Geneva: World Health Organization.

This page intentionally blank.

Chapter 11

Klebsiella

Edwin E. Geldreich

DESCRIPTION OF THE AGENT

The genus *Klebsiella* includes at least seven currently recognized species and 72 serotypes. Most of these organisms are of environmental origin without significance to human health, while other strains of the same genus originate in the intestinal tract of warm-blooded animals. They are found as human pathogens, commensals in humans, in soil and water, and as plant pathogens. Five of these (*K. pneumoniae*, *K. oxytoca*, *K. rhinoscleromatis*, *K. planticola*, and *K. ozaenae*) are known to be clinically significant. Like other coliform bacteria, *Klebsiella* are lactose fermenting, nonmotile, gram-negative bacilli. Under certain conditions they form a gelatinous encapsulation.

Klebsiella typically use citrate and give a negative methyl red and positive Voges-Proskauer reaction, although some strains have atypical biochemical reactions, such as fermenting glucose at 5° C or lactose fermentation at 44.5° C (fecal *Klebsiella*). An estimated 60 to 85 percent of all *Klebsiella* isolated from feces and clinical specimens are positive in the fecal coliform test and identify as *K. pneumoniae*. As a consequence, classification of these bacteria into a clear-cut scheme has been difficult.

DESCRIPTION OF THE DISEASE

K. pneumoniae, particularly antibiotic-resistant serotypes, can cause human infections of the respiratory system, genito-urinary tract, nose, and throat, and occasionally meningitis and septicemia. *Klebsiella*-caused infection is sometimes a primary etiology agent but more often is found in mixed infection or as an opportunistic invader. Virulence does not appear to depend on capsule formation. In a study of 94 hospitals, the infection rate (16.7 infections per 100 patients) for pathogenic *K. pneumoniae* was the cause of 1.1 percent of all nosocomical deaths. Infections of the urinary system, lower respiratory tract, and surgical wounds were the most frequent cause of *Klebsiella*-associated illness or deaths.

RESERVOIRS FOR THE AGENT

Approximately 30 to 40 percent of all warm-blooded animals, humans included, have *Klebsiella* in their intestinal tract, with individual densities ranging up to 10^8 *Klebsiella* per gram of feces. *K. planticola* and *K. terrigena* have their origins in the environment, being found on fruit and vegetables, dairy products, seed embryos, internal and external tree tissues, hay, and cotton. Wood pulp, paper mills, textile finishing plants, and sugar cane processing operations may release 10[illegible] to 10^6 *Klebsiella* per millilitre of effluent and account for about 50 to 90 percent of the total coliform population of such effluents. Water storage tanks constructed from fresh redwood lumber have been shown to be a source of *Klebsiella* in the distribution network.

MODE OF TRANSMISSION

Transmission is often from body contact with water supply during bathing, ingestion, or by person-to-person contact through poor hand-washing habits in hospitals or senior citizen care institutions. Inhalation of moisture from vaporizers using drinking water contaminated with *Klebsiella* should also be considered a risk to some individuals.

METHODS FOR DETECTING THE AGENT

The public health significance of *Klebsiella* can be very difficult to interpret unless the available information is supplemented by data on key growth responses and antibiotic resistance characteristics. Fortunately, the biochemical characteristics of commercial multi-test systems provide speciation for most isolates purified from coliform colonies on M-Endo agar cultures. A more desirable approach is the use of the differential medium M-Kleb agar in connection with the membrane filter (MF) procedure. This approach provides quantitative information on total *Klebsiella* density in the sample and, in conjunction with a biochemical multi-testing of positive (dark blue or dark gray) colonies, yields identification of species.

OCCURRENCE OF THE AGENT IN PEOPLE, ANIMALS, AND THE ENVIRONMENT

Surface water and unprotected groundwater receive *Klebsiella* from both environmental and fecal sources. Environmental strains are introduced to the source of raw water intake from urban and rural runoff and by discharges of wood, paper, and textile processing wastes. Fecal *Klebsiella* enter the water in point source discharges from municipal sewage and meat processing works and in nonpoint source discharges from farm animal waste runoff.

SURVIVAL OF THE AGENT IN THE ENVIRONMENT

Densities of *Klebsiella* in surface waters are influenced by available nutrients and seasonal water temperatures. For example, *Klebsiella* may survive for 20 days in laboratory "pure water" as a consequence of trace organics introduced to the supply as contaminates from the air. Those strains of *Klebsiella* that persisted in this environment developed into a mucoid mutant that dominated over time.

DOCUMENTED WATERBORNE OUTBREAKS

No community waterborne outbreaks have been reported to be caused by *Klebsiella* in public water supplies. The lack of evidence of increased illness in a community during coliform biofilm events involving *Klebsiella* may relate to difficulties in gathering reports of water-related illness cases among susceptible people at home, in the work environment, and the hospital setting. Furthermore, most of the *Klebsiella* waterborne occurrences do not involve fecal strains. In those infrequent situations in which the laboratory analyses reveal fecal *Klebsiella* in the distribution system, the colonization sites must be destroyed to avoid more frequent releases of this opportunistic pathogen at higher densities into the water supply. Infective dose (ID_{50}) values for environmental and clinical isolates of *Klebsiella* have been reported to be between 3.5×10^1 to 7.9×10^5 cells per mL. Therefore, ingestion of 100 mL of drinking water (approximately one glass of water) containing 3.5×10^1 *Klebsiella* per mL could present a risk to susceptible individuals.

EFFECTIVENESS OF WATER TREATMENT PROCESSES

Many of the water systems reporting coliform occurrences in their distribution networks have noted that the predominate organism was a member of the *Klebsiella* genus. Although klebsiellae can be controlled effectively by adequate disinfection in a clean pipe environment, these organisms can be protected by particulate material, porous pipe sediments, biological debris, macroinvertebrates, and disinfection demand products. Furthermore, *Klebsiella* can encapsulate, which provides some protection from disinfectants. As the organisms become established in this type of environment, growth beyond meager subsistence can result in the periodic sloughing of cells into water flowing past the sites. This condition can persist until elevated disinfectant residuals penetrate the protective habitat and inactivate the microbes. Systematic flushing of the entire system, sanitizing of all new line extensions, cross-connection control, cleaning of storage reservoirs and standpipes, and corrosion control in iron pipes are often effective in suppressing the seasonal reoccurrence of these biofilm events.

NATIONAL OR INTERNATIONAL GUIDELINES AND MONITORING RECOMMENDATIONS

Klebsiella organisms are coliform bacteria and as such are included in the national and international guidelines for total coliform occurrences. Generally these standards limit total coliforms to less than one organism or their absence in 100 mL of treated drinking water. World Health Organization guidelines have established a limit of less than 10 total coliforms per 100 mL of untreated groundwater, provided no fecal coliforms are detected in the sample.

INFORMATION SOURCES

Clancy, C.F. 1989. Enterobacteriaceae. In *Practical Handbook of Microbiology.* pp. 71–86. O'Leary, W., ed. Boca Raton, Fla.: CRC Press.

Geldreich, E.E. 1996. *Microbial Quality of Water Supply in Distribution Systems.* Boca Raton, Fla.: CRC Lewis Publishers.

Geldreich, E.E., and Rice, E.W. 1987. Occurrence, Significance and Detection of *Klebsiella* in Water Systems. *Jour. AWWA*, 79:74–80.

Kelly, M.T., D.J. Brenner, and J.J. Farmer, III. 1985. Enterobacteriaceae. In *Manual of Clinical Microbiology*, 4th ed. pp. 263–277. Lennette, E.H., A. Balows, W.J. Hausler, Jr., and H.J. Shadomy, eds. Washington, D.C.: ASM Press.

Chapter 12

Legionella

Nancy H. Hall

DESCRIPTION OF THE AGENT

Legionella are bacteria of the family Legionellaceae. They are facultative, gram-negative, non–spore-forming small bacilli (from 0.2 to 0.8 µm wide by 2 to 20 µm or more in length) that do not grow on ordinary laboratory media. The genus *Legionella* is composed of at least 36 different species, 4 subspecies of *Legionella pneumophila*, and 5 sets of serogroups. *Legionella* bacteria are ubiquitous in the aquatic environment and as biofilm organisms. They are able to colonize hot-water tanks, cooling towers, distribution systems, and other water sources. Probably all *Legionella* species can cause illness, but only about half of the known species have been implicated in human disease. The species *Legionella pneumophila* causes most *Legionella* infections.

DESCRIPTION OF THE DISEASE

The disease caused by *Legionella* bacteria is called legionellosis. The two forms of legionellosis are Legionnaires' disease and Pontiac fever. In the United States, the frequency of Legionnaires' disease is estimated to be 17,000 to 23,000 cases a year, although public health officials suspect this is a low estimate. The occurrence of Pontiac fever is estimated to be 2 to 100 times more frequent than Legionnaires' disease.

Legionnaires' disease is a severe respiratory illness characterized by pneumonia. Incubation period for Legionnaires' disease is 2 to 10 days, with an attack rate of 1 to 6 percent. The risk of contracting Legionnaires' disease is greater for individuals with underlying disease and immunosuppression. Additional risk factors include being a male over 50 years of age, cigarette smoking, excessive use of alcohol, and surgery.

Pontiac fever is a self-limiting, nonpneumonic, influenza-like illness. No known cases of pneumonia or deaths with Pontiac fever are documented. The incubation period of Pontiac fever usually ranges between 20 and 48 hours, with a mean of 36 hours and an attack rate of nearly 100 percent.

Five methods of diagnosis for legionellosis are culture isolation from respiratory secretions or tissues, direct fluorescent antibody test on respiratory secretions or tissues, indirect fluorescent antibody test performed on acute and convalescent sera, nucleic acid hybridization for detection of *Legionella* rRNA, and urinary antigen detection by radioimmunoassay, enzyme-linked immunosorbent assay, or agglutination assay.

RESERVOIRS FOR THE AGENT

Legionella bacteria are ubiquitous in aquatic environments, both natural and artificial. These organisms have been found in lakes, rivers, and streams, and have colonized artificial environments such as cooling towers, evaporative condensers, and hot-water tanks, with and without association of disease. These artificial environments are thought to act as either amplifiers or disseminators of legionellae. The temperature of the water appears to be a major determinant of *Legionella* colonization in artificial settings. Legionellae are most often isolated from environmental water sources between 35 and 45° C, and killed at temperatures above 60° C.

MODE OF TRANSMISSION

The mode of transmission is by inhalation of moist aerosols contaminated with *Legionella* bacteria. *Legionella* in the environment is amplified in a water system, cooling tower, whirlpool spa, and other sources. The bacteria are transmitted through water vapor (aerosalization) to a susceptible host. In immunosuppressed individuals, the bacteria can cause legionellosis.

METHODS FOR DETECTING THE AGENT

The three primary methods used to detect legionellae in environmental samples are culture, direct fluorescent antibody test, and polymerase chain reaction (PCR). Culture has been the method of choice for detection of legionellae from environmental samples but is sometimes difficult because of interference or overgrowth by other organisms. Selective media and pretreatment techniques (acid and heat treatment) are usually necessary to enhance recovery and reduce overgrowth. Sample concentration by either filtration or centrifugation before culture may be necessary to detect low numbers of legionellae in relatively clean samples. Environmental samples may also contain legionellae that are viable but nonculturable; any culture method will typically underestimate the total population density.

The direct fluorescent antibody test has been used to see legionellae in its natural habitat and is a very useful diagnostic tool. This technique does not provide absolute specificity and does not allow viable and nonviable cells to be differentiated unless secondary staining with tetrazolium dyes is performed.

The PCR test kits (EnviroAmp® *Legionella* kit*) amplifies gene sequences and uses probes to detect deoxyribonucleic acid (DNA) from organisms of the genus *Legionella* and the species *Legionella pneumophila* in environmental water samples. This process is helpful when viable, nonculturable legionellae are thought to be present. The major limitations of this method are cost, presence of inhibitory substances, and necessity of a dedicated PCR laboratory.

---

*Perkin Elmer, Branchburg, N.J.

OCCURRENCE OF THE AGENT IN PEOPLE, ANIMALS, AND THE ENVIRONMENT

Legionella are ubiquitous in the environment and are found in water, both natural and treated, as well as in water distribution and storage systems.

SURVIVAL OF THE AGENT IN THE ENVIRONMENT

Legionella bacteria thrive in the freshwater environment under a wide range of temperatures (about 5 to 63° C) and pH (5.5 to 9.2). Several studies have shown a unique association between legionellae and protozoa in the environment. *Legionella* bacteria have the capacity to survive inside free-living protozoa (e.g., amoebas), which may explain how these bacteria evade water purification systems. Legionellae are more readily isolated from warm than from ambient sites, as demonstrated by their frequent occurrence in domestic hot-water tanks and hot-water plumbing systems. Other factors that encourage *Legionella* growth include pH, stagnation, sediment formation, presence of nutrients in natural-rubber sealing washers and gaskets, and presence of protozoa.

DOCUMENTED WATERBORNE OUTBREAKS

Some of the more notable outbreaks caused by *Legionella* bacteria are listed in Table 12-1. The largest outbreak of Legionnaires' disease occurred among persons attending the American Legion convention held in Philadelphia, Pa., in July 1976, where over 220 cases and 34 deaths were reported. Since this outbreak, the majority of nosocomial legionellosis cases have been linked to contaminated hospital water distribution systems. The reservoirs that have been associated with community-acquired legionellosis have been cooling tower or evaporative condensers, and more recently, whirlpool spas. Most community-acquired cases occur in the summer months, whereas nosocomial legionellosis occurs year-round. Although *Legionella* bacteria have been implicated in numerous outbreaks, the recovery of legionellae from environmental sources does not constitute proof of the source of the infecting agent. Four criteria must be met to confirm the source of the *Legionella* outbreak: (1) association between exposure to a potential source, (2) identification of the mechanism of aerosol production, (3) occurrence of disease established, and (4) isolation of similar *Legionella* subtypes from patient and suspected environmental site.

Table 12-1 Notable outbreaks of legionellosis

Location	Setting	Date	Cases/Deaths	Source
Pontiac, Mich.	Health Dept.	August 1968	144/0	Evap. condenser
Philadelphia, Pa.	Hotel	August 1976	221/34	Unknown
Los Angeles, Calif.	Hospital	1977–1980	175+/28	Potable water
Pittsburgh, Pa.	Hospital	1979–1981	100+/?	Potable water
Seattle, Wash.	Hospital	1984–1988	21/9	Nebulizer
Staffordshire, England	Hospital	1985	163/39	Cooling system
South Australia	Statewide	1987-1989	30/0	Potting soil mixes
Bogalusa, La.	Grocery Store	November 1989	34/2	Produce mister
Bermuda	Cruise Ship	1994	50/0	Whirlpool

EFFECTIVENESS OF WATER TREATMENT PROCESSES

Strategies for prevention of legionellosis in the absence of disease are based on outbreak investigations and control. Although routine maintenance procedures for water systems may not prevent legionellosis, the following measures have been shown to reduce the prevalence of legionellae in water systems:

- maintain hot water at 50° C or higher in the return and cold water below 20° C
- limit thermal stratification in central hot-water storage equipment
- periodically clean and remove sediment in central hot-water storage tanks and cooling towers
- maintain hot-water tank temperature between 71 and 77° C
- remove obstructions to flow or conditions of stagnation
- consistently provide adequate maintenance and disinfection control procedures, especially for whirlpools and cooling towers

Additional control measures used after outbreaks include the following: cleaning of scale or sediment accumulation or replacement of faucets and showerheads, and supplemental chlorination of the heated water to achieve 1 to 2 mg/L of free residual chlorine. If outbreaks of legionellosis are to be prevented, control methods must focus not just on legionellae but the whole microbial community, particularly biofilm. The accumulation of microbial slime and sludge that supports and protects *Legionella* bacteria in these systems must be reduced.

NATIONAL OR INTERNATIONAL GUIDELINES AND MONITORING RECOMMENDATIONS

The Surface Water Treatment Rule (SWTR) requires a treatment technique (filtration and disinfection for surface water supplies) rather than a maximum contaminant level (MCL) for *Legionella* to significantly reduce the transport and potential for colonization in the distribution system. Following the outbreak linked to a grocery store mist machine, the US Food and Drug Administration (FDA) issued cleaning and maintenance guidelines for the use of ultrasonic vegetable misters. The Centers for Disease Control (CDC) Guidelines for Prevention of Nosocomial Pneumonia state that only sterile fluids should be used in nebulizers or humidifiers in the hospital setting. The CDC Recommendation for Cruise Ship Prevention of Sea-Associated Legionnaires' Disease states that existing health guidelines should be followed for whirlpool maintenance and vigorous filter cleaning and maintenance should be performed frequently. Guidelines for the control and prevention of legionellosis for cooling towers have been established in many countries (e.g., Australia, New Zealand, and United Kingdom). The Australian standards are the most restrictive, requiring tower registration and submission of building plans, site surveys, maintenance procedures, and other documentation to regulatory authorities.

The value of routine monitoring for legionellae of water sources not implicated in disease remains questionable, since legionellae are ubiquitous and long-term decontamination is difficult. Most public health investigators recommend environmental sampling for legionellae only after two or more epidemiologically linked cases have been identified. Currently, environmental sampling is not recommended after individual community-acquired cases because of the considerable time and expense required to collect samples from the many potential sources in the environment.

INFORMATION SOURCES

Blackmon, J.A., et al. *Legionellosis: Review Article*. Atlanta, Ga.: Centers for Disease Control, US Department of Health and Human Services.

Broadbent, C.R. 1993. *Legionella* in Cooling Towers: Practical Research, Design, Treatment, and Control Guidelines. In *Legionella: Current Status and Emerging Perspectives*. Barbaree, J.W., R.F. Breiman, and A.P. Dufour, eds. Washington, D.C.: American Society of Microbiology.

Dennis, P.J. 1993. Potable Water Systems: Insights into Control. In *Legionella: Current Status and Emerging Perspectives*. Barbaree, J.W., R.F. Breiman, and A.P. Dufour, eds. Washington, D.C.: American Society of Microbiology.

Fliermans, C.B. 1995. *Legionella* Ecology. In *Bioaerosals: Indoor Air Research Series*. Burge, H.A., ed. Boca Raton, Fla.: Lewis Publishers.

Guidelines for Prevention of Nosocomial Pneumonia Recommendations and Report. 1997. *MMWR*, 46:28–34. Atlanta, Ga.: Centers for Disease Control.

Hoge, C.W., and R.F. Breiman. 1991. Advances in the Epidemiology and Control of *Legionella* Infections. *Epidemiologic Reviews*, 13:329–340.

Jernigan, D.B., et al. 1996. Outbreak of Legionnaires' Disease among Cruise Ship Passengers Exposed to a Contaminated Whirlpool Spa. *Lancet*, 347:494–499.

Memorandum from a WHO Meeting. 1990. Epidemiology, Prevention, and Control of Legionellosis. Bulletin of the World Health Organization. Geneva: WHO.

This page intentionally blank.

Chapter 13

Mycobacterium avium Complex

Mark W. LeChevallier

DESCRIPTION OF THE AGENT

Members of the *Mycobacterium avium* complex (i.e., *M. avium* and *intracellulare*) are acid-fast, rod-shaped bacteria 0.2 to 0.6 by 1.0 to 10.0 µm in size. Mycobacteria are aerobic, nonmotile bacilli that do not form spores. The cell walls of the bacteria contain high levels of lipid (waxy) material and are not affected by staining procedures that use acid alcohol. Therefore, they are described as acid fast.

DESCRIPTION OF THE DISEASE

Members of the *M. avium* complex (MAC) are opportunistic human pathogens and can infect the lungs, producing cough, fatigue, weight loss, low-grade fever, and night sweats similar to *M. tuberculosis*. From the lungs, the organism can be disseminated throughout the body. The greatest increase in MAC infections is seen in acquired immunodeficiency syndrome (AIDS) patients. Approximately 25 to 50 percent of these patients suffer debilitating and life-threatening infection.

RESERVOIRS FOR THE AGENT

M. avium complex are ubiquitous in the environment and have been found in soil, house dust, water (wastewater, surface and groundwater water, and drinking water), animals, and poultry. *M. avium* levels can be hundreds or thousands times higher in soils than in treated drinking water.

MODE OF TRANSMISSION

M. avium complex can be transmitted through inhalation or ingestion of contaminated water, soil, or other materials. Evidence for environmental transmission, especially in immunocompromised individuals include (1) the frequency of gastrointestinal colonization increases as the stage of human immunodeficiency virus (HIV) advances, (2) higher frequency of isolation of MAC from the gut than from the respiratory tract, and (3) gastrointestinal symptoms, e.g., nausea, vomiting, and diarrhea.

METHODS FOR DETECTING THE AGENT

Isolation of MAC organisms from water or biofilm samples is difficult because of their very slow growth (i.e., greater than seven days for colony formation). Optimum growth temperature is 37° C. Disinfection is required to kill nonmycobacteria that can overgrow the mycobacterial colonies. As an alternative, mycobacterial selective media can be used. These media permit direct isolation and enumeration of MAC without decontamination.

Identification of MAC isolates is achieved through application of chemical or molecular techniques. Characteristic mycolic acids and other cell wall lipids of *M. avium* can be identified using capillary gas chromatography (GC) or high-performance liquid chromatography (HPLC) methods. Deoxyribonucleic acid (DNA) probes are commercially available for identification of MAC, as well as multiplex polymerase chain reaction (PCR) techniques.

OCCURRENCE OF THE AGENT IN PEOPLE, ANIMALS, AND THE ENVIRONMENT

Members of the MAC (i.e., *M. avium* and *intracellulare*) are found in natural waters and drinking water distribution systems throughout the United States. Table 13-1 summarizes the number of MAC colony-forming units (cfu) per 100 mL of drinking water samples reported by different authors.

The differences in the numbers may reflect different pretreatment steps used in the processing of environmental samples, different isolation media, and variations in water quality.

SURVIVAL OF THE AGENT IN THE ENVIRONMENT

Members of the MAC are resistant to chlorination and are able to grow in water samples to which no additional nutrient substrate had been added. Further, they grow over a wide range of temperatures (e.g., 15 to 45° C) and salinities (e.g., 0 to

Table 13-1 Summary of reports on *Mycobacterium avium* complex in water

Study	Sample Types	*M. avium*, *cfu / 100 mL*
Haas et al. (1983)	Distribution System	0.08–0.14
Carson et al. (1988a)	Hospitals	14.5–195
duMoulin et al. (1988)	Hospitals	141
Fischeder et al. (1991)	Distribution System	10–45,000
von Reyn et al. (1993)	Distribution System and Hospitals	20–10,000
Glover et al. (1994)	Distribution System and Dwelling	0.20–2

2 percent NaCl). *M. avium* complex organisms are found in highest numbers in waters of low dissolved oxygen, of high organic matter, and of high zinc concentrations. Recent evidence suggests that the level of biodegradable organic material can influence the growth of mycobacteria in drinking water. DNA fingerprinting studies have shown that single, unique strains can persist as long as 41 months in a water distribution system.

Because of their lipid cell walls, MAC organisms are hydrophobic and readily colonize surfaces. The reported resistance of mycobacteria to zinc and copper may aid the development of biofilms of these organisms on plastic, copper, or galvanized (i.e., zinc-coated) pipes.

DOCUMENTED WATERBORNE OUTBREAKS

M. avium strains have been detected in nebulizer reservoirs, ice machines, hot- and cold-water faucets, toilets, sinks, and other water sources in patient care sites. The strains were serologically similar to clinical isolates. *M. avium* strains from infected AIDS patients were shown to be genetically related to isolates recovered from water to which the patients were exposed through drinking or bathing. An epidemiological study of 290 homes of HIV patients found MAC in 0.76 percent (4 of 528) water samples, 1 of 397 (0.25 percent) food samples, but in 55 percent of 157 soil samples taken from potted plants. Some of the soil isolates were similar by serotyping and multilocus enzyme electrophoresis analysis. Other environmental mycobacteria may be of health concern. *M. xenopi* was detected in drinking water faucets and showers from 5 of 11 apartments of patients infected with the organism.

EFFECTIVENESS OF WATER TREATMENT PROCESSES

Most species of mycobacteria survive treatment with 1 mg/L free chlorine. *Mycobacterium marinum* was reported to be resistant to 10 mg/L free chlorine. No reduction in mycobacterial numbers was found following chlorination in the water treatment plant examined. Distribution system data suggest that use of chloramines as a postdisinfectant may select for the presence of mycobacteria, although many systems that convert to chloramines do so because of high levels of organic carbon in the water supply. Institutional plumbing systems (such as hospitals and office buildings) can be disinfected for mycobacteria using hot water. Treatment of *M. avium* suspensions at 60° C for 4 minutes reduced viable counts by 90 percent (1 log).

NATIONAL OR INTERNATIONAL GUIDELINES AND MONITORING RECOMMENDATIONS

There are no national or international guidelines for mycobacteria in water. *M. avium* and *M. intracellulare* have been included in a list of candidate contaminants for possible regulation by the US Environmental Protection Agency (USEPA). The World Health Organization declined to consider mycobacteria in their 1997 revisions of the WHO guidelines for drinking water quality.

INFORMATION SOURCES

Carson, L.A., L.A. Bland, L.B. Cusick, M.S. Favero, G.A. Bolan, A.L. Reingold, and R.C. Good. 1988a. Prevalence of Nontuberculous Mycobacteria in Water Supplies of Hemodialysis Centers. *Appl. Environ. Microbiol.,* 54:3122–3125.

Carson, L.A., L.B. Cusick, L.A. Bland, and M.S. Favero. 1988b. Efficacy of Chemical Dosing Methods for Isolating Nontuberculous Mycobacteria From Water Supplies of Dialysis Centers. *Appl. Environ. Microbiol.*, 54:1756–1760.

Carson, L.A., N.J. Petersen, M.S. Favero, and S.M. Aguero. 1978. Growth Characteristics of Atypical Mycobacteria in Water and Their Comparative Resistance to Disinfectants. *Appl. Environ. Microbiol.*, 36:839–846.

Collins, C.H., J.M. Grange, and M.D. Yates. 1984. Mycobacteria in Water. *J. Appl. Bacteriol.*, 57:193–211.

duMoulin, G.C., and K.D. Stottmeier. 1986. Waterborne Mycobacteria: An Increasing Threat to Health. *Am. Soc. Microbiol. News*, 52:525–529.

duMoulin, G.C., K.D. Stottmeier, P.A. Pelletier, A.Y. Tsang, and J. Hedley-Whyte. 1988. Concentration of *Mycobacterium avium* by Hospital Hot Water Systems. *J. Am. Med. Assoc.*, 260:1599–1601.

Falkinham, J.O., III, B.C. Parker, and H. Gruft. 1980. Epidemiology of Infection by Nontuberculous Mycobacteria. I. Geographic Distribution in the Eastern United States. *Am. Rev. Respir. Dis.*, 121:931–937.

Fischeder, R., R. Schulze-Röbbecke, and A. Weber. 1991. Occurrence of Mycobacteria in Drinking Water Samples. *Zbl. Hyg.*, 192:154–158.

George, K.L., and J.O. Falkinham, III. 1986. Selective Medium for the Isolation and Enumeration of *Mycobacterium avium-intracellulare* and *M. scrofulaceum*. *Can. J. Microbiol.*, 32:10–14.

Glover, N., A. Holtzman, T. Aronson, S. Froman, O.G.W. Berlin, P. Dominguez, K.A. Kunkel, G. Overturf, G. Stelma, Jr., C. Smith, and M. Yakrus. 1994. The Isolation and Identification of *Mycobacterium Avium* Complex (MAC) Recovered from Los Angeles Potable Water, a Possible Source of Infection in AIDS Patients. *Intern. J. Environ. Health Res.*, 4:63–72.

Haas, C.N., M.A. Meyer, and M.S. Paller. 1983. The Ecology of Acid-fast Organisms in Water Supply, Treatment, and Distribution Systems. *Jour. AWWA*, 75:139–144.

Horsburgh, C.R. 1991. *Mycobacterium avium* Complex Infection in the Acquired Immunodeficiency Syndrome. *New England J. Med.*, 324:1332–1338.

Kulski, J.K., C. Khinsoe, T. Pryce, and K. Christiansen. 1995. Use of Multiplex PCR to Detect and Identify *Mycobacterium avium* and *M. Intracellulare* in Blood Culture Fluids of AIDS Patients. *J. Clin. Microbiol.*, 33:668–674.

Pelletier, P.A., E.M. Carney, and G.C. duMoulin. 1991. Comparative Resistance of *Mycobacterium avium* Complex and Other Nontuberculous Mycobacteria to Chloramine. In *Proc. AWWA Water Quality Technology Conference*. pp. 47–58. Denver, Colo.: American Water Works Association.

Ratledge, C. 1976. The Physiology of the Mycobacteria. *Adv. Microb. Physiol.*, 13:115–224.

Schulze-Röbbecke, R., and R. Fischeder. 1989. Mycobacteria in Biofilms. *Zbl. Hyg.*, 188:385–390.

Singh, N., and V. Lu. 1994. Potable Water and *Mycobacterium avium* Complex in HIV Patients: Is Prevention Possible? *Lancet*, 343:1110–1111.

von Reyn, C.F., R.D. Waddell, T. Eaton, R.D. Arbeit, J.N. Maslow, T.W. Barber, R.J. Brindle, C.F. Gilks, J. Lumio, J. Lähdevirta, A. Ranki, D. Dawson, and J.O. Falkinham, III. 1993. Isolation of *Mycobacterium avium* Complex from Water in the United States, Finland, Zaire, and Kenya. *J. Clin. Microbiol.*, 31:3227–3230.

von Reyn, C.F., J.N. Maslow, T.W. Barber, J.O. Falkinham, III, and R.D. Arbeit. 1994. Persistent Colonisation of Potable Water as a Source of *Mycobacterium avium* Infection in AIDS. *Lancet*, 343:1137–1141.

Yajko, D.M., D.P. Chin, P.C. Gonzalez, P.S. Nassos, P.C. Hopewell, A.L. Reingold, R. Horsburgh, M.A. Yakrus, S.M. Ostroff, and W.K. Hadley. 1995. *Mycobacterium avium* Complex in Water, Food, and Soil Samples Collected from the Environment of HIV-Infected Individuals. *J. Acquired Immun. Deficiency Syndromes and Human Retroviol.*, 9:176–182.

Chapter 14

Pseudomonas

Edwin E. Geldreich

DESCRIPTION OF THE AGENT

The genus *Pseudomonas* includes over 29 species. Pseudomonads are gram-negative rods that may be motile because of polar flagella. Highly mucoid strains may lack motility. No spores are produced and metabolism is rapid in a variety of aerobic environments at ambient temperatures. These organisms are often glucose-nonfermenting, but tests for acid production from various other carbohydrates are not clear-cut, leading to ambiguities in species interpretation. Most fluorescent pseudomonads, including *P. aeruginosa*, *P. fluorescens*, and *P. putida*, produce water-soluble pigments (yellow, green, and red), while other strains (e.g., some *P. aeruginosa*) form a nonfluorescent water-soluble blue pigment. Development of these pigments (which may be an erratic trait of some strains) are influenced by nutritional factors, choice of media for cultivation, and incubation temperatures between 20 and 42° C.

DESCRIPTION OF THE DISEASE

The ability of *P. aeruginosa* to rapidly colonize a variety of environments, including the susceptible human, makes it a major opportunistic pathogen, particularly *P. aeruginosa* serogroup 11 and possibly serogroup 9. Infection with *P. aeruginosa* is usually associated with hospitalized patients as a secondary infection (nosocomial infections). Also susceptible are infants, individuals with suppressed immune systems from chemical therapy, and older people with reduced natural barriers to infection. Bacteremia attributable to *Pseudomonas* has become a major concern in the management of trauma as well as in the management of susceptible patients recovering from burns, intensive surgery, and others exposed to cancer therapy. *P. aeruginosa* is a cause of severe epidemic diarrhea of infants, ocular infections, cystic fibrosis, spa- and whirlpool-associated folliculitis, osteomyelitis, and malignant external otitis.

RESERVOIRS FOR THE AGENT

Pseudomonas species are ubiquitous bacteria able to flourish in a wide variety of habitats, e.g., surface water, aquifers, bottled water, distilled water, seawater, soils, and vegetation. *P. aeruginosa* has been isolated from cold waters only following storms, suggesting soil and vegetation may be reservoirs of these bacteria found in surface waters.

MODE OF TRANSMISSION

The route of exposure to *Pseudomonas* may be ingestion of food or water, body contact with water supply during bathing, or person-to-person contact in hospitals.

METHODS FOR DETECTING THE AGENT

Most species can grow in mineral base medium without growth factors. Growth is often optimal at 15 to 30° C, although *P. aeruginosa* grows well at 41.5° C. Membrane filtration and multiple tube fermentation (MTF) techniques are available for the enumeration of *P. aeruginosa* in water samples. M-PA agar is used in the membrane filter procedure with incubation at 41.5° C for 72 hours. Typical colonies are flat in appearance with light outer rims and brownish to green–black centers. Confirmation involves milk agar incubated at 35° C for 24 hours. *P. aeruginosa* hydrolyzes casein and produces a yellowish to green diffusible pigment. Asparagine broth is used in the MTF test with incubation at 35° C for 24 hours. Production of a greenish fluorescent pigment constitutes a positive presumptive test. Confirm positive tubes in acetamide broth for a purple color within 36 hours at 35° C incubation.

OCCURRENCE OF THE AGENT IN PEOPLE, ANIMALS, AND THE ENVIRONMENT

The infrequent occurrence (3 to 19 percent) of *Pseudomonas* in the human intestinal tract suggests that colonization of the gastrointestinal system rarely occurs in healthy adults, possibly due to potent host-defense mechanisms against this group of bacteria. Because municipal sewage contains a mixture of domestic wastes, industrial discharges, and intermittent stormwater runoff, *P. aeruginosa* will be found in 90 percent of sewage samples. While *P. aeruginosa* is the most significant species in some drinking water supplies, others found in the distribution system include *P. cepacia*, *P. fluorescens*, *P. mallei*, *P. maltophilia*, *P. putida*, and *P. testosteroni*. *P. stutzeri*, *P. diminuta*, and *P. acidovorans* have been found in bottled waters.

Some pseudomonads are among the prominent denitrifiers. Others grow prodigiously in sand or carbon filtration beds and on tertiary treatment devices, such as reverse osmosis and electrodialysis membranes. Biofilm development in distribution system sediments and home water treatment devices attached to public water supplies are also important contributors. Water supply attachments used with dental equipment and poorly maintained whirlpools are also potential sources of these organisms.

SURVIVAL OF THE AGENT IN THE ENVIRONMENT

Densities of *P. aeruginosa* in surface waters receiving waste and stormwater discharges may range from 1×10^1 to 1×10^4 cells per 100 mL and are influenced by available nutrients and seasonal water temperatures. Low-density subsistence of pseudomonads in bottled water and distilled water may continue for months because of the organism's ability to slow down metabolism and survive on trace amounts of carbon and nitrogen sources in the product water.

DOCUMENTED WATERBORNE OUTBREAKS

P. aeruginosa found in a contaminated water supply has been linked to one waterborne outbreak that occurred in a newborn nursery. The groundwater supply had become contaminated by seepage of sewage and infiltration of contaminated surface water.

EFFECTIVENESS OF WATER TREATMENT PROCESSES

Pseudomonas organisms may grow prodigiously in the water–air interfaces of process basins, sand filters, granular activated carbon (GAC) beds, and distribution system sediments unless proper measures are taken to control their colonization. Frequent removal of scum, careful control of backwashing procedures, and sediment removal in the pipe network are essential. This implies that distribution systems must be adequately flushed to maintain a disinfectant residual above 0.5 mg/L at the distal ends of the system. Home water treatment devices using carbon filters or reverse osmosis and electrodialysis membranes can also be amplifiers of these organisms unless attention is given to careful maintenance of these units.

NATIONAL OR INTERNATIONAL GUIDELINES AND MONITORING RECOMMENDATIONS

Because *P. aeruginosa* is the most prevalent *Pseudomonas* in human disease, its occurrence has been limited to less than one organism in 250 mL of bottled drinking water by the European Community. There are no federal regulations on restricting *Pseudomonas* in drinking water supplies.

INFORMATION SOURCES

Geldreich, E.E. 1996. *Microbial Quality of Water Supply in Distribution Systems*. Boca Raton, Fla.: CRC Lewis Publishers.

Gilardi, G.L. 1985. *Pseudomonas*. In *Manual of Clinical Microbiology*. 4th ed. pp. 350–372. Lennette, E.H., A. Balows, W.J. Hausler, Jr., and H.J. Shadomy, eds. Washington, D.C.: ASM Press.

Palleroni, N.J. 1989. *Pseudomonas*. In *Practical Handbook of Microbiology*. pp. 55–86. O'Leary, W., ed. Boca Raton, Fla.: CRC Lewis Press.

Prier, J.E., and H. Friedman, eds. 1974. *Opportunistic Pathogens*. Baltimore, Md.: University Park Press.

Young, V.M., ed. 1977. *Pseudomonas aeruginosa*. New York: Raven Press.

This page intentionally blank.

Chapter 15

Salmonella

Terry C. Covert

DESCRIPTION OF THE AGENT

The genus *Salmonella* is included in the family Enterobacteriaceae, which is a large and diverse group of bacteria found in soil, water, wastes, plants, and the normal flora of animals. Over 2,000 *Salmonella* serotypes are listed by the Kauffmann-White antigenic scheme. Salmonellae are facultatively anaerobic, non–spore-forming, gram-negative bacilli, 2 to 5 µm long and 0.8 to 1.5 µm wide, usually motile by peritrichous flagella, except *S. pullorum* and *S. gallinarum*. Gas is usually produced from glucose, nitrates are reduced to nitrites, citrate is used, and most *Salmonella* produce hydrogen sulfide. Salmonellae are positive for lysine decarboxylase and ornithine decarboxylase, with the important exceptions of *S. paratyphi A* and *S. typhi*. Lactose is usually not fermented, with the exception of *S. arizonae*. Salmonellae yield negative Voges-Proskauer and positive methyl red tests and do not produce cytochrome oxidase.

DESCRIPTION OF THE DISEASE

The genus *Salmonella* includes a wide variety of serotypes pathogenic for humans or animals, and usually for both. Three clinically distinguishable forms of salmonellosis occur in humans, including gastroenteritis, enteric fever, and septicemia. Gastroenteritis is an infection of the colon usually occurring 18 to 48 hours after ingestion of the organism. It is characterized by diarrhea, fever, and abdominal pain. The infection is usually self-limiting, lasting two to five days. Enteric fever is most often caused by *S. typhi* (typhoid fever) and the paratyphoid bacilli, *S. paratyphi A*, *B*, and *C*. Enteric fever from *S. typhi* is more prolonged and has a higher mortality rate than paratyphoid fever. Symptoms include sustained fever, diarrhea, abdominal pain, and may involve fatal liver, spleen, respiratory, and neurological damage. Typhoid fever symptoms persist for two to three weeks. Enteric fevers from other than *S. typhi* have a shorter incubation period, 1 to 10 days, compared to 7 to 14 days for typhoid fever, and the symptoms are less severe. *Salmonella* septicemia is characterized by chills, high remittent fever, anorexia, and bacteremia. Organisms may localize in any organ of the body and produce focal lesions resulting in meningitis, endocarditis, pneumonia, or osteomyelitis.

RESERVOIRS FOR THE AGENT

Reservoirs of *Salmonella* are domestic and wild animals, including poultry, swine, cattle, birds, rodents, and pets such as tortoises, turtles, chicks, dogs, and cats. Humans also serve as a reservoir, e.g., convalescent carriers and those with asymptomatic infections. The occurrence of chronic carriers is rare in humans, but is common in birds and animals.

MODE OF TRANSMISSION

Infection from *Salmonella* occurs through ingestion of food, milk, or water contaminated with feces from infected hosts or by ingestion of the infected meat products. *S. typhi* and *S. paratyphi* only colonize humans, therefore, infection with these organisms indicates exposure to human feces. Most often this involves ingestion of the organisms from food or water contaminated with human excreta. Unlike *S. typhi* and *S. paratyphi*, nontyphoidal *Salmonella* spp. are widely distributed in nature and closely associated with animals. Consumption of contaminated poultry and meat products are the most common sources of transmission. Meat products can become contaminated with fecal matter during slaughter. Improper storage or undercooking allows the organisms to proliferate. *Salmonella* infection is also widespread in rodents. When the bacteria are excreted in the feces, contamination of food and water permits transmission of the infection to humans. Person-to-person, fecal–oral transmission does occur and has been a problem in health care facilities traced to inadequate hand washing.

METHODS FOR DETECTING THE AGENT

Selective enrichment is needed for isolation of salmonellae from samples containing mixed bacterial flora (i.e., feces, food, and environmental). Enrichment increases the ratio of *Salmonella* to other bacterial cells. Three selective enrichment media commonly used are tetrathionate broth, selenite broth, and Rappoport-Vassiliadis (RV) medium. Numerous selective plating media have been used to isolate *Salmonella*. These media are differential and vary from highly selective to low selectivity. Laboratories should include a highly selective medium along with low and or moderately selective media when isolating salmonellae. Salmonellae grow readily on routine selective, differential media forming 2- to 3-mm diameter colonies in 24 to 48 hours. Colonies may be circular with a smooth surface and an even edge, or flat with a uneven surface and serrated edge. The temperature range of growth is from 10 to 43° C, with an optimum temperature of 37° C. Elevated incubation temperatures, including 40, 41.5, and 43° C, help suppress background growth and may improve detection of salmonellae but also suppress growth of some serotypes, including *S. typhi*.

After primary isolation on selective media, presumptive *Salmonella* isolates can be tested with commercial identification systems or screened with triple sugar iron agar, urea broth, and lysine iron agar. Isolates with *Salmonella* biochemical profiles should be tested with commercial polyvalent O group, H, and Vi antisera. With environmental samples, a large sample volume usually should be examined (1 L or more). Concentration of the organisms can be accomplished using Moore Swabs, membrane filtration, diatomaceous earth, or large-volume samplers.

OCCURRENCE OF THE AGENT IN PEOPLE, ANIMALS, AND THE ENVIRONMENT

Salmonellosis represents a major communicable worldwide disease problem. The annual occurrence of typhoid fever is estimated at 17 million cases, with 600,000 deaths. In contrast to typhoid fever, with humans being the sole source of the organism, animals and animal products are major sources of other *Salmonella*. Animal husbandry studies have shown approximately 50 percent of US chickens are culture positive for *Salmonella*. Cold-blooded animals such as turtles are also carriers and sources of infection. Large numbers of *Salmonella* may be present in contaminated surface water and waste treatment plant influents and effluents. Studies have shown that 80 percent of activated sludge effluents and 58 percent of contaminated surface waters may contain *Salmonella*.

SURVIVAL OF THE AGENT IN THE ENVIRONMENT

Bacterial survival in aquatic ecosystems is affected by numerous factors, including protozoa, antibiosis, organic matter, algal toxins, dissolved nutrients, ultraviolet (UV) light, heavy metals, and temperature. Recent studies of survival of enteric pathogens in aquatic environments have shown these organisms may enter a viable but nonculturable physiological state. Because the vast majority of detection and enumeration techniques require culturing using selective media, the detection of viable organisms may be compromised. Salmonellae are frequently isolated in polluted waters and can persist in high-nutrient waters. Wastewater treatment reduces but does not eliminate indicator bacteria and *Salmonella*. Reported *Salmonella* levels range from 1 to 1,100/100 mL from nonchlorinated wastewater effluents. *Salmonella* discharged in the effluents from municipal wastewater treatment plants were reported to survive for an extended time in the nutrient-rich water of the Red River of North Dakota during the sugar beet processing season.

DOCUMENTED WATERBORNE OUTBREAKS

The vast majority of waterborne outbreaks of salmonellosis are classified as acute gastrointestinal illness of unknown etiology. Waterborne outbreaks in the United States usually involve poor-quality source water, inadequate treatment, or contamination of the distribution system (e.g., cross-connections). Large outbreaks of waterborne salmonellosis have not been reported in the United States, with the exception of the Riverside, Calif., *S. typhimurium* gastroenteritis outbreak in 1965, which affected 18,000 people. The water supply was implicated, but the source of contamination was not determined. During 1976 to 1980, 223 cases of waterborne salmonellosis were reported from small water suppliers and private wells. In 1993 a waterborne outbreak of *S. typhimurium* in Gideon, Mo., affected more than 650 persons and resulted in 7 deaths. Contamination was traced to a water storage tower with defective roof vent covers that allowed free access by birds.

EFFECTIVENESS OF WATER TREATMENT PROCESSES

Disinfection is an important barrier in prevention of human exposure to pathogens in drinking water. Chlorination is effective for inactivating *Salmonella* in properly maintained distribution systems using conventional treatment (coagulation, sedimentation, filtration, and disinfection). Chlorine residuals need to be at least 0.2 mg/L at the distal ends of the distribution system. Early studies have shown that *S. typhi* is as susceptible to chlorine disinfection as *Escherichia coli*.

NATIONAL OR INTERNATIONAL GUIDELINES AND MONITORING RECOMMENDATIONS

There are no permissible levels of *Salmonella* in drinking water. Because many waterborne pathogens are difficult to detect or enumerate in water and the methods are often impractical to use for routine monitoring, the US Environmental Protection Agency (USEPA) and World Health Organization have adopted total coliform, fecal coliform, and *Escherichia coli* microbiological standards for drinking water. These organisms are used as indicators of water treatment efficacy, distribution system integrity, and recent fecal contamination. The coliform group of organisms are present in the normal intestinal flora of humans and warm-blooded animals and are eliminated in large numbers in fecal wastes. The presence of fecal coliform or *E. coli* in a drinking water supply usually is interpreted as evidence of the presence of enteric bacterial pathogens. Implicitly, routine coliform monitoring is to provide an alert against treatment barrier failure.

INFORMATION SOURCES

Angulo, F.J., et al. 1997. A Community Waterborne Outbreak of Salmonellosis and the Effectiveness of a Boil Water Order. *Amer. J. Public Health*, 87(4):580–584.

Craun, G.F. 1986. Statistics of Waterborne Outbreaks in the U.S. In *Waterborne Diseases in the United States*. Boca Raton, Fla.: CRC Press.

Craun, G.F., P.S. Berger, and R.L. Calderon. 1997. Coliform Bacteria and Waterborne Disease Outbreaks. *Jour. AWWA*, 89(3):99–104.

Geldreich, E.E. 1996a. Waterborne Pathogen Invasions: A Case for Water Quality Protection in Distribution. In *Microbial Quality of Water Supply in Distribution Systems*. Boca Raton, Fla.: CRC Press.

———. 1996b. Pathogenic Agents in Freshwater Resources. *Hydrological Processes*, 10:315–333.

Gray, L.D. 1995. *Escherichia*, *Salmonella*, *Shigella*, and *Yersinia*. In *Manual of Clinical Microbiology*, 6th ed. pp. 450–456. Murray, P.R., E.J. Baron, M.A. Pfaller, F.C. Tenover, and R.H. Yolken, eds. Washington, D.C.: ASM Press.

Miller, S.I., E.L. Hohmann, and D.A. Pegues. 1995. *Salmonella* (Including *Salmonella typhi*). In *Principles and Practice of Infectious Diseases*, 4th ed. pp. 2013–2032. Mandell, G.L., J.E. Bennett, and R. Dolin, eds. New York: Churchill Livingstone Inc.

Ross, E.C., K.W. Campbell, and H.J. Ongerth. 1966. *Salmonella typhimurium* Contamination of Riverside, Calif., Supply. *Jour. AWWA*, 58(2):165–174.

Smith, J.J., J.P. Howington, and G.A. McFeters. 1994. Survival, Physiological Response, and Recovery of Enteric Bacteria Exposed to a Polar Marine Environment. *Appl. Environ. Microbiol.*, 60:2868–2875.

Chapter 16

Serratia

Edwin E. Geldreich

DESCRIPTION OF THE AGENT

The *Serratia* genus is composed of small, gram-negative, motile, coccobacilli that characteristically give positive reactions for citrate, motility, Voges-Proskauer, ONPG (see glossary), and fermentation of mannitol and trehalose. Lactose is fermented slowly or not at all. *Serratia marcescens* is the type species and produces a nondiffusible red pigment that is more pronounced when incubated at temperatures between 25 and 30°C. Most pathogenic *Serratia* strains isolated in clinical laboratories are nonpigmented. Other strains are plant pathogens found in the environment.

DESCRIPTION OF THE DISEASE

S. marcescens, *S. odorifera*, *S. rubidaea*, and the sub-group *S. liquefaciens* are recognized as potential opportunistic pathogens that may spread in epidemic proportions causing nosocomial infections in hospital patients. *S. marcescens* is a frequent cause of infections ranging from cystitis to life-threatening bloodstream and central nervous system infections. In one case, *Serratia* was isolated from the feces of a two-month-old infant who had developed diarrhea. The antibody titer to this organism in the feces increased eight-fold while the antibody titers against five "O" groups of *Escherichia coli* remained unchanged, indicating *Serratia* was the causative agent. Because many hospitals harbor multiple antibiotic-resistant strains of *S. marcescens*, resistance may be transferred to various pathogens in the clinical environment.

RESERVOIRS FOR THE AGENT

Serratia strains are considered to be ubiquitous in the environment. They may be found in surface and groundwater, soil, decaying vegetation, insects, decaying meat, and spoiled milk.

MODE OF TRANSMISSION

Serratia strains are spread by person-to-person contact and by contaminated water from sumps in hospital equipment. *S. marcescens* infections have been transmitted via medical solutions and peritoneal-dialysis effluents. Two studies on the contribution of water-supply-associated bacteria and patient or consumer illness suggest that water-supply-derived organisms are part of the problem, but not necessarily the major source of nosocomial infections in the hospital environment or in the drinking water at the home tap.

METHODS FOR DETECTING THE AGENT

Heterotrophic plate count (HPC) media will often reveal the presence of *Serratia* in water samples when incubated on a nondifferential medium (i.e., R2A medium) in the range of 20 to 30° C using either the membrane filtration (MF) procedure or a spread plate technique. There are no differential media specifically for detecting *Serratia*.

OCCURRENCE OF THE AGENT IN PEOPLE, ANIMALS, AND THE ENVIRONMENT

Serratia and other pigmented bacteria appear to occur seasonally in high-quality waters (such as private wells, distribution systems, finished reservoir supplies, and bottled water). Colonization may occur in a variety of attachment devices, including drinking water fountains, ice machines, point-of-use treated water, laboratory high-quality water systems, humidifying units, and hemodialysis equipment. *Serratia* have also been found in the heterotrophic bacterial population on media substrate in granular activated carbon (GAC) filters. Densities in water are variable, most often being less than 100 organisms/mL unless predominate colonization occurs in a biofilm.

SURVIVAL OF THE AGENT IN THE ENVIRONMENT

Decaying vegetation is often a niche for the survival of *Serratia* in the watershed. Cannibalism of *Serratia* cells may continue for months, with rises and falls of the population. Persistence in tap water is about 100 days, and much longer in contaminated well water. In distilled water, *Serratia* may survive for 48 days at room temperature.

DOCUMENTED WATERBORNE OUTBREAKS

While over 50 hospital outbreaks of infection have been due to *S. marcescens*, no waterborne outbreaks have been documented in the literature.

EFFECTIVENESS OF WATER TREATMENT PROCESSES

Serratia frequently can be isolated from treated water because these organisms are more chlorine-resistant than many nonpigmented aerobic, heterotrophic bacteria. They may also enter the distribution system via soil contamination during line breaks and their repairs. Since this organism passes through conventional treatment barriers, control is best achieved by reducing sediment accumulations in pipe networks and water storage reservoirs. Removing scum around process basins will suppress habitat sites for *Serratia* and many other organisms.

NATIONAL OR INTERNATIONAL GUIDELINES AND MONITORING RECOMMENDATIONS

No national or international guidelines limit the occurrence of *Serratia* in water supply.

INFORMATION SOURCES

Clancy, C.F. 1989. Enterobacteriaceae. In *Practical Handbook of Microbiology.* pp. 71–90. O'Leary, W., ed. Boca Raton, Fla.: CRC Press.

Farmer III, J.J., and D.J. Brenner. 1977. Concept of a Bacterial Species: Importance to Writers of Microbiological Standards for Water. In *Bacterial Indicators/Health Hazards Associated with Water.* pp. 37–47. Hoadley, A.W., and B.J. Dutka, eds. Philadelphia, Pa.: American Society for Testing and Materials.

Kelly, M.T., D.J. Brenner, and J.J. Farmer, III. 1985. Enterobacteriaceae. In *Manual of Clinical Microbiology,* 4th ed. pp. 263–277. Lennette, E.H., A. Balows, W.J. Hausler, Jr., and H.J. Shadomy, eds. Washington, D.C.: ASM Press.

This page intentionally blank.

Chapter 17

Shigella

Nelson P. Moyer

DESCRIPTION OF THE AGENT

The genus *Shigella* of the family Enterobacteriaceae consists of the four species (serogroups) *S. dysenteriae* (serogroup A), *S. flexneri* (serogroup B), *S. boydii* (serogroup C), and *S. sonnei* (serogroup D). Serogroups A, B, and C are subdivided into 12, 13, and 18 serotypes, respectively.

Shigella species have been taxonomically related to *Escherichia coli* by DNA–DNA hybridization studies. *Shigella*e are facultatively anaerobic, chemoorganotrophic, nonsporulating, nonmotile, oxidase negative, gram-negative rods, 0.3 to 1 µm in diameter and 1 to 6 µm in length, appearing singly, in pairs, and in short chains. The optimum temperature for growth is 37°C. When grown on blood agar, colonies are translucent, circular, convex, and measure 1 to 2 mm in diameter.

DESCRIPTION OF THE DISEASE

Shigella species cause acute gastroenteritis and dysentery in humans by invading the intestinal mucosa. Shigellosis is characterized by diarrhea, fever, nausea, vomiting, and cramps. Illness ranges from mild, self-limiting diarrhea to toxic megacolon and hemolytic uremic syndrome. Most cases in the United States are caused by *S. sonnei*. The incubation period for shigellosis is usually one to three days. While mild cases of shigellosis are self-limiting, antibiotic treatment is necessary in severe cases. Antimicrobial susceptibility tests must be performed before therapy, because multiple drug-resistant strains are becoming prevalent in the United States. Organisms are detectable in stool for up to one week after symptoms resolve. Immunity from natural infection is short-lived and no effective vaccine is available.

RESERVOIRS FOR THE AGENT

Infected humans are the only significant reservoir.

MODE OF TRANSMISSION

Transmission occurs primarily through direct or indirect fecal–oral contact with patients or carriers. The infective dose is low, between 10 to 100 bacteria. Fecally contaminated water, food, and milk also transmit disease. Flies can transfer bacteria from feces to foods.

METHODS FOR DETECTING THE AGENT

Methods for the reliable recovery of shigellae from the environment are not yet available. Membrane filtration (MF) and centrifugation have been used to concentrate environmental samples, with and without subsequent broth enrichment cultures. GN broth enrichment (see glossary) has been used to recover *Shigella* from stools and other samples where they may be present in low numbers. Recently, polymerase chain reaction (PCR) has shown promise for detection of shigellae in environmental samples. Diagnosis of shigellosis is made by recovery of the shigellae from stool or rectal swabs on differential and selective culture media such as MacConkey agar or xylose lysine deoxycholate (XLD) agar. Clear colonies from MacConkey agar and colorless to pinkish colonies from XLD agar plates are inoculated into triple sugar iron (TSI) and lysine iron agar (LIA) slants that are incubated for 18 hours at 35° C. Presumptive *Shigella* cultures appear as nonmotile, gas negative, hydrogen negative isolates producing alkaline slants and acid butts in TSI and LIA agar. A small amount of growth from the LIA slant is suspended in normal saline and used to conduct slide agglutination tests with homologous antisera for serogroups A, B, C, and D. Serotyping is usually restricted to outbreak investigations. *Shigella* species are biochemically differentiated from *E. coli* by the lysine and motility tests.

OCCURRENCE OF THE AGENT IN PEOPLE, ANIMALS, AND THE ENVIRONMENT

Shigellosis occurs worldwide and is most common in areas where sewage treatment and personal hygiene are poor to nonexistent. Most cases in the United States occur in children, and secondary transmission to household contacts is common. Outbreaks of shigellosis occur in institutional settings, such as day-care centers, mental hospitals, nursing homes, and refugee camps, from contamination of food and water, and by person-to-person contact. Shigellosis is associated with travel to developing countries where sanitation is lacking. Shigellosis outbreaks may also occur in hogans (Native American dwellings) and colonies (Latin America border communities) where flowing water supply is not available.

SURVIVAL OF THE AGENT IN THE ENVIRONMENT

Shigellae do not survive well at acid pH, so buffered transport media at pH 7.4 to 7.6 are required if clinical specimens are not processed immediately after they are collected. Shigellae are sensitive to chlorination at normal levels, and they do not compete favorably with other organisms in the environment. They persist up to four days in river water. Viable but nonculturable forms have been reported in estuarine waters, but the infectivity of nonculturable shigellae is unknown.

DOCUMENTED WATERBORNE OUTBREAKS

Waterborne outbreaks of shigellosis most commonly result from fecal contamination of nonchlorinated private and noncommunity water supplies. Treatment deficiencies, septic tank contamination of wells, or cross-connections between wastewater and potable water lines are most commonly implicated in drinking water outbreaks. The availability of running water in the home is key to reducing the spread of cases through poor personal hygiene habits. Outbreaks are also associated with recreational exposure to fecally contaminated swimming and wading pools, and polluted surface water such as lakes and ponds. Sewage contamination of shellfish beds has caused outbreaks of foodborne disease associated with oysters. Shigellae caused 17 of 21 (81 percent) of drinking water associated outbreaks, and 12 of 71 (17 percent) of recreational water associated outbreaks reported to the Centers for Disease Control and Prevention (CDC) between 1985 and 1994. Sixteen states reported waterborne shigellosis outbreaks during this 10-year period. Drinking water outbreaks occur year around, while recreational water outbreaks typically occur in summer months between May and September. *S. sonnei* was implicated in 11 of 12 drinking water outbreaks, and 16 of 17 recreational water outbreaks. One outbreak each in drinking and recreational water was caused by *S. flexneri*, and *S. boydii* was recovered from victims of one of the recreational water outbreaks (Mississippi River near Dubuque, Iowa) caused by *S. sonnei*.

EFFECTIVENESS OF WATER TREATMENT PROCESSES

Isolation of cases, stool precautions, hand washing, and proper diaper and sewage disposal are the primary control mechanisms for prevention of shigellosis. Water and wastewater treatment processes incorporating disinfection are sufficient for inactivation of shigellae.

NATIONAL OR INTERNATIONAL GUIDELINES AND MONITORING RECOMMENDATIONS

Shigella species are enteric pathogens of humans, and should be absent from the environment. No occurrence of this pathogenic agent in food or water is considered safe.

INFORMATION SOURCES

Centers for Disease Control and Prevention. 1996. Surveillance for Waterborne Disease Outbreaks—United States, 1993–1994. *MMWR*, 45(SS-1):1–33.

Watanabe, H., and N. Okamura. 1992. The Genus *Shigella*. In *The Prokaryotes*, 2nd ed., Vol. 3. pp. 2754–2759. Balows, A., H.G. Trüper, M. Dwarkin, W. Harder, and K.H. Schleifer, eds. New York: Springer-Verlag.

This page intentionally blank.

Chapter 18

Staphylococcus

Edwin E. Geldreich

DESCRIPTION OF THE AGENT

Staphylococci are gram-positive cocci that may occur as single cells, in pairs, packet clusters, or as short chains of several individual cells. Species in this genus are usually nonmotile, catalase positive, and ferment glucose. Some strains encapsulate or form a slime layer. While most species are facultative anaerobes, some strains of *Staphylococcus aureus* grow more favorably in aerobic environments. All strains of this species are potential pathogens. *S. aureus* strains are coagulase positive and often form a yellow to orange pigmentation on some media after two to three days of incubation, although certain antibiotic resistant strains may vary in the intensity of color development. Of the coagulase negative species, *S. epidermis* and *S. saprophyticus* have been associated with human infections.

DESCRIPTION OF THE DISEASE

S. aureus, *S. epidermis*, and *S. saprophyticus* may be the opportunistic pathogens associated with infections of the skin (cellulitis, pustules, boils, carbuncles, and impetigo), bacteremia, peritonitis associated with dialysis, genitourinary infections, and postoperative wound infections. *S. aureus* may also cause meningitis, osteomyelitis, and violent diarrhea and vomiting from ingestion of the enterotoxin caused by the organism growing in food. *S. aureus* concentrations in drinking water can be a health concern for individuals in contact with water for extended periods, such as from dishwashing, whirlpool therapy, and dental hygiene. Densities of 200 to 400 cocci per mL have been shown to set up a carrier state in the nose of 50 percent of newborn infants, and an *S. aureus* density of a few hundred cells per mL in a water contact may induce infection in traumatized skin.

RESERVOIRS FOR THE AGENT

Major reservoirs of staphylococci include warm-blooded animals (in the skin, nose, ear, and mucous membranes), sewage, and stormwater runoff. *S. aureus* and other species of this genus are a major component of the normal human flora of the skin and to a lesser extent in fecal wastes.

MODE OF TRANSMISSION

The major concern with *S. aureus* in water transmission is contact with cuts and scratches on the skin, infecting the ears or the eyes during bathing, or in water used to prepare uncooked foods. Ingestion is the pathway for gastrointestinal infections from contaminated foods, or for individuals on intensive antibiotic therapy.

METHODS FOR DETECTING THE AGENT

Pigmented *Staphylococcus* colonies can be seen on heterotrophic plate count (HPC) cultures done on samples taken from the water distribution system. A better characterization of the extent of these organisms in drinking water will require the use of more selective media and procedures such as described in *Standard Methods for the Examination of Water and Wastewater.* The recovery of *S. aureus*, *S. epidermis*, and *S. saprophiticus* should be emphasized rather than total staphylococci in the heterotrophic bacteria population. Unfortunately, no specific media are available for these three opportunistic pathogens. Some success has been reported for the use of M-staphylococcus broth in a modified multiple-tube procedure or Baird-Parker agar in the membrane filter (MF) procedure. Presumptive results are verified by placing pure cultures from the MF into a commercial multi-test system for biochemical reactions. Any turbid tubes in the multiple-tube test are confirmed in Lipovitellin-salt-mannitol agar streak plates.

OCCURRENCE OF THE AGENT IN PEOPLE, ANIMALS, AND THE ENVIRONMENT

The density of coagulase-positive *Staphylococcus* (i.e., *S. aureus*) ranges from 10^2 to 10^4 per gram in the normal human fecal flora, but occurrence is quite variable (10 to 93 percent). Coagulase-negative strains of *Staphylococcus* may be found in 31 to 59 percent of feces from healthy people. Because of their presence in feces and on human skin, staphylococci are not surprisingly the most numerous bacteria shed by swimmers in natural bathing waters and chlorinated swimming pools. In one study, approximately two thirds of the staphylococci in bathing waters were *S. aureus*. Densities of *S. aureus* in both studies ranged from a few to several hundred cells per 100 mL. *S. aureus* was found to be one of the two most concentrated opportunistic pathogens in urban stormwater, ranging from 10 to 1,000 organisms per mL. In a study of private water supplies in Oregon, *S. aureus* was isolated from over 6 percent of 320 rural water supplies. Inspection of HPC data on these samples suggested a 63 percent *S. aureus* occurrence for HPC above 300 organisms per mL. Colonization sites of these and other opportunistic pathogens in public and private water supplies are most often aerator screens on faucets. In public and private water systems, persistence or growth may be localized in slow-flow pipe sections and dead ends where sediments accumulate.

SURVIVAL OF THE AGENT IN THE ENVIRONMENT

In drinking water, *Staphylococcus* may persist at 20° C for 20 to 30 days, provided trace amounts of organic nutrients are available. Growth in water is slow at temperatures below 20° C, and merely at subsistence rate below 10° C.

DOCUMENTED WATERBORNE OUTBREAKS

S. aureus and several other staphylococci species are opportunistic pathogens in the hospital environment and water supply may play a subordinate role in disease transmission. However, no waterborne outbreaks caused by staphylococci, or *S. aureus* in particular, have been documented. The health risk of staphylococci associated with exposure to poor-quality small water systems and private water supplies is undocumented.

EFFECTIVENESS OF WATER TREATMENT PROCESSES

Numerous reports suggest the staphylococci are more resistant to ultraviolet light (UV) radiation at ambient temperature than *Salmonella* and *Escherichia coli*, and require 45 minutes or more contact time. Filtration of surface waters may entrap significant numbers of these heterotrophic bacteria but some will pass through water treatment barriers. Systematic flushing of distribution systems to reduce the nutrient source for these and other opportunistic bacteria is important. Hospital maintenance crews must periodically flush the building water supply lines and clean all water supply attachment devices on a scheduled basis to suppress colonization of staphylococci and other opportunistic bacteria.

NATIONAL OR INTERNATIONAL GUIDELINES AND MONITORING RECOMMENDATIONS

No national or international guidelines limit this opportunistic pathogen in water supply.

INFORMATION SOURCES

American Public Health Association, American Water Works Association, and Water Environment Federation. 1995. *Standard Methods for the Examination of Water and Wastewater.* Eaton, A.D., L.S. Clesceri, and A.E. Greenberg, eds. Washington, D.C.: American Public Health Association.

Evans, J.B. 1977. Coagulase Positive Staphylococci as Indicators of Potential Health Hazards from Water. In *Bacterial Indicators/Health Hazards Associated with Water.* pp. 126–130. Hoadley, A.W., and B.J. Dutka, eds. ASTM STP 635. Philadelphia, Pa.: American Society for Testing and Materials.

Geldreich, E.E. 1996. *Microbial Quality of Water Supply in Distribution Systems.* Boca Raton, Fla.: CRC Press.

Kloos, W.E., and J.H. Jorgensen. 1985. *Staphylococci.* In *Manual of Clinical Microbiology.* 4th ed. pp. 143–153. Lennette, E.H., A. Balows, W.J. Hausler, Jr., and H.J. Shadomy, eds. Washington, D.C.: ASM Press.

This page intentionally blank.

Chapter 19

Vibrio cholerae

Gary A. Toranzos and Alan Toro

DESCRIPTION OF THE AGENT

The recent Latin American cholera outbreak has reawakened interest in this disease as well as the need for water utilities and public health workers to become familiar with the ecology and the isolation techniques for the characterization of the etiological agent *Vibrio cholerae* in water.

V. cholerae is divided into two major serogroups, the 01 and the non-01. Furthermore, the 01 group is divided into El Tor and classical biotypes. The 01 strains have been further divided into three serotypes: the *Inaba*, *Ogawa*, and *Hikojima*. The three serotypes seem to be variants of the same strain as a result of genetic switching. Serotype conversion has been shown to take place both *in vivo* and *in vitro*. It is important to note that the first six pandemics seem to have been caused by the classical biotype, whereas the seventh pandemic was caused by the El Tor biotype. El Tor has some intrinsic differences from the classical biotype. It seems to be sturdier and may be more prone to transportation by patients who have a mild or asymptomatic infection, as it is known to be excreted for longer periods of time by infected individuals.

Over 130 serogroups of *V. cholerae* have been reported. However, until 1992 only the toxigenic 01 serogroup had been associated with cholera epidemics and pandemics. The non-01 serogroup was mainly associated with extraintestinal infections and limited outbreaks of gastroenteritis. A newly described non-01 serogroup, the 0139 (Bengal), recently caused outbreaks of cholera in India and Bangladesh. The 0139 serogroup has been isolated from only certain areas of the world, such as Bangladesh, India, Thailand, Malaysia, Pakistan, and Nepal. Thus, *V. cholerae* non-01 isolates from patients affected by cholera-like symptoms should be tested against 0139 antiserum in those areas. The same would apply to isolates from patients known to have been in these areas in the recent past. Areas of the world not known to be affected by 0139 should not necessarily be alarmed by the isolation of *V. cholerae* non-01 from the environment.

DESCRIPTION OF THE DISEASE

V. cholerae causes infections ranging from asymptomatic to very serious profuse watery diarrhea known as "rice water stools," and vomiting, which lead to rapid and severe dehydration and possibly death within one to five days. Under extreme circumstances, death may occur within 2 to 24 hours. Under these conditions, rehydration therapy is absolutely necessary. Death occurs as a result of loss of fluids and electrolyte imbalance, thus intravenous as well as oral rehydration therapy must be administered. There is a genetic predisposition towards a more serious cholera infection in those individuals belonging to the blood group O, than in individuals belonging to other blood groups. This phenomenon was demonstrated by the severity of the disease during the cholera epidemic in Latin America, where the type O is the predominant blood group.

RESERVOIRS FOR THE AGENT

V. cholerae has been shown to survive for extended periods of time in environmental waters, and tropical fresh waters may also serve as reservoirs if contaminated with the feces of infected individuals. Ship ballast water has been implicated in the dissemination of *Vibrio* spp. around the world.

In nature, *V. cholerae* may be found in association with zooplankton, sediments, and shellfish. Shellfish grown and harvested in fecal polluted waters may act as reservoirs. As a result of the long survival rates of *V. cholerae*, it is possible to assume that the microorganism has the ability to become part of the aquatic microbiota and to become endemic in certain areas of the world. This has been demonstrated in the United States and Australia, where toxigenic 01 strains were shown to survive in aquatic environments for years in the total absence of fecal contamination; thus, these environments may serve as reservoirs. The most important reservoir may still be asymptomatic human carriers and diseased people who shed the microorganisms in their feces.

In the United States, studies have shown that Gulf Coast marshes may be the environmental reservoir for *V. cholerae* 01.

MODE OF TRANSMISSION

Contaminated food seems to be the most prevalent mode of transmission for *V. cholerae*. Nonetheless, the importance of water as a direct or an indirect vehicle cannot be underestimated. This is because contaminated water used to wash foodstuffs can serve as the starting point of an epidemic, as the microorganisms will grow better in cooked foods than in raw foods as a result of other microorganisms which may be killed during cooking. Such was the case in an oil rig off the coast of Texas where contaminated water apparently used to wash cooked rice led to an outbreak.

Most other cases of cholera in the United States have been associated with the consumption of raw shellfish and partially cooked seafood, especially oysters. No person-to-person transmission has been documented, possibly as a result of the high infectious dose of *V. cholerae*. However, contaminated hands, if not washed, may contaminate food, and the microorganism may grow to sufficient concentrations (e.g., in low-acid foods, as was the case of rice in the oil rig example) for infection to occur.

Polluted drinking water as a vector for *V. cholerae* is a problem in areas of the world that do not practice drinking water disinfection, or where treated water is susceptible to posttreatment contamination. For this reason, the monitoring of residual disinfectant in the distribution system is important. Water stored in tanks that allow the insertion of hands is also a risk, since the hands will contaminate the water.

METHODS FOR DETECTING THE AGENT

The most commonly used medium for the isolation of *V. cholerae* is a nonselective medium, alkaline peptone water (APW) at a pH value of 8.4. APW is only partially inhibitory, because the pH goes acidic rather rapidly as microorganisms grow in this medium. For this reason modifications were made to this medium to make it more selective for *Vibrio* spp. by adding NaCl at 1 or 3 percent, plus 0.05M Tris buffer (pH 8.4). These modifications were shown to be sufficiently selective to inhibit the interfering microbiota and to make the isolation of *Vibrio* spp. easier. Results have actually shown that these modifications allow for a more efficacious isolation of *V. cholerae* from untreated sewage.

It is very unlikely that *V. cholerae* would be present in large concentrations in environmental waters, thus the first step in the detection of this pathogen is the concentration of at least a 1-L volume, which can be accomplished by membrane filtration (MF) in the case of low-turbidity waters. In the case of high-turbidity waters, a gauze pad (Moore swab) is placed in the stream and left for approximately 48 hours. The filter or gauze pad is then placed into APW and incubated at 35° C. After 6, 15, and 18 hours, aliquots are obtained from the upper portion of the APW and streaked onto thiosulfate-citrate-bile salts-sucrose agar (TCBS). Typical *V. cholerae* shows up as yellow colonies as a result of the sucrose fermentation in this selective medium. However, caution should be exercised, because not all yellow colonies indicate the presence of *V. cholerae*. In fact, it is possible that most of the yellow colonies belong to other bacterial genera. Any yellow colony should be tested either with *V. cholerae* polyvalent sera or subjected to further biochemical testing before drawing conclusions as to the presence of this microorganism.

Although the culturing methods are still the most widely used, research is being carried out to develop molecular techniques for the detection of toxigenic strains of *V. cholerae*. However, at the present time, the molecular techniques are being used more as a strain characterization tool, rather than as a detection tool. The use of molecular techniques is still rather new for the detection of pathogens in the environment, thus, specially trained personnel are necessary to carry out the latter procedures. Several reports on the use of the polymerase chain reaction (PCR) for the characterization of *V. cholerae* isolates have proven to be very efficient in the determination of toxigenicity. It is advised that if molecular techniques such as the PCR are going to be used, they should only be used for the detection of *V. cholerae* after preenrichment growth in media such as those described above. The direct detection of *V. cholerae* from the environment has so far eluded investigators, possibly as a result of the presence of compounds present in environmental samples that may inhibit detection by molecular methods.

OCCURRENCE OF THE AGENT IN PEOPLE, ANIMALS, AND THE ENVIRONMENT

Most data on the occurrence of *V. cholerae* in the environment have been presented in terms of its presence–absence, since most data were obtained using either the Moore swab or MF followed by identification of a few typical colonies. Neither technique will allow for enumeration of the microorganisms. It is known that acutely ill patients afflicted with cholera excrete about 10^5 to 10^9 vibrios per mL of stool, thus large numbers of this microorganism will be excreted to the environment. However, it is very likely that many of these microorganisms cannot withstand negative environmental conditions, such as low pH, thus, only low concentrations of *V. cholerae* are likely to remain in the environment. Concentrations ranging from 10^2 to 10^5 *V. cholerae* cells/mL raw sewage were observed in Peru. However, concentrations of up to 5×10^5 and 5×10^7 *V. cholerae*/mL raw sewage were observed in a hospital treating several cholera-afflicted patients.

SURVIVAL OF THE AGENT IN THE ENVIRONMENT

As previously mentioned, these microorganisms can survive for long periods of time under certain environmental conditions. Low pH will rapidly inactivate the microorganisms, however, neutral to alkaline pH will protect *V. cholerae*. High humidity will protect the microorganisms against inactivation. For example, *V. cholerae* seeded into dry soils were inactivated more rapidly than when the microorganisms were seeded into soils kept moist by the addition of sewage, as would be the case of sewage irrigation.

In aquatic environments, *V. cholerae* is rapidly inactivated in fresh waters. These microorganisms seem to have a requirement for Na^+, thus they will survive better in saline waters than in fresh waters. Studies have shown that 90 percent of seeded microorganisms are inactivated after 18 hours in fresh, unsterile surface waters, whereas it takes up to 95 hours to inactivate the same percentage in unsterile seawater.

Low-acid foods seem to be a propitious medium for the survival of *V. cholerae*. In fact, foods contaminated after cooking (such as cooked rice, mentioned previously) have been shown to be the source of several outbreaks.

DOCUMENTED WATERBORNE OUTBREAKS

Cholera is typically a disease spread by poor sanitation. High population densities also add to the danger of disease outbreaks. Waterborne outbreaks of cholera have been documented, and probably water was involved in all the large epidemics that have occurred in the last century. Unfortunately, in most epidemics it is difficult, if not impossible, to determine if water or food is primarily responsible for the outbreak. In Portugal, contaminated bottled spring water was responsible for over 2,000 cases of cholera. The same plant also bottled carbonated water, which was not documented to have been involved in the outbreak. This is because *V. cholerae* is not stable at low pH values, such as that of carbonated water. The outbreak also points to the fact that as bottled water becomes more widely used, there may be a higher risk of cholera and other diseases, unless there are strict microbiological controls at the bottling plants. The occurrence of an outbreak linked to commercially bottled water in a US territory also underlines the importance of maintaining proper microbiological controls in bottled water.

Several other waterborne cholera outbreaks have occurred, but in every case, either untreated or nondisinfected water was the vehicle. This points to the importance of maintaining residual disinfectant in the potable water distribution network—untreated or poorly treated municipal water may result in large outbreaks.

In areas of the world where outbreaks have occurred, it is likely that environmental reservoirs of *V. cholerae* exist. In industrialized regions of the world, there is little chance of waterborne cholera infections. This is due to such safeguards as collection of sewage, sewage treatment, natural self-purification of streams, protected aquifers, water supply treatment, and protected water supply in the distribution system. However, even in developed countries, rural areas may be susceptible to cholera if the drinking waters are not properly disinfected. Special attention should be paid to untreated groundwaters. The importance of the presence of residual chlorine in the drinking water cannot be overemphasized. An already well-known episode took place during the last outbreak of cholera in Latin America. Chlorination was stopped in some areas because of the fear of formation of disinfection by-products, which are thought to be carcinogenic. The fact that water disinfection was stopped may have made the outbreak even more serious than it should have been.

In Africa, waterborne outbreaks have been traced to the consumption of untreated well or surface water. Contamination of water kept in containers has also been described as the source of several waterborne outbreaks. Similarly, during the Latin American outbreak, water played an important role in the transmission of the disease. Field investigations demonstrated that the consumption of either unboiled municipal water or water that had been stored in containers in which hands had been introduced, was responsible for the transmission of *V. cholerae* 01.

EFFECTIVENESS OF WATER TREATMENT PROCESSES

As previously mentioned, virtually all waterborne outbreaks of cholera have been caused by untreated or improperly treated waters. Chlorine disinfection, such as the one used during conventional drinking water treatment, is extremely effective, as are other types of disinfection. However, posttreatment contamination is still very dangerous. If the population has access to chlorinated waters, and there is a boil water order issued, the heat actually will drive off residual chlorine from the water and contamination by inserting contaminated hands into water vessels is still possible.

Although *V. cholerae* is very sensitive to low levels of chlorine, certain strains have been found to be more resistant. Certain isolated strains with a "rugose" colony morphology seem to be more resilient to chlorine disinfection. Data are still scant on this last point and more research needs to be done on the prevalence of these strains of *V. cholerae*.

Sewage treatment is effective in eliminating *V. cholerae*. Although chlorination of wastewater effluents is helpful, *V. cholerae* has not been shown to survive for long periods of time under the conditions of treated effluents, thus, proper treatment of the wastes is more important than disinfection.

NATIONAL OR INTERNATIONAL GUIDELINES AND MONITORING RECOMMENDATIONS

Cholera is an internationally reportable disease. According to the International Health Regulations, every member country has to notify the World Health Organization immediately of any cases of the disease. However, this has not always occurred due to fear of border closings and trade restrictions. The latter fear is not completely unfounded, however, and border closings and other such measures have proven to be destructive and not at all beneficial in controlling cholera. Extensive travel, along with the difficulty in spotting asymptomatic individuals, makes control of infection rather ineffective. As far as cholera is concerned, the best control still lies with the proper disposal of sewage and the efficient treatment of drinking water. Countries where cholera is endemic should participate actively in programs such as the World Health Organization's Control of Diarrheal Diseases Program. In any case, monitoring of domestic sewage should be carried out in affected areas by using Moore swabs. Active surveillance of clinical cases should be an ongoing effort and information on cases or probable cases of cholera should be exchanged at the local, national, and international levels.

It is very unlikely that disinfected water supplies will contain *V. cholerae*, thus efforts to monitor drinking water for the presence of this microorganism are not warranted. It would be more useful to monitor the potable water distribution network for the presence of residual chlorine. This will protect the population against outbreaks transmitted by municipal water supplies. However, during emergencies, such as those during an outbreak linked to water, it is absolutely necessary to modify the treatment of existing water sources or to use alternative sources. Disinfection of source water or rechlorination of community supplies during distribution should be established.

INFORMATION SOURCES

American Public Health Association, American Water Works Association, and Water Pollution Control Federation. 1989. *Standard Methods for the Examination of Water and Wastewater.* 17th ed. pp. 9.145–9.147. Washington, D.C.: APHA.

Centers for Disease Control and Prevention/National Center for Infectious Diseases. 1992. Laboratory Methods for the Diagnosis of *Vibrio cholerae*. pp. ix–x. Atlanta, Ga.: CDC.

———. 1996. Surveillance for Waterborne Disease Outbreaks in the United States. 1993–1994. Centers for Disease Control Surveillance Summaries. Vol. 45/No. SS1. Atlanta, Ga.: CDC.

Colwell, R.R., and J. Kaper. 1977. *Vibrio* Species as Bacterial Indicators of Potential Health Hazards Associated with Water. In *Bacterial Indicators/Health Hazards Associated with Water.* Hoadley, A.W., and B.J. Dutka, eds. Tallahassee, Fla.: ASTM Press.

Colwell, R.R., and W.M. Spira. 1992. The Ecology of *Vibrio cholerae*. In *Cholera*. Barua, D., and W.B. Greenough, III, eds. New York: Plenum Medical Book Co.

Craun, G., D. Swerdlow, R. Tauxe, R. Clark, K. Fox, E. Geldreich, D. Reasoner, and E. Rice. 1991. Prevention of Waterborne Cholera in the United States. *Jour. AWWA*, 83:40–45.

DePaola, A., et al. 1992. Isolation of Latin American Epidemic Strain of *Vibrio cholerae* 01 from U.S. Gulf Coast. *Lancet*, 339–624.

Fields, P.I., T. Popovic, I.K. Wachsmuth, and O. Olsvik. 1922. Use of Polymerase Chain Reaction for Detection of Toxigenic *Vibrio cholerae* Strains from the Latin American Cholera Epidemic. *J. Clin. Microbiol.*, 30:2118–2121.

Kaysner, C.A., and W.E. Hill. 199[illegible]. Toxigenic *Vibrio cholerae* 01 in Food and Water. In *Vibrio Cholerae and Cholera. Molecular to Global Perspectives.* Wachsmuth, I.K., P.A. Blake, and O. Olsvik, eds. Washington, D.C.: ASM Press.

Khan, M., W.H. Mosley, J. Chakraborty, A.M. Sarder, and M.R. Khan. 1981. The Relationship of Cholera to Water Source and Use in Rural Bangladesh. *Int. J. Epidemiol.*, 10:23–25

Khan, M.U., and M.D. Shahidullah. 1982. Role of Water and Sanitation in the Incidence of Cholera in Refugee Camps. *Trans. Royal Soc. Trop. Med. Hyg.*, 76:373–377.

Manning, P.A., U.H. Stroeher, and R. Morona. 1994. Molecular Basis for O-antigen Biosynthesis in *Vibrio cholerae* 01: Ogawa-Inaba Switching. In *Vibrio Cholerae and Cholera. Molecular to Global Perspectives.* Wachsmuth, I.K., P. Blake, and O. Olsvik, eds. Washington, D.C.: ASM Press.

McCarthy, S.A., and F.M. Khambaty. 1994. International Dissemination of Epidemic *Vibrio cholerae* by Cargo Ship Ballast and Other Nonpotable Waters. *Appl. Environ. Microbiol.*, 60:2597–2601.

Morris, J.G., and the Cholera Laboratory Task Force. 1994. *Vibrio cholerae* 0139 Bengal. In *Vibrio Cholerae and Cholera. Molecular to Global Perspectives.* Wachsmuth, I.K., P.A. Blake, and O. Olsvik, eds. Washington, D.C.: ASM Press.

Perez-Rosas, N., and T.C. Hazen. 1989. In Situ Survival of *Vibrio cholerae* and *Escherichia coli* in a Tropical Rain Forest Watershed. *Appl. Environ. Microbiol.*, 55:495–499.

Tauxe, R., L. Seminario, R. Tapia, and M. Libel. 1994. The Latin American Epidemic. In *Vibrio Cholerae and Cholera. Molecular to Global Perspectives.* Wachsmuth, I.K., P.A. Blake, and O. Olsvik, eds. Washington, D.C.: ASM Press.

Toro, A., N. González, J. Torres, E. Dvorsky, and G.A. Toranzos. 1995. Modified Culture Methods for the Detection of *Vibrio* spp. from Estuarine Waters. *Wat. Sci. Tech.*, 31:5–6.

Vugia, D.J. 1994. Cholera Surveillance. In *Vibrio Cholerae and Cholera. Molecular to Global Perspectives.* Wachsmuth, I.K., P.A. Blake, and O. Olsvik, eds. Washington, D.C.: ASM Press.

World Health Organization. 1992. *Guidelines for Drinking Water Quality.* 2nd ed., Vol. 1, pp. 142–143. Geneva: World Health Organization.

This page intentionally blank.

Chapter 20

Yersinia

Colin R. Fricker

DESCRIPTION OF THE AGENT

The genus *Yersinia*, family Enterobacteriaceae, was named after the French bacteriologist Yersin. It is composed of at least 11 species at present, the type species of which is *Y. pestis*. However, the taxonomy is confused and further work is required to establish the exact taxonomic position of several members of the genus. As with other members of the Enterobacteriaceae, the yersinias are facultatively anaerobic, gram-negative, non-sporulating, oxidase-negative rods that ferment glucose with production of acid. The cells are 0.5 to 0.8 µm in diameter and 1 to 3 µm in length, in some ways resemble *Pasteurellaceae*, and can be pleomorphic depending on the age of culture and the medium on which it was grown. All species are nonmotile when grown at 37° C, but motile by means of peritrichous flagella when grown below 30° C, except for *Y. pestis* which is never motile. The yersinias will grow on simple media and tolerate bile salts.

DESCRIPTION OF THE DISEASE

The yersinias are responsible for a plethora of diseases in man and animals. In humans the disease may occasionally be present as enteritis or enterocolitis, but more frequent symptoms are a septicemia and generalized disease or more commonly acute inflammation of the mesenteric lymph glands (referred to as pseudoappendicitis). *Y. enterolitica* was first isolated from a human skin ulcer in 1939 and is now recognized as an important cause of gastrointestinal disease in human beings. The spectrum of disease in animals is similar to that encountered with *Y. pseudotuberculosis* and the organism has been associated with abortion in sheep. *Y. enterocolitica* can be responsible for acute septicemias not unlike those caused by *Y. pseudotuberculosis* but is far more commonly associated with gastroenteritis. The disease is usually found in children under the age of seven, tends to occur mainly in autumn and winter, and is characterized by fever, diarrhea, abdominal cramps, and sometimes vomiting. The symptoms often last for about two weeks but the disease is usually self-limiting, although secondary immunological complications occur fairly frequently.

In older children and adults, *Y. enterocolitica* usually causes a terminal ileitis and the pseudoappendicitis syndrome.

RESERVOIRS FOR THE AGENT

While *Y. pestis* and *Y. pseudotuberculosis* are specific pathogens of man and animals, *Y. enterocolitica* and some other species are normally saprophytic and can be found in animal feces where they occur as part of the normal flora and in soil and water. In addition, many foods may be contaminated with *Y. enterocolitica*, pork and unpasteurized milk in particular have been implicated as causes of outbreaks of disease. The yersinias certainly occur as saprophytes in freshwater systems and they have been isolated from slow sand filter beds where they appear to be capable of growth. Essentially, the yersinias can be found where one might expect to encounter coliform organisms.

MODE OF TRANSMISSION

Y. enterocolitica is transmitted by the fecal–oral route and various foodstuffs, milk, and water have been implicated as vehicles of disease. In addition, increasing evidence shows that gastrointestinal disease due to these organisms may be a zoonosis. Sick puppies were implicated as the source of an outbreak in the United States.

METHODS FOR DETECTING THE AGENT

Most yersinias will grow on laboratory culture media designed for the growth of coliform bacteria but cannot easily be differentiated from other coliforms. They ferment carbohydrates with the production of acid (but seldom gas) and are oxidase negative and catalase positive. For example, some strains are positive for ONPG (see glossary) and will grow well in media designed to detect coliforms. Identification of isolates growing in Colilert® from treated water samples in the United Kingdom has shown that the incidence of yersinias in such waters is negligible.

The preferred medium for detecting yersinias from water is by membrane filtration (MF) followed by incubation on CIN agar at 32° C for 24 hours. Typical colonies of *Yersinia* will develop as a dark-red bull's-eye surrounded by a zone of transparency. Some strains of *Yersinia* fail to grow and some coliforms may also give this bull's-eye appearance. Considerable care should be taken in identifying any colonies that form. An alternative approach is to use an enrichment culture. Test portions can first be incubated in a preenrichment medium at pH 8.3 at low temperature, either 15° C for two days or 4° C for seven days, followed by enrichment in bile-oxalate-sorbose broth, which should be incubated at 25° C for three to five days. Methods for the detection of yersinias using polymerase chain reaction (PCR) have also been developed, but these have not been widely used and are of doubtful benefit.

OCCURRENCE OF THE AGENT IN PEOPLE, ANIMALS, AND THE ENVIRONMENT

Yersinia have been isolated from a wide variety of different water sources and no particular seasonal difference is seen in the frequency of their isolation. Furthermore, in the limited number of studies that have looked at other water parameters, such as pH, dissolved oxygen, biochemical oxygen demand (BOD), chemical oxygen demand (COD), and salt concentration, no correlation was seen. Additionally, yersinias were present in the absence of "coliform" organisms, although some strains of *Yersinia* are regarded as coliforms (e.g., UK definition). Yersinias have also been found fairly frequently in chlorinated drinking water supplies, particularly in Europe, where in most cases they were present together with fecal coliforms. From the limited serotyping data available, strains most often found in water are not those commonly associated with human disease.

SURVIVAL OF THE AGENT IN THE ENVIRONMENT

Many strains of *Yersinia* are able to grow at low temperatures (e.g., 4° C) and in laboratory experiments they were shown to survive periods in excess of one year at 4° C. They will also survive and in some cases grow in waters up to 25° C, reaching levels as high as 10^3 colony-forming units (cfu)/mL. Their presence has been demonstrated in a wide variety of water types with different levels of eutrophication and salinity, and in sewage. They are often found in samples of sewage sludge and, although the major pathogenic strains are not frequently encountered, some strains survive for periods greater than one year.

DOCUMENTED WATERBORNE OUTBREAKS

Yersinias are recognized mainly as foodborne pathogens, but may often be found in water. The low occurrence of yersinias in treated (chlorinated) drinking water has meant that disease associated with consumption of fully treated drinking water has not been reported. Apparent outbreaks of yersinia-related disease have occasionally been associated with consumption of untreated water, the largest of which occurred in Montana in 1977. In this outbreak, no clinical evidence of *Yersinia* infection was demonstrated and no yersinias were isolated from patient stools. The tentative diagnosis of *Yersinia* infection was based solely on the finding of various strains of yersinias in water that had been consumed by those affected. The likelihood of detecting small outbreaks of yersinia-related disease is low because most laboratories do not specifically look for yersinias in patient stools. If a low incidence of waterborne yersiniosis occurs, it is likely to be unrecognized. Larger waterborne outbreaks associated with treated water are unlikely since the organisms are mostly removed by water treatment. If water were contaminated after treatment, e.g., by cross-connection, other etiological agents would be far more likely to be recognized than yersinias.

EFFECTIVENESS OF WATER TREATMENT PROCESSES

Yersinias appear to have a similar sensitivity to chlorine as *Escherichia coli*, thus routine chlorination should be adequate for control of the presence of yersinias in treated drinking water and distribution systems. Strain-to-strain variation in chlorine sensitivity has been seen but this has not been shown to present a significant risk. As with other bacteria, there is a relationship between chlorine concentration, water temperature, and rate of inactivation, with higher temperatures resulting in more rapid cell death. Suboptimal chlorine treatment has been shown to yield cells that will grow in liquid media but not on agar substrates. However, the chlorine susceptibility of these organisms suggests that routine water treatment, including an adequate level of chlorination, is likely to prevent the risk of *Yersinia* infection.

NATIONAL OR INTERNATIONAL GUIDELINES AND MONITORING RECOMMENDATIONS

While no regulatory standards have been established specifically for yersinias in the United States or elsewhere, depending on the definition used, some yersinias may be detected as coliforms. Because the procedures for detecting yersinias specifically are so poor, a regulation covering yersinias will not likely be implemented in the foreseeable future.

INFORMATION SOURCES

Christie, A.B. 1990. *Topley and Wilson's Principles of Bacteriology, Virology and Immunity.* Vol. 2. Systematic Bacteriology. Parker, M.T., and L.H. Collier, eds. London: Edward Arnold.

Eden, K.V., M.L. Rosenberg, M. Stoopler, B.T. Wood, A. Highsmith, P. Skaily, J.G. Wells, and J.C. Feeley. 1977. Waterborne Gastrointestinal Illness at a Ski Resort—Isolation of *Yersinia enterocolitica* from Drinking Water. *Public Health Report*, 92:245–250.

Schiemann, D.A. 1990. *Yersinia enterocolitica* in Drinking Water. In *Drinking Water Microbiology.* pp. 322–3[illegible]9. McFeters, G.A., ed. New York: Springer-Verlag.

Introduction to Parasitic Pathogenic Agents

Acanthamoeba spp.	*Gnathostoma spinigerum*
Ascaris lumbricoides	*Isospora belli*
Balantidium coli	Microsporidia
Blastocystis hominis	*Naegleria fowleri*
Cryptosporidium parvum	Schistosomatidae
Cyclospora cayetanensis	*Spirometra mansonoides*
Dracunculus medinensis	*Taenia solium*
Entamoeba histolytica	*Toxoplasma gondii*
Giardia lamblia	*Trichuris trichiura*

Waterborne parasites are acknowledged to be the leading identifiable agents of diseases acquired from drinking water. While bacteria usually have been cited as the major problem since Koch's 1836 observations, waterborne parasitic diseases date back to biblical times, with *Dracunculus medinensis* recorded as the "fiery serpent of Moses." Parasites causing waterborne diseases such as giardiasis and cryptosporidiasis were regarded as normal fauna of the human intestines. *Giardia lamblia* was first observed by von Leewonhoek in 1681 from his stools, using his newly invented microscope, but it was not until the 1960s that *Giardia* was recognized as a significant cause of human disease. *Cryptosporidium parvum* was first described by Tyzzer in 1912, but was not acknowledged as a significant threat to human health until the 1990s.

Worldwide, waterborne parasites have played a major role in shaping history, and they continue to make their mark on human endeavor. For example, flat worms cause resort customers swimmer's itch. In Africa, Asia, and Central and South America, close relatives of organisms responsible for swimmer's itch cause serious human disease. Were it not for *Schistosoma haemotobium*, Napoleon's soldiers may not have languished in the African campaign. Parasites will continue to play a major economic and social role in human life. The water treatment industry must always aspire to mitigate against parasites such as those described in this section, illustrated in Figure III-1, as well as those that will be recognized in the future.

Figure III-1 Parasitic pathogenic agents discussed in section III

Organism	Diagnostic or Infective Stage	Physical Appearance	Occurrence	Treatment and Contact Time
Acanthamoeba spp.	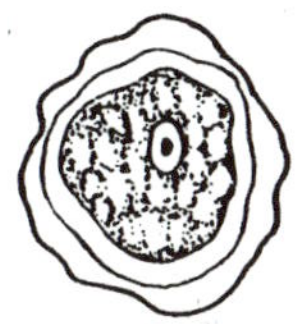	15–20-µm star-shaped, hexagonal, polygonal, or spherical cyst	Ubiquitous; worldwide; Keratitis syndrome per recreational water activities and contact lens wearers	Temperature, pH, biological and biochemical demands influence contact time with chlorine
Ascaris lumbricoides	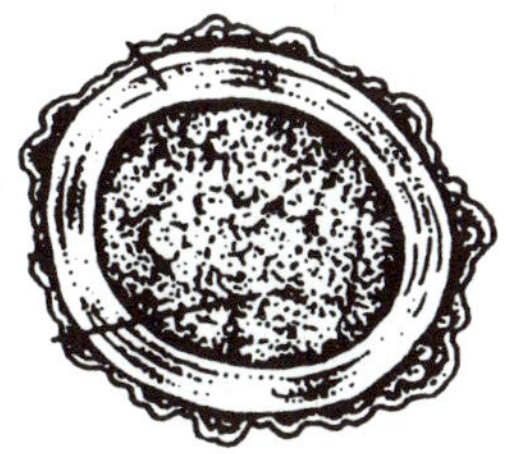	Ellipsoid 35–50 × 50–70-µm fertilized egg with knobby albuminous coat	Worldwide; most common in warm countries and where sanitation is poor	Coagulation and filtration; resistant to chlorine
Balantidium coli	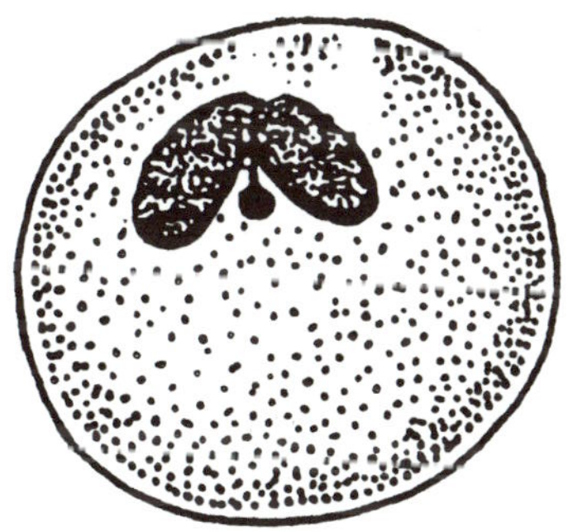	Spherical or oval 50–70-µm cyst. Macronucleus and micronucleus can be obscured. The largest intestinal protozoan of man	Worldwide; incidence of infection in human host is low	Unknown
Blastocystis hominis	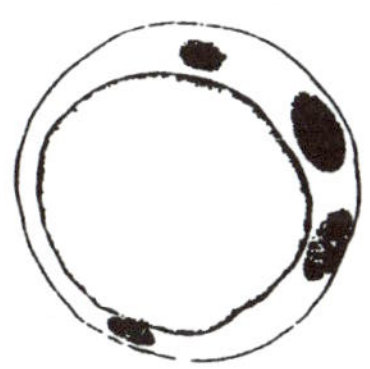	6–40-µm spherical cyst, characterized by a large, central body surrounded by small, multiple nuclei	Worldwide	Unknown

Figure III-1 Parasitic pathogenic agents discussed in section III *(continued)*

Organism	Diagnostic or Infective Stage	Physical Appearance	Occurrence	Treatment and Contact Time
Cryptosporidium parvum	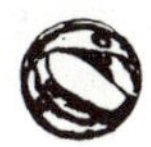	Spherical, thick-walled, 4–6-µm oocyst containing 4 sporozoites	Worldwide	Filtration; resistant to standard chlorine disinfection; some ultraviolet (UV) light and ozone treatments appear promising
Cyclospora cayetanensis	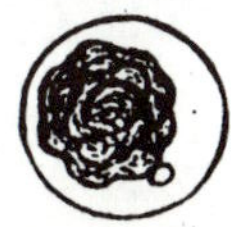	Spherical 8–10-µm oocysts unsporulated and sporulated. The sporulated oocyst is the infectious stage	Worldwide	Filtration; resistant to standard chemical disinfection
Dracunculus medinensis	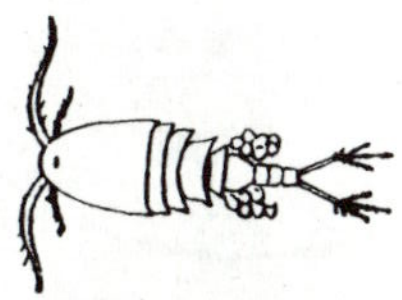	*Cyclops* spp. containing the infective stages	Africa, Middle East, Indian subcontinent	Unknown
Entamoeba histolytica	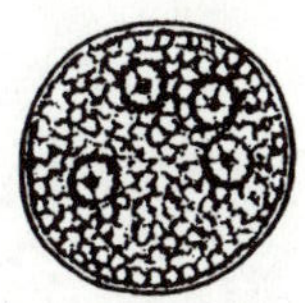	Spheroid 10–20-µm cyst with a refractive hyaline cell wall containing 4 nuclei; may contain chromatoid body	Worldwide	Coagulation and rapid sand filtration or slow sand filtration; resistant to chlorine disinfection
Giardia lamblia	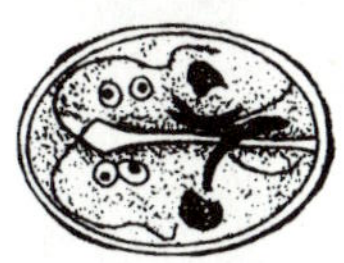	Round to oval 8–18-µm long × 5–16-µm wide cyst containing 2 to 4 nuclei and distinctive axoneme	Worldwide	Multibarrier filtration; free chlorine, chloramine, chlorine dioxide, and ozone are known to inactivate cysts. $C \times T$ (chlorine) required to inactive cysts range from 9 to 342
Gnathostoma spinigerum	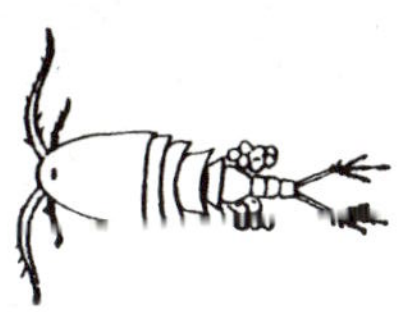	*Cyclops* spp. or other copepods containing the infective stages	Southeast Asia, Japan, Thailand, Ecuador, Argentina, and Mexico	Unknown

Figure III-1 Parasitic pathogenic agents discussed in section III *(continued)*

Organism	Diagnostic or Infective Stage	Physical Appearance	Occurrence	Treatment and Contact Time
Isospora belli	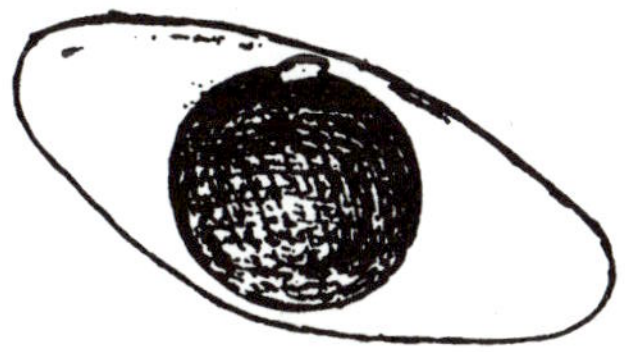	Ellipsoidal unsporulated and sporulated oocyst 20–30-μm long × 10–19-μm wide	Worldwide; tropical regions of the Western Hemisphere	Unknown
Microsporidia *Enterocytozoon bieneusi Encephalitozoon (Septata) intestinalis*		Spore size ranging from 1.5 to 2.5 μm	Ubiquitous; worldwide	Chlorine $C \times T$ near 32 with *in vitro* assay
Naegleria fowleri	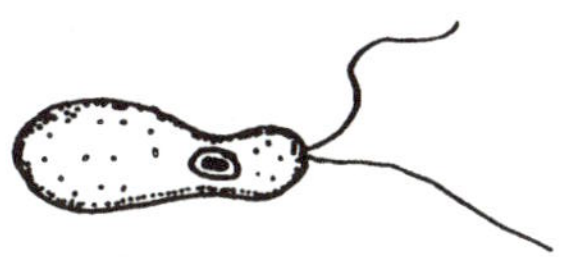	10–35-μm limax-like amoeba trophozoite	Worldwide; associated with aquatic activities	Susceptible to chlorine at 1 mg/L
Family Schistosomatidae	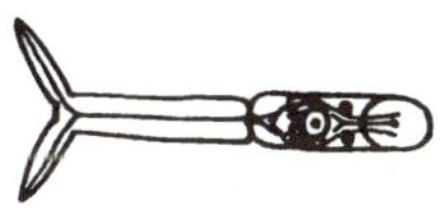	Cercaria breaks out of snails into water	Cosmopolitan; United States, Canada, Europe, Mexico, Central America, Japan, Malaya, and Australia	Molluscicide
Spirometra mansonoides	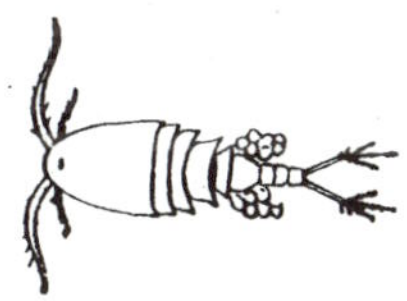	*Cyclops* spp. or other copepods containing the infective stages	Worldwide; frequently in Southeast Asia. Cases have been reported in the southeastern United States	Unknown

Figure III-1 Parasitic pathogenic agents discussed in section III *(continued)*

Organism	Diagnostic or Infective Stage	Physical Appearance	Occurrence	Treatment and Contact Time
Taenia solium	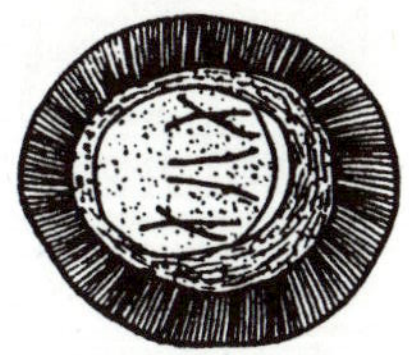	30–40-μm egg indistinguishable from that of *T. saginata*	United States, Mexico, Central and South America	Unknown
Toxoplasma gondii	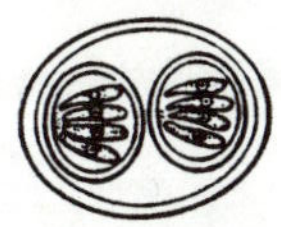	10-μm × 12-μm mature oocysts with 2 sporocysts containing 4 sporozoites each	Worldwide	Resistant to chlorine
Trichuris trichiura	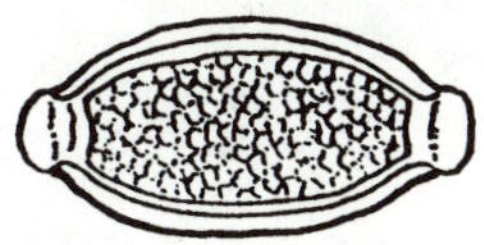	22–25-μm × 50–55-μm ovoid fertilized egg; at each tip is a translucent plug.	Worldwide	Coagulation and filtration; resistant to chlorine

Chapter 21

Acanthamoeba spp.

Govidina S. Visvesvara and Hercules de Moura

DESCRIPTION OF THE AGENT

Small free-living amoebas belonging to the genus *Acanthamoeba* are mitochondria-bearing eukaryotic protozoa that normally live in soil, fresh water, brackish water, and even in sewage and sludge. They feed on bacteria and multiply in their environmental niche as free-living organisms. They cause infections of the human brain, skin, and eye and feed on human tissue. Because of their ability to live as free-living organisms in nature and as pathogens living within their hosts, they are also called *amphizoic amoebas*. Because they cause a fatal disease of the central nervous system (CNS) called *granulomatous amebic encephalitis* (GAE) in humans, especially in immunocompromised patients, they are often referred to as opportunistic pathogens. The genus *Acanthamoeba* consists of as many as 20 species which are placed in three groups based on their morphology. Unlike *Naegleria fowleri*, the only species of *Naegleria* that causes human disease, several species of *Acanthamoeba* (e.g., *A. castellanii*, *A. culbertsoni*, *A. divionensis*, *A. healyi*, *A. rhysodes*, *A. hatchetti*, *A. polyphaga*, etc.) are known to cause infection in humans.

Acanthamoeba has two stages in its life cycle—the trophozoite and the cyst. Acanthamoeba trophozoites measure 15 to 45 µm and are characterized by the presence of fine, tapering, spine-like projections, called *acanthapodia*, from the surface of the body, which are periodically protruded and retracted. The trophozoites usually have one nucleus with a large, dense nucleolus. *Acanthamoeba* divide by conventional mitosis, in which the nucleolus and the nuclear membrane disappear during cell division. Numerous mitochondria, ribosomes, and vacuoles are present within the cytoplasm. *Acanthamoeba* does not have a flagellated stage, but differentiates into a cyst during adverse conditions. The cysts are uninucleate and double-walled with a wrinkled, proteinaceous outer ectocyst and an inner cellulose-containing endocyst that may be stellate, polygonal, oval, triangular, or round. Pores or ostioles are present at the point of contact between the ecto- and the endocyst and the pores are usually covered by an operculum.

DESCRIPTION OF THE DISEASE

Several species of *Acanthamoeba* (*A. castellanii*, *A. culbertsoni*, *A. rhysodes*, *A. polyphaga*, *A. divionensis*, and *A. healyi*) cause a chronic and usually fatal GAE and skin lesions that may last for several weeks to even months. GAE is a slowly progressive CNS disease with no clear-cut incubation period. It has an insidious onset, lasting from a few days to several weeks or months. The most common clinical symptoms include headache, irritability, confusion, seizures, dizziness, drowsiness, and sometimes diplopia, lethargy, and hemiparesis. Some patients, especially those with human immunodeficiency virus/acquired immunodeficiency syndrome (HIV/AIDS), develop skin lesions, abscesses, or erythematic nodules. Microscopically, the lesions consist of hemorrhagic necrosis of CNS parenchyma, with variable amounts of subacute and chronic inflammatory reaction, with amoebic trophozoites and cysts around and within the walls of blood vessels. Because of a granulomatous reaction, the disease caused by *Acanthamoeba* is called granulomatous amoebic encephalitis. Trophozoites and cysts may be found in liver, lungs, kidneys, prostate, lymph nodes, skin, and other organs, suggesting hematogenous dissemination.

As many as 103 cases (72 in the United States) of granulomatous disease caused by *Acanthamoeba* with and without the involvement of skin lesions have been reported from around the world. Though many of these patients have been treated with a number of antiviral, antibacterial, antimycotic, and antiprotozoal therapeutic agents, except in three documented cases, all have died.

Acanthamoeba spp. also cause a painful vision-threatening disease of the cornea, *Acanthamoeba* keratitis (AK). If the infection is not treated promptly it may lead to a chronic ulceration of the cornea, loss of visual acuity, and eventual blindness and enucleation. More than 700 cases of *Acanthamoeba* keratitis have been reported worldwide. The principal risk factor for AK is the use of soft contact lenses and nonsterile homemade saline.

Acanthamoeba keratitis is characterized by severe ocular pain, a 360° or partial paracentral stromal ring infiltrate, recurrent corneal breakdown of the epithelial, and a corneal lesion refractory to commonly used ophthalmic antibacterial medication. Although *Acanthamoeba* is resistant to commonly used chemotherapeutic agents, especially in the cyst stage, even at very high concentrations some patients with *Acanthamoeba* keratitis have been treated successfully with topical application of a combination of drugs, including propamidine isethionate (Brolene), clotrimazole, neosporin suspensions, and polyhexamethylene biguanide.

RESERVOIRS FOR THE AGENT

No human or animal reservoir for *Acanthamoeba* spp. has been identified, possibly because no survey has been conducted to identify sources of such reservoir hosts. Both invertebrates, such as aquatic insects and their larvae, mollusks, and crustaceans, and all classes of vertebrates need to be surveyed for their ability to act as reservoirs for these amoebas.

MODE OF TRANSMISSION

Unlike *N. fowleri*, no clear-cut and direct evidence shows that *Acanthamoeba* GAE can be directly acquired from water, though this is quite likely. The portal of entry in the case of GAE is probably through the lower respiratory tract, ulceration of the skin or mucosa, or any open wounds. CNS disease is probably acquired by hematogenous spread from a primary site, such as the respiratory tract or skin lesion. Recent cases of GAE in AIDS patients who first developed skin abscesses and later developed CNS symptoms strongly suggests secondary dissemination to the CNS from a primary location, such as skin.

Acanthamoeba keratitis, however, has been directly traced to the use of contaminated saline solution made by dissolving salt tablets with commercially available unsterile bottled water. There are also indications that AK has been acquired from recreational water, e.g., hot tubs, swimming pools, and lakes.

METHODS FOR DETECTING THE AGENT

Acanthamoeba spp. can be easily detected and isolated from the suspected source, such as soil, water, sewage, cerebrospinal fluid, and small pieces of tissue (e.g., brain, lungs, skin, and cornea). Samples should be collected aseptically and can be stored for short periods at room temperature, but never frozen. Personnel handling specimens should take appropriate precautions, such as wearing gloves, surgical masks, and working in a biological safety cabinet. Water samples should be sent to a qualified reference laboratory for testing.

Acanthamoeba spp. have also been known to harbor *Legionella*, *Mycobacteria*, and certain viruses, which accentuate the public health importance of these organisms.

OCCURRENCE OF THE AGENT IN PEOPLE, ANIMALS, AND THE ENVIRONMENT

GAE due to *Acanthamoeba* is a chronic illness that occurs primarily in immunosuppressed, chronically ill, or otherwise debilitated persons with no history of exposure to fresh water. A few cases, however, have occurred in healthy persons with no known immunodeficiency or risk factors for HIV. *Acanthamoeba* is also known to cause CNS and other organ infections in canines, ovines, bovines, monkeys, kangaroos, rabbits, and even in fish and reptiles.

Members of the genus *Acanthamoeba* are ubiquitous and occur worldwide. They have been isolated from soil; freshwater lakes and ponds; sewage and sludge; dust in air; thermal effluents of power plants; swimming pools; hot springs; brackish water and seawater; ocean sediments; frozen water; tap water; bottled water; heating, ventilating, and air conditioning units; bacterial, mycotic, and mammalian cell cultures; vegetables; and mushrooms.

SURVIVAL OF THE AGENT IN THE ENVIRONMENT

Acanthamoebae can survive indefinitely in the environment as cysts that are resistant forms able to withstand adverse conditions. For example, *Acanthamoeba* has been isolated from bottled water, ocean sediments, antarctic soil, and frozen swimming areas in Norway.

DOCUMENTED WATERBORNE OUTBREAKS

No definite outbreaks of *Acanthamoeba* encephalitis have been described; however, as agents of keratitis, *Acanthamoeba* have been shown to be transmitted through hot tub water, bottled water, and contact lens cleaning and holding solutions, particularly homemade saline solution.

EFFECTIVENESS OF WATER TREATMENT PROCESSES

Several factors, including pH, temperature, and biological and biochemical demands that influence the growth of amoebas also influence the amoebicidal effects of chlorine and other disinfectants. Scattered reports based on experimental laboratory data suggest that *Acanthamoeba* spp. are more resistant to chlorine than *Naegleria* spp. Isolated reports of resistance of *A. culbertsoni* to high levels (40 mg/L) of chlorine exist; however, other reports indicate that chlorine levels of 1.25 mg/L chlorine is enough to kill *Acanthamoeba*, including *A. culbertsoni*. Of the four disinfectants used, deciquam 222 (a quarternary ammonium compound) was found to be the most effective amoebicide, followed by chlorine, chlorine dioxide, and ozone. Another compound, Baquacil (a 20 percent solution of polyhexamethylene biguanide [PHMB]), used in the disinfection of swimming pools in New Zealand, has been found to be a good amoebicidal agent. Purified PHMB is now being used therapeutically in AK cases.

INFORMATION SOURCES

Brown, T.J., and R.T.M. Cursons. 1987. Prophylaxis. In *Amphizoic Amoebae Human Pathology*. pp. 217–236. Rondanelli, E.G., ed. Padua, Italy: Piccin.

John, D.T. 1993. Opportunistically Pathogenic Free-Living Amebae. In *Parasitic Protozoa*. Vol. 3. pp. 143–246. Krier, J.P., and J.R. Baker, eds. New York: Academic Press, Inc.

Ma, P., G.S. Visvesvara, A.J. Martinez, F.H. Theodore, P.M. Daggett, and T.K. Sawyer. 1990. *Naegleria* and *Acanthamoeba* Infections: Review. *Rev. Infect. Dis.*, 12:490–513.

Martinez, A.J. 1985. *Free-Living Amebas: Natural History, Prevention, Diagnosis, Pathology, and Treatment of the Disease*. Boca Raton, Fla.: CRC Press.

Page, F.C. 1985. *A New Key to Fresh Water and Soil Gymnamoebae*. Cumbria, England: Fresh Water Biological Association.

Visvesvara, G.S. 1995. Pathogenic and Opportunistic Free-Living Amebae. In *Manual of Clinical Microbiology*. 6th ed. pp. 1196–1203. Murray, P.R., E.J. Baron, M.A. Pfaller, F.C. Tenover, and R.H. Yolken, eds. Washington, D.C.: ASM Press.

Visvesvara, G.S., and J.K. Stehr-Green. 1990. Epidemiology of Free-Living Ameba Infections. *J. Protozool*, 37:25S–33S.

Chapter 22

Ascaris lumbricoides

Huw Smith, Tony Grimason, and Celia Holland

DESCRIPTION OF THE AGENT

Ascaris lumbricoides, superfamily Ascaridoidea, is a large roundworm found in humans. The parasite exists in three distinct forms: the egg or ovum; the larva, which migrates through various organs of the body; and the adult, which resides in the intestinal tract. The sexes are separate. Similar species are parasites in pigs, horses, dogs, and cats. Parasitic nematodes have five consecutive developmental stages in their life cycle. The fertile egg develops into the first-stage larva, which molts to become the second-stage larva. The second-stage larva molts two times, to become the third- and fourth-stage larva, before it becomes adult.

Adult females are fertilized in the intestine by adult males. One adult female can lay more than 200,000 ova daily, and more than 25 million eggs total. Fertilized eggs are excreted in the host feces. Embryonation occurs when the fertilized, unsegmented embryo develop into a larvae in the environment. A moist microclimate, ambient temperature, and protection from ultraviolet light (UV) encourage embryonation. The second-stage (L2) larva develops within the eggshell in 10 to 14 days under ideal conditions. If ingested, the L2 is stimulated to hatch in the intestine. Hatched L2 penetrate the wall of the jejunum and, within a few days, migrate to the liver through the vasculature and/or lymphatics. The larvae migrate through the heart to the pulmonary capillaries, where they remain for about two weeks and molt into third-stage (L3) larvae. Third-stage larvae migrate into the alveolar spaces, up the respiratory tree, and are then swallowed. Acid-resistant L3 worms pass through the stomach, molting into the L4 larvae in the intestine, where they grow rapidly. After about eight weeks, adult female worms mate with mature males and lay fertile eggs. The cycle from infection to egg-laying adult normally takes 10 to 16 weeks.

The transmissive stage is the fertilized egg, and the infective stage is the fully embryonated egg containing the L2 larva. The two commonly identified stages are fertilized or unfertilized eggs, and adult male and female worms. Fertilized ova differ in morphology from unfertilized eggs. Eggs are oval to spherical in shape. Voided ova are generally a yellowish brown in color, ellipsoid (ovoid) to circular, measuring 35–50 × 50–70 µm. The fertile ovum is encased in a knobbly (mammilated), bile-stained outer albuminous coat that protects developing larva in the environment and, being sticky, adheres to a variety of surfaces. Unfertilized eggs are elongated and larger than fertilized eggs, measuring 43–47 × 85–95 μm, and have thin shells with a grossly irregular mammilated layer.

DESCRIPTION OF THE DISEASE

The prepatent period (two to three months) is the interval of time between ingesting infectious eggs and the first appearance of ova in the stool. The incubation period is the time between ingesting infectious eggs and the development of recognized symptoms or signs of illness. This can vary from a few days to several months depending on the number of infectious ova ingested and the susceptibility of the individual. In light infections, individuals may remain asymptomatic.

Symptoms can be due to migrating larvae, adult worms, or both. Symptoms are more severe with more larval or adult worms, or both. Pulmonary and intestinal infection, allergy to *Ascaris* allergens, and other complications can all give rise to symptoms. Adult worms may produce mild abdominal pain; however, individuals infected with low doses often only become aware of infection when ova are found in the stool. *A. lumbricoides* is responsible for 35 percent of intestinal obstruction in endemic areas. Chronic ascariasis is widely recognized as a contributory factor to impaired nutritional status; infected children who receive antihelminthic treatment show increases in weight-for-age and height-for-age.

RESERVOIRS FOR THE AGENT

Humans are the reservoir of *A. lumbricoides*. Coprophagous animals such as pigs, dogs, cats, and chickens that feed on human feces, act as transport hosts by dispersing or redistributing fertile ova to other sites associated with human activities. *Ascaris* ova have been found in surface water, groundwater, and seawater, but not in treated drinking water. They have also been detected in night soil (fertilizer); sewage; sludge; soil, particularly in the vicinity of houses; and on crops, utensils, and beaches.

MODE OF TRANSMISSION

Transmission can occur by any route where infective ova are ingested by a susceptible human host. This necessitates the external maturation of ova to infectivity in the environment, thus contact with recently voided feces is not a risk. In endemic areas, major routes of transmission include the following:

- defecation by infected individuals, especially children, in backyards or compounds that leads to the contamination of soil, fingers, hands, and cooking utensils
- use of untreated human feces as fertilizer (night soil), especially for crops that receive minimal heating before consumption
- defecation by agricultural workers in or near fields where they work (defecating in or near flowing water is often believed to be more sanitary than defecating into latrines where water may be unavailable for handwashing)
- use of untreated sewage effluent for irrigating crops that receive minimal heating before consumption

- consumption of contaminated unfiltered drinking water or communal drinking water
- redistribution of fertile ova to other uncontaminated sites associated with human activities by coprophagous animals such as pigs, dogs, cats, and chicken that feed on human feces

METHODS FOR DETECTING THE AGENT

Detection of *Ascaris* ova is by microscopic morphological and morphometric examination of suspect organisms by bright field microscopy. Microscopic examination of a fecal smear or concentrate (e.g., formalin-ether or salt flotation) can reveal the presence of either fertile or unfertilized ova. A concentration technique is recommended for diagnosing light infections. Single-sex infection by adult male worms or immature or old female adult worms cannot be diagnosed microscopically by fecal examination because no ova are produced.

OCCURRENCE OF THE AGENT IN PEOPLE, ANIMALS, AND THE ENVIRONMENT

A. lumbricoides appears to be specific to humans; however, mature worms can occur in nonhuman primates, and mammals can be infected experimentally. Human infections with *Ascaris suum* (from pigs) cannot be ruled out in endemic areas where pigs and humans live closely together. Recent evidence from Central and North America indicates that cross-infection could occur even though the two parasite populations appear to be reproductively isolated.

The most recent estimates for the worldwide prevalence of ascariasis are 1,273 million infections (24 percent prevalence). Infections are generally acquired during the first or second year of age, peak in children 5 to 15 years old, and then stabilize across the adult ages. Climate can influence egg survival and embryonation; the prevalence of ascariasis is lower in arid African countries than in those with higher rainfall. The prevalence of ascariasis is intimately linked to socioeconomic conditions. The poorer the conditions, the higher the prevalence of ascariasis. Factors such as housing type, water source, and availability of latrines show a significant relationship with *Ascaris* prevalence. In contrast to prevalence, *Ascaris* intensity (mean number of worms per person) peaks in the 5- to 15-year-olds and declines markedly in adults. The number of worms per person within a host population are not normally distributed but follow an aggregated or overdispersed frequency distribution. Thus, the majority of hosts harbor few or no worms and the minority of hosts harbor heavy worm burdens. Clearly, the most heavily parasitised individuals are more at risk from morbidity and mortality, and contribute the most to environmental contamination and the transmission of infection.

SURVIVAL OF THE AGENT IN THE ENVIRONMENT

Ascaris ova occur commonly in the environment. Densities of the ova depend on the level of infection in the indigenous population. *Ascaris* ova can be found in surface water, groundwater, and seawater, but not in treated drinking water. They can also be present in feces, night soil, sewage (see Table 22-1), sludge, soil, and on crops and beaches.

Densities of *Ascaris* sp. ova can vary greatly in raw wastewaters and are indicators of endemic disease within the human population. Other factors include the size and socioeconomic status of the population, the percentage of the population sewered, shock loadings from the discharge of pit latrine tankers, the provision of separate or combined sewers, and seasonal and sampling factors.

Ascaris ova are among the most environmentally resistant of intestinal pathogens. Because the embryo develops into the infective larva outside the body of the host, Ascaris ova are well-suited to prolonged survival in the environment. The development of the embryo into the infective larva and its survival in the environment depend on aerobic metabolism, but these ova can also survive in anaerobic conditions. *Ascaris* ova remain viable for months without oxygen, although their development is interrupted. Under conditions of ambient temperature (22 to 35° C), moisture, shade from UV light, and oxygen, embryonation to infectivity takes 12 to 14 days for *Ascaris* ova. At lower temperatures, embryonation takes longer. Infective ova of *Ascaris* can remain viable for several years. In temperate climates, *Ascaris* ova can remain viable for seven years in moist, loose soils with moderate shade. Ova survive longer when buried in soil, and clay soils that retain moisture enhance survival. *Ascaris* ova do not embryonate below 18° C, can remain viable for 43 days at –23° C, and can continue development when the temperature is elevated. In arctic tundra, *Ascaris* ova may remain viable for up to 100 years. *Ascaris* ova are resistant to cold desiccation and chemicals such as strong salt solutions and moderate concentrations of formalin and hypochlorite. However, exposure for short periods of time (hours) to temperatures above 37° C will kill developing embryos.

DOCUMENTED WATERBORNE OUTBREAKS

While associated with foodborne outbreaks of disease, no waterborne outbreak of ascariasis associated with treated public drinking water supplies has been documented.

EFFECTIVENESS OF WATER TREATMENT PROCESSES

Effective coagulation and filtration processes remove *Ascaris* ova. Chlorine and chloramine disinfectants are ineffective against *Ascaris* ova. Exposure to UV light early in embryonation destroys the developing embryo. Conventional sewage treatment processes are not effective in destroying ova. Ova need to be retained for 10 to 12 months in septic tanks, cesspools, or other sewage detention facilities before they are destroyed.

Table 22-1 Occurrence of *Ascaris* spp. ova in raw sewage

Country	*Ascaris* (*ova/L*)
Russia	60
United States	30
India	59.3–838
India	6×10^7–1.6×10^9
India	488–838
India	4–120
Nigeria	≤1,400
Morocco	17

INFORMATION SOURCES

Anon. 1989. Health Guidelines for the Use of Wastewater in Agriculture and Aquaculture. *Technical Report Series No. 778*. Geneva: World Health Organization.

Chan, M.-S. 1997. The Global Burden of Intestinal Nematode Infections—50 years on. *Parasitol. Today*, 13(11):438–443.

Crompton, D.W.T. 1994. *Ascaris lumbricoides*. In *Parasitic Diseases and Infectious Diseases Epidemiology and Ecology*. pp. 175–196. Scott, M.E., and G. Smith, eds. San Diego, Calif.: Academic Press.

Feacham, R.G., D.J. Bradley, H. Garelick, and D.D. Mara. 1982. *Sanitation and Disease. Health Aspects of Excreta and Wastewater Management*. Chichester, UK: John Wiley & Sons.

This page intentionally blank.

Chapter 23

Balantidium coli

Lynne S. Garcia

DESCRIPTION OF THE AGENT

While many of the organisms in the phylum Ciliophora are free-living, members of the genus *Balantidium* are parasites found in the intestinal tract of invertebrate and vertebrate hosts. *B. coli* is the only pathogenic ciliate of humans and is the largest of the protozoa that are parasites in humans (Table 23-1). Both the trophozoite and cyst forms are found. Trophozoite is quite large, approximately 50 to 100 µm in width, oval in shape, and covered with short cilia. The anterior end is somewhat pointed and is provided with a cytostome. The posterior end is broadly rounded. The cytoplasm has many vacuoles containing bacteria and debris. The trophozoite has two nuclei, one very large bean-shaped macronucleus and a small round micronucleus. The

Table 23-1 Characteristics of *Balantidium coli*

Species	Shape and Size	Motility	Number of Nuclei	Other Features
Balantidium coli Trophozoite	Ovoid with tapering anterior end; 50–100 µm in length; 40–70 µm in width; usual range: 40–50 µm	Ciliates: rotary, boring; may be rapid	One large kidney-shaped macronucleus, one small round micronucleus, which is difficult to see even in the stained smear; macronucleus may be visible in unstained preparation	Body covered with cilia, which tend to be longer near cytostome; cytoplasm may be vacuolated
Cyst	Spherical or oval, 50–70 µm; usual range: 50–55 µm		One large macronucleus visible in unstained preparation; micronucleus difficult to see	Macronucleus and contractile vacuole are visible in young cysts; in older cysts, internal structure appears granular; cilia difficult to see within the cyst wall

organisms normally live in the large intestine where the trophozoites feed on cell debris, starch grains, bacteria, and mucus. The cilia beat in a sequence, producing waves along the surface of the trophozoite. The organisms move in a spiral motion, and can move backward by reversing the cilia.

The cyst is formed as the trophozoite moves down the intestine. Nuclear division does not occur in the cyst; therefore, only two nuclei are present—the macronucleus and the micronucleus. The cysts measure from 50 to 70 µm and are the infective form to humans. The parent multiplies asexually by transverse binary fusion; conjugation has also been documented, but is rare.

DESCRIPTION OF THE DISEASE

Some individuals with *B. coli* infections are asymptomatic, others develop symptoms of severe dysentery similar to those caused by amoebiasis. Symptoms usually include diarrhea or dysentery, tenesmus, nausea, vomiting, anorexia, and headache. Insomnia, muscular weakness, and weight loss have also been reported. The diarrhea may persist for weeks to months before dysentery develops. Tremendous fluid loss may occur, characteristic of a type of diarrhea similar to that seen in cholera or in some coccidial infections. In healthy individuals, the infection may resolve spontaneously or may become latent.

B. coli has the potential to invade intestinal tissue by mechanical and enzymatic action on the mucosal surface. *B. coli* may penetrate the mucosa with cellular infiltration in the area of the developing ulcer. Some of the abscess formations may extend to the muscular layer. The ulcers may vary in shape, and the ulcer bed may be full of pus and necrotic debris.

The organism can be identified in routine stool examinations, particularly wet preparation examinations of fresh and concentrated material, using low-power (10×) or high-power (40×) microscopes. The organism can easily be seen in a wet preparation on low power. Organism recognition and identification on a permanent stained smear may be very difficult. The protozoa are so large that stains obscure any internal morphology. *B. coli* organisms may even be confused with helminth eggs because of their size, particularly when the cilia are not visible.

Tetracycline is the current drug of choice for treatment of *B. coli*, although it is considered investigational for this infection. The dosage is 500 mg four times daily for 10 days. Iodoquinol or metronidazole may be used as alternatives.

RESERVOIRS FOR THE AGENT

The natural habitat for *B. coli* is the large intestine of humans, monkeys, and pigs. *B. coli* is widely distributed in hogs, particularly in warm and temperate climates, and in monkeys in the tropics. Human infection is found in warmer climates, sporadically in cooler areas, and in institutionalized groups with low levels of personal hygiene.

MODE OF TRANSMISSION

Infections with *B. coli* are transmitted through infective cysts by the fecal–oral contamination of food or water. A patient who is symptomatic with diarrhea is passing the trophozoite (noninfectious form). However, an individual who is an asymptomatic carrier without diarrhea will be passing the infectious cyst form. The usual source of infection for humans is the pig.

METHODS FOR DETECTING THE AGENT

The same direct microscopic examination approach used for other protozoan parasites (amoebas and flagellates), can be used for *B. coli*; however, the same potential problems exist. These problems include lack of specific monoclonal-based reagents for high specificity and recovery problems related to low organism numbers. Many species of ciliates live in water and can be found in fecal specimens contaminated by water containing these organisms. They usually belong to the genera *Chilodon* or *Cyclidium* and can be confused with *B. coli* when compared morphologically.

EPIDEMIOLOGY

Although *B. coli* has been reported from many different simian hosts, domestic hogs probably serve as the most important reservoir host for human infection. In areas where pigs are the main domestic animal, the incidence of human infection can be quite high. Particularly susceptible to infection are persons working as pig farmers or in slaughterhouses (e.g., 28 percent infection in New Guinea). Human infection is fairly rare in temperate areas, although once the infection is established, it can develop into an epidemic, particularly where poor environmental sanitation and personal hygiene are found. This situation has been seen in mental hospitals in the United States. Because the mode of transmission is ingestion of infective cysts through contaminated food or water, preventive measures involve increased attention to personal hygiene and sanitation.

SURVIVAL OF THE AGENT IN THE ENVIRONMENT

Cysts in feces remain viable in stool for one to two days at room temperature and disappear in approximately one week. Like most intestinal protozoa, the cysts are relatively resistant to environmental conditions, but will rapidly die when exposed to drying or direct sunlight.

INFORMATION SOURCES

Abramowicz, M., ed. 1995. Drugs for Parasitic Infections. *Med. Lett.,* 37:99–108.

Beaver, P.C., R.C. Jung, and E.W. Cupp. 1984. *Clinical Parasitology.* 9th ed. Philadelphia, Pa.: Lea & Febiger.

Garcia, L.S., and D.A. Bruckner. 1997. *Diagnostic Medical Parasitology.* 3rd ed. Washington, D.C.: ASM Press.

Garcia, L.S., S. Bullock-Iacullo, J. Palmer, and R.Y. Shimizu. 1995. Diagnosis of Parasitic Infections: Collection, Processing and Examination of Specimens. In *Manual of Clinical Microbiology.* 6th ed. Murray, P.R., E.J. Baron, M.A. Pfaller, F.C. Tenover, and R.H. Yolken, eds. American Society for Microbiology.

Garcia-Laverde, A., and L. De Bonilla. 1975. Clinical Trials with Methonidazole in Human Balantidiasis. *Am. J. Trop. Med. Hyg.,* 24:781–783.

National Committee for Clinical Laboratory Standards. 1993. Procedures for the Recovery and Identification of Parasites from the Intestinal Tract, Proposed Guideline, M28-P. Villanova, Pa.: National Committee for Clinical Laboratory Standards.

This page intentionally blank.

Chapter 24

Blastocystis hominis

Lynne S. Garcia

DESCRIPTION OF THE AGENT

Blastocystis hominis was classified as an organism related to *Blastomyces* spp., a cyst form of a flagellate, or a yeast of the genus *Schizosaccharomyces*. However, this organism has been reclassified as a protozoan. Analysis of 10 stocks of *B. hominis* isolated from human stools revealed two distinct groups of organisms. Other studies on 61 isolates suggest that there may be four separate serologic groups. Further studies will be needed to determine whether or not these groups should be classified as separate species and whether or not they have epidemiologic significance. More recent biochemical studies have revealed at least two variant strains.

B. hominis is capable of pseudopod extension and retraction, reproduces by binary fission or sporulation, and has a membrane-bound central body that takes up 90 percent of the cell (Table 24-1). The organism is strictly anaerobic, normally requires bacteria for growth, and ingests bacteria and other debris. The classic form usually seen in the human stool specimen varies in size from 6 to 40 µm and is characterized by the large central body that may be involved with carbohydrate and lipid storage. The more amoebic form can occasionally be seen in diarrheal fluid but may be extremely difficult to recognize. *B. hominis* is usually identified by the more typical round form with the central body.

Table 24-1 Morphologic criteria used to identify *Blastocystis hominis*

Species	Shape and Size	Other Features
Blastocystis hominis	Organisms are generally round, measure approximately 6 to 40 µm, and are usually characterized by a large, central body (looks like a large vacuole) surrounded by small, multiple nuclei; central body area can stain various colors (trichrome) or remain clear	The more amoebic form can be seen in diarrheal fluid, but will be difficult to identify; due to variation in size, may be confused with various yeast cells

DESCRIPTION OF THE DISEASE

When *B. hominis* is present in large numbers in the absence of other parasites bacteria, or viruses, it may cause diarrhea, cramps, nausea, fever, vomiting, and abdominal pain and require therapy. In patients with other underlying conditions the symptoms may be more pronounced. Incidence of this organism appears to be higher than suspected in stools submitted for parasite examination. *B. hominis* should certainly be considered the possible pathogen in patients with symptoms, but in whom no other etiologic agent has been identified. Other recent studies suggest that when a symptomatic *B. hominis* infection responds to therapy, the improvement probably represents elimination of some other undetected pathogenic organism, such as *Entamoeba histolytica, Giardia lamblia,* and *Dientamoeba fragilis*. Data from other geographic areas indicate that *B. hominis* is commonly seen in stool samples, although likely nonpathogenic. Consequently, the true role of this organism in terms of colonization or disease is still somewhat controversial.

In a recent study from Germany, the prevalence and clinical significance of *B. hominis* in a large group of HIV patients was investigated. The data from this study of 262 patients suggest that the isolation of *B. hominis* does not justify treatment, even in symptomatic, severely immunocompromised patients. Symptoms will go away without therapy in most patients, or other infectious or noninfectious etiologies will be identified. Therapy should be limited to patients with persistent, unexplained symptoms after a thorough evaluation, screening, and examination of multiple stools.

RESERVOIRS FOR THE AGENT

B. hominis has been confirmed in humans, monkeys, apes, pigs, and possibly guinea pigs, and multiple species are likely involved. *B. hominis* is also widespread in avian hosts. In Australia, the organism has been found in dogs, cattle, sheep, horses, pigs, chickens, geese, ducks, ostriches, alpacas, llamas, koala, and wombat. However, it is still unclear whether the organism is a zoonosis or if different species of *Blastocystis* invade specific hosts.

MODE OF TRANSMISSION

B. hominis infections are transmitted through infective cysts (central body forms) found in fecal–oral contamination of food or water. Stages other than the cyst form will be destroyed on contact with water. The presence of thin- and thick-walled cysts have been reported. Thin-walled cysts are thought to be autoinfectious, leading to multiplication of the organism in the intestinal tract. The thick-walled cysts are responsible for external transmission via the fecal–oral route. This life cycle might explain the high percentage of positive carriers in many studies where the percentage of patients with *B. hominis* is often much higher than those infected with other intestinal protozoa.

METHODS FOR DETECTING THE AGENT

Methods used to detect other protozoan parasites (amoebas and flagellates) can be used. However, the lack of specific monoclonal-based reagents for high specificity and recovery of low organism numbers and small organism size are problems to be aware of. Morphologically, these organisms can resemble large yeast forms, or even artifacts.

Routine stool examinations are very effective in recovering and identifying *B. hominis*, although the permanent stained smear is the procedure of choice.

Examination of wet preparations may not easily reveal the organism. If the fresh stool is rinsed in water before fixation (for the concentration method), *B. hominis* organisms, other than the cysts, will be destroyed, thus possibly yielding a false-negative report.

Both enzyme-linked immunosorbent assay (ELISA) and fluorescent antibody tests (FA) have been developed for detection of serum antibody to *B. hominis* infections. Demonstration of a strong antibody response is consistent with the ability of this organism to cause symptoms. In a second study using FA, serum antibody production both during and following *B. hominis* symptomatic disease is immunological evidence for the pathogenic role for this protozoan.

OCCURRENCE OF THE AGENT IN PEOPLE, ANIMALS, AND THE ENVIRONMENT

B. hominis is likely transmitted via the fecal–oral route through contaminated food or water. Although other possible modes of transmission are not defined, the incidence and apparent worldwide distribution indicate the traditional route of infection. Prevention would probably involve improved personal hygiene and sanitary conditions.

SURVIVAL OF THE AGENT IN THE ENVIRONMENT

Because prevalence numbers of *B. hominis* in human stool samples are often reported to be higher than other protozoans, infective cyst forms have been shown to remain viable at least as long as the other protozoa. Like most intestinal protozoa, the cysts are relatively resistant to environmental conditions, but will die when dried or exposed to direct sunlight.

DOCUMENTED WATERBORNE OUTBREAKS

No information on documented waterborne outbreaks is available.

EFFECTIVENESS OF WATER TREATMENT PROCESSES

No information on effective water treatment processes is available.

INFORMATION SOURCES

Albrecht, H., H.J. Stellbrink, K. Koperski, and H. Greten. 1995. *Blastocystis hominis* in Human Immunodeficiency Virus-Related Diarrhea. *Scandinavian Journal of Gastroenterology,* 30:2:909–914.

Boreham, P.F.L., J.A. Upcroft, and L.A. Dunn. 1992. Protein and DNA Evidence for 2 Demes of *Blastocystis hominis* from Humans. *Int. J. Parasitol.,* 22:49–53.

Garavelli, P.L., C.H. Zierdt, T.A. Fleisher, H. Liss, and B. Nagy. 1995. Serum Antibody Detected by Fluorescent Antibody Test in Patients with Symptomatic *Blastocystis hominis* Infection. *Recenti Progressi in Medicina,* 86:398–400.

Garcia, L S., and D.A. Bruckner. 1997. *Diagnostic Medical Parasitology.* 3rd ed. Washington, D.C.: ASM Press.

Garcia, L.S., S. Bullock-Iacullo, J. Palmer, and R.Y. Shimizu. 1995. Diagnosis of Parasitic Infections: Collection, Processing and Examination of Specimens. In *Manual of Clinical Microbiology,* 6th ed. Murray, P.R., E.J. Baron, M.A. Pfaller, F.C. Tenover, and R.H. Yolken, eds. American Society for Microbiology.

Mansour, N.S., E.M. Mikhail, N.A. Elmasry, A.G. Sabry, and E.W. Mohareb. 1995. Biochemical Characterization of Human Isolates of *Blastocystis hominis. J. Med. Microbiol.,* 42:304–307.

Markell, E.K., and M.P. Udkow. 1986. *Blastocystis hominis*: Pathogen or Fellow Traveler? *Am. J. Trop. Med. Hyg.,* 35:1023–1026.

Muller, H.E. 1994. Four Serologically Different Groups Within the Species *Blastocystis hominis. Zentralblatt Fur Bakteriologie—Intl. J. Med. Microbiol, Virol, Parasit, and Inf. Dis.,* 280:403–408.

Shlim, D.R., C.W. Hoge, R. Rajah, J.C. Rabold, and P. Echeverria. 1995. Is *Blastocystis hominis* a Cause of Diarrhea in Travellers? A Prospective Controlled Study in Nepal. *Clin. Infect. Dis.,* 21:97–101.

Singh, M., K. Suresh, L.C. Ho, G.C. Ng, and E.H. Yap. 1995. Elucidation of the Life Cycle of the Intestinal Protozoan *Blastocystis hominis. Parasitology Research,* 81:446–450.

Yoshikawa, H., J. Satoh, and Y. Enose. 1995. Light and Electron Microscopic Localization of Lipids in *Blastocystis hominis. J. Electron Microscopy,* 44:100–103.

Zierdt, C.H., W.S. Zierdt, and B. Nagy. 1995. Enzyme-Linked Immunosorbent Assay for Detection of Serum Antibody to *Blastocystis hominis* in Symptomatic Infections. *J. Parasitol.,* 81:127–129.

Chapter 25

Cryptosporidium parvum

Charles R. Sterling and Marilyn M. Marshall

DESCRIPTION OF THE AGENT

Tyzzer described the morphology and life cycle of *Cryptosporidium parvum* in 1912. The parasite remained relatively obscure until 1971 when it was found to be associated with bovine diarrhea. In 1976 two independent groups reported the first cases of human cryptosporidiosis. In 1982 physicians reported to the Centers for Disease Control (CDC) cases of severe diarrhea associated with acquired immune deficiency syndrome (AIDS) patients in which the causative agent was *Cryptosporidium*. Since 1984 when the first waterborne outbreak associated with *Cryptosporidium* was reported, to the massive Milwaukee, Wis., outbreak in 1993, medical, public health, and water treatment personnel have become increasingly aware of this parasite and its potential for causing infectious disease.

Cryptosporidium is in suborder Eimeriorina and family Cryptosporidiidae. The suborder Eimeriorina also contains the medically important coccidian parasites *Isospora belli* and *Toxoplasma gondii*. The transmissible stage parasite is a mature, thick-walled oocyst, 4 to 6 µm in size. When oocysts are ingested along with food or water, the cyst membrane opens (excystation) in the small intestine releasing sporozoites that attach to and invade epithelial cells of the gastrointestinal tract. Excystation usually requires reducing conditions, pancreatic enzymes, and bile salts; however, it may occur in warm aqueous solutions without any special stimuli.

Sporozoites that have penetrated enterocytes develop into trophozoites. The trophozoite stage divides by asexually forming meront stages containing merozoites. These merozoites can infect neighboring cells or produce stages that will initiate the sexual cycle where zygotes are formed after fertilization and then develop into environmentally resistant, thick-walled oocysts. Oocysts are released in feces and can transmit infection from one host to another. Approximately 20 percent of zygotes develop into thin-walled, oocysts-autoinfective life cycle forms that can maintain the parasite life cycle in the host. This stage and the type I meronts of the asexual cycle are believed to be largely responsible for the continuation of life-threatening disease in immunodeficient persons who do not have repeated exposure to environmentally resistant forms.

DESCRIPTION OF THE DISEASE

Profuse and watery diarrhea is the most common symptom of cryptosporidiosis. Other symptoms include abdominal pain, nausea, fever, and fatigue. The incubation period is from 5 to 28 days, with a mean of 7.2 days. The duration of the symptom varies according to the immune status of the host. In patients with compromised immune systems, the illness may be life-threatening. Most other hosts with intact immune systems are able to clear the infection. Patients with late-stage AIDS, regardless of age, are highly susceptible to cryptosporidiosis and after exposure, most immunocompromised individuals develop prolonged, severe life-threatening diarrhea. Individuals may be infected with as few as 30 oocysts.

RESERVOIRS FOR THE AGENT

Experiments and anecdotal information indicate that *C. parvum* is likely to be infectious to all species of mammals including humans. The young of most animal species are particularly prone to infection and diarrhea.

MODE OF TRANSMISSION

Close personal contact appears to be an important source of transmission. This most likely occurs with person-to-person contact between family and household members, sexual partners, health-care personnel, and day-care employees and attendees. Another route is animal-to-person (zoonosis), involving pets, farm animals, and laboratory animals. Water is the largest potential common source of transmission.

METHODS FOR DETECTING THE AGENT

Detection methods for *Cryptosporidium*, such as those specified in the Information Collection Rule (ICR), require that large volumes of water be concentrated and the retentate eluted and then concentrated by centrifugation. Pelleted material is separated from debris by flotation on a Percol sucrose gradient. A portion of this material is placed on a membrane filter and stained with a fluorescent antibody. Oocysts are confirmed by size, shape, and internal morphological characteristics. Variations in sample collection, turbidity, and weather conditions may influence results, as explained in chapter 3. Efforts to improve sampling, processing, and detection of enteric parasitic protozoans have been published by the US Environmental Protection Agency (USEPA).

In method 1622, direct immunomagnetic separation technology is used to selectively remove the oocyst from other particulates in the sample. The recovered parasites are stained with fluorescent antibodies and then confirmed with the fluorescent DAPI stain. Other detection techniques are being developed, such as fluorescence-activated cell sorting (FACS) coupled with fluorescent *in situ* hybridization (FISH).

OCCURRENCE OF THE AGENT IN PEOPLE, ANIMALS, AND THE ENVIRONMENT

Cryptosporidium oocysts are widely distributed in water and were reported in 87 percent of source water samples and 27 percent of drinking water samples. In the massive Milwaukee outbreak, investigators found that the severity of illness in Milwaukee residents, as defined by more frequent abdominal cramping, nausea, vomiting, and fever, was greater than in previously described sporadic cases. In addition, the severity of illness was greater in visitors to Milwaukee than its residents. Of both visitors and residents with laboratory-confirmed cryptosporidiosis, 39 percent had recurrent bouts of watery diarrhea that lasted an average of 2 days after having had normal stools for 2 to 14 days. Outbreaks of cryptosporidiosis associated with swimming pools have also been reported.

Not all US states require cases of cryptosporidiosis to be reported to local and state health departments. Recent awareness, however, has prompted some states to require that their cryptosporidiosis cases be reported to the CDC. Many physicians, however, are still unfamiliar with the parasite and many persons do not seek medical attention for diarrheal illness. The mean prevalence rate for *Cryptosporidium* infection is between 1 and 3 percent in Europe and North America, but is considerably higher in underdeveloped countries, where levels of infection range from 5 percent in Asia to approximately 10 percent in Africa.

SURVIVAL OF THE AGENT IN THE ENVIRONMENT

As long as the thick two-layered wall remains intact, *Cryptosporidium* oocysts are resistant to environmental elements such as cold and water. Oocysts can survive for months in cold moist environments, such as lakes and streams. Oocysts in water can retain viability and infectivity even after freezing at –15° C for 8 to 24 hours; however, oocysts can be rendered noninfectious when water temperatures of 64.2° C or higher are held for 2 minutes or longer. They are also susceptible to drying at 18 to 28° C for more than 4 hours.

DOCUMENTED WATERBORNE OUTBREAKS

Outbreaks associated with *Cryptosporidium* have been documented in the United States since 1984. These outbreaks have occurred in water systems using well and spring water treated solely by chlorination and in filtered surface water systems. *Cryptosporidium* is the etiological agent that has caused the greatest number of individuals to become ill from waterborne disease in recent times. Outbreaks caused by this organism are often unrecognized. In the Milwaukee outbreak that occurred in 1993, the organism was first identified from stool samples of ill patients. This information, along with the treatment plant records, pointed to the water supply as a likely source of infection.

EFFECTIVENESS OF WATER TREATMENT PROCESSES

Utilities should consider all surface water to be contaminated with *Giardia* or *Cryptosporidium*. Watersheds should be managed to limit the introduction of *Cryptosporidium* into drinking water supplies. Continuous optimization of plant performance for turbidity and particle removal are key monitoring parameters that should be used by utilities to signal possible problems. Treatment conditions (e.g., sedimentation, coagulation, and filtration) should be optimized to produce a filter effluent turbidity of 0.1 ntu or less. When filter effluent turbidity ranged between 0.1 and 0.3 ntu, *Cryptosporidium* presence was as much as 90 percent (1 log) greater than when filter effluent turbidity was 0.1 ntu or less.

INFORMATION SOURCES

Addiss, D.G., M.J. Arrowood, E.B. Mary, D.G. Colley, D.D. Juranek, and J.E. Kaplan. 1995. Assessing the Public Health Threat Associated With Waterborne Cryptosporidiosis: Report of a Workshop. RR-6:1–19. Atlanta, Ga.: Centers for Disease Control and Prevention.

American Society of Testing Materials. 1992. Proposed Test Method for *Giardia* and *Cryptosporidium Oocysts.* In *Low Turbidity Water by a Fluorescent Antibody Procedure. A Book of ASTM Standards.* pp. 925–935. Philadelphia, Pa.: ASTM.

Crockett, C.S., and C.N. Haas. Understanding Protozoa in Your Watershed. *Jour. AWWA,* 89(9):62–73.

Fayer, R. 1994. Effect of High Temperature on Infectivity of *Cryptosporidium parvum* Oocysts in Water. *Appl. Environ. Microbiol.,* 64:2732–2735.

Fayer, R., and N. Thomas. 1996. Effects of Low Temperature on Viability of *Cryptosporidium parvum* Oocysts. *Appl. Environ. Microbiol.,* 62:1431–1433.

LeChevallier, M.W., W.D. Norton, and R.G. Lee. 1991a. Occurrence of *Giardia* and *Cryptosporidium* spp. in Surface Water Supplies (published erratum appears in *Appl. Environ. Microbiol.,* 1992. 58(2):780). *Appl. Environ. Microbiol.,* 57:2610–2616.

———. 1991b. *Giardia* and *Cryptosporidium* spp. in Filtered Drinking Water Supplies. *Appl. Environ. Microbiol.,* 57:2617–2621.

Mackenzie, W.R., N.J. Hoxie, M.E. Proctor, M.S. Gradus, K.A. Blair, D.E. Peterson, J.J. Kazmierczak, D.G. Addiss, K.R. Fox, J.B. Rose, and J.P. Davis. 1994. A Massive Outbreak in Milwaukee of *Cryptosporidium* Infection Transmitted Through the Public Water Supply. *New England J. Med.,* 331:161–167.

Mackenzie, W.R., W.L. Schell, K.A. Blair, D.G. Addiss, D.E. Peterson, N.J. Hoxie, J.J. Kazmierczak, and J.P. Davis. 1995. Massive Outbreak of Waterborne *Cryptosporidium* Infection in Milwaukee, Wisconsin: Recurrence of Illness and Risk of Secondary Transmission. *Clin. Infect. Dis.,* 21:57–62.

McAnulty, J.M., D.W. Fleming, and A.H. Gonzalez. 1994. A Community-Wide Outbreak of Cryptosporidiosis Associated with Swimming at a Wave Pool. *JAMA,* 272:1597–1600.

Meisel, J.L., D.R. Perera, C. Meligro, and C.E. Rubin. 1976. Overwhelming Water Diarrhea Associated with *Cryptosporidium* in an Immunosuppressed Patient. *Gastroenterology,* 70:1156–1160.

Nime, F.A., J.D. Burek, D.L. Page, M.A. Holscher, and J.H. Yardley. 1976. Acute Enterocolitis in a Human Being Infected with the Protozoan *Cryptosporidium. Gastroenterology,* 70:592–598.

Panciera, R.J., R.W. Thomassen, and F.M. Gardner. 1971. Cryptosporidial Infection in a Calf. *Vet. Pathol.,* 8:479–484.

Patania, N.L., J.G. Jacangelo, L. Cummings, A. Wilczak, K. Riley, and J. Oppenheimer. 1995. Optimization of Filtration for Cyst Removal. Denver, Colo.: American Water Works Association Research Foundation and American Water Works Association.

Roberston L.J., A.T. Campbell, and H.V. Smith. 1992. Survival of *Cryptosporidium parvum* Oocysts under Various Environmental Pressures. *Appl. Environ. Microbiol.,* 58:3494–3500.

Sterling, C.R, and M.J. Arrowood. 1993. Cryptosporidia. In *Parasitic Protozoa,* 2nd ed., Vol. 6. pp. 159–225. Kreier, J.P., ed. New York: Academic Press.

USEPA. 1996. *ICR Microbial Labor Manual.* Publication EPA/600/R-951/178. Office of Research and Development. Washington, D.C.: Government Printing Office.

———. 1997. Method 1622: *Cryptosporidium* in Water by Filtration/IMS/FA. EPA 821-R-97-021. USEPA.

Chapter 26

Cyclospora cayetanensis

Ynés Ortega

DESCRIPTION OF THE AGENT

Cyclospora belongs to the family Eimeriidae. The species name *cayetanensis* was derived from the university where it was initially studied, Cayetan (Universidad Peruana Cayetano Heredia), and -ensis (Latin, belonging to). In 1979 *Cyclospora*-like organisms were first observed in Papua New Guinea. The organisms were thought to represent a new species of *Isospora* because of the structure of its sporocysts. From 1985 on, organisms 8 to 10 µm in size, staining red with modified acid-fast stains, and autofluorescing under ultraviolet (UV) light were reported with increasing frequency in humans worldwide. They were described as CLBs (coccidian-like bodies, cyanobacter-like bodies), or blue–green algae, and held responsible for diarrheal illness. Researchers eventually showed that CLBs belonged to the coccidian genus *Cyclospora*. *Cyclospora* was linked to previous reports of CLB infections based on the organism's biological characteristics and patients' symptoms and response to treatment.

Noninfectious *Cyclospora* oocysts are passed in the feces of infected individuals. These unsporulated oocysts require about 7 to 15 days to sporulate and become infectious. Unsporulated and sporulated oocysts measure 8 to 10 µm in diameter. Intracellular stages of the parasite have been observed in the cytoplasm of jejunal enterocytes of infected individuals. Asexual stages have been observed by electron and light microscopy. An animal model and an *in vitro* cultivation system for *Cyclospora* will help confirm the life cycle and identify possible mechanisms of pathogenesis.

DESCRIPTION OF THE DISEASE

Onset of illness caused by *Cyclospora* has been reported as abrupt in 68 percent and gradual in 32 percent of adult patients. Infections typically last an average of seven weeks, up to four months in acquired immune deficiency syndrome (AIDS) patients. Symptoms mimic those caused by cryptosporidiosis, including mild nausea, anorexia, abdominal cramping, and watery diarrhea. Most adult patients reported weight losses of up to 5 to 10 percent. Diarrhea alternating with constipation is commonly reported. Some patients have had flatulence, joint pain, and night sweats. Infection in children is less severe, and is usually asymptomatic. *Cyclospora* was detected in 12 percent of Nepalese children between 18 months and 5 years old.

RESERVOIRS FOR THE AGENT

Humans may be the only natural host, although organisms similar to CLBs have been observed in chimpanzees and baboons.

MODE OF TRANSMISSION

Epidemiological evidence strongly suggests water can transmit *Cyclospora*, especially because of the one- to two-week sporulation time. Most reports of infection have come from predominantly coastal cities or regions. Consumption of untreated water or reconstituted milk has led to infection. Indigenous *Cyclospora* infections in many countries including the United States have been described in patients with no travel history.

Accidental ingestion of contaminated water while siphoning water from a tank or cleaning a flooded basement were reported as possible sources of infection. Epidemiological evidence suggested that water from a rooftop reservoir was responsible for an outbreak involving 20 individuals, most of whom were physician residents in a Chicago hospital. In another instance, 12 of 14 British soldiers and dependents stationed in Nepal developed diarrhea. Examination of the chlorinated drinking water, consisting of river and municipal water, at the camp demonstrated the presence of *Cyclospora* oocysts.

During May and June of 1996, approximately 850 cases of cyclosporiasis were confirmed in the United States and Canada, nearly all in areas east of the Rocky Mountains. Epidemiological investigation suggested the infections were due to eating strawberries and raspberries. During 1997 *Cyclospora* outbreaks were reported in Virginia, Maryland, the District of Columbia, and Canada. These outbreaks were associated with the consumption of raspberries and basil. In 1998 importation of G18S ribosomal RNA Guatamalan raspberries was not permitted in the United States and no cases of cyclosporiasis were reported during that year. Canada reported some cases of *Cyclospora* that were associated with imported Guatamalan raspberries. Infections have been observed in the hot and humid season.

METHODS FOR DETECTING THE AGENT

Light microscopy of wet mounts, modified acid-fast staining, and autofluorescence are currently used for identifying *Cyclospora*. The nested polymerase chain reaction (PCR) may provide specificity and sensitivity to some laboratories and will be useful in population and environmental studies. Restriction fragment length polymorphism (RFLP) analysis of the PCR amplified products (18S ribosomal RNA) does differentiate *Cyclospora* from *Eimeria* strains. *Cyclospora* oocysts stain variably using a modified acid-fast technique and measure 8 to 10 μm in diameter. They stain best using the modified carbolfuchsin technique. Specific detection tests based on the use of monoclonal antibodies or other probe-specific technologies are being developed to better define the epidemiology of this organism and determine the extent to which water and other routes can transmit the organism.

OCCURRENCE OF THE AGENT IN PEOPLE, ANIMALS, AND THE ENVIRONMENT

Organisms similar in appearance to *Cyclospora* have now been described from patients with protracted diarrheal illness in North, Central, and South America; the Caribbean; Africa; Southeast Asia; Australia; England; and Eastern Europe. *Cyclospora* and *Cryptosporidium* oocysts have been detected in vegetables purchased from some markets in Lima, Peru. Other sources of infection include travelers or natives infected with *Cyclospora*, contaminated food, and possibly insects as transport hosts. Epidemiological studies will be invaluable in helping to sort the mechanisms of transmission and to define control against infection with *Cyclospora*.

INFORMATION SOURCES

Ashford, R.W. 1979. Occurrence of an Undescribed Coccidian in Man in Papua New Guinea. *Ann. Trop. Med. Parasit.*, 73:497–500.

Ashford, R.W., D.C. Warhurst, and G.D.F. Reid. 1993. Human Infection with Cyanobacterium-Like Bodies. *Lancet,* 341:1034.

Bendall, R.P., S. Lucas, A. Moody, G. Tovey, and P.L. Chiodini. 1993. Diarrhoea Associated with Cyanobacterium-Like Bodies: A New Coccidian Enteritis of Man. *Lancet,* 341:590–92.

CDC. 1996. Update: Outbreaks of *Cyclospora cayetanensis* Infection—United States and Canada. *MMWR*, 45(28):611–612.

Connor, B.A., D.R. Shlim, J.V. Scholes, J.L. Rayburn, J. Reedy, and R. Rajah. 1993. Pathologic Changes in the Small Bowel in Nine Patients with Diarrhea Associated with a Coccidia-Like Body. *Annals Intern. Med.*, 119:377–82.

Hale, D., W. Aldeen, and K. Carroll. 1994. Diarrhea Associated with Cyanobacteria-Like Bodies in an Immunocompetent Host. An Unusual Epidemiological Source. *JAMA,* 271:144–145.

Hoge, C.W., D.R. Shlim, R. Rajah, J. Triplett, M. Shear, J.G. Rabold, and P. Echevarria. 1993. Epidemiology of Diarrhoeal Illness Associated with Coccidian-like Organism among Travelers and Foreign Residents in Nepal. *Lancet*, 341:1175–1179.

Hoge, C.W., P. Echevarria, R. Rajah, J. Jacobs, S. Malthouse, E. Chapman, L.M. Jimenez, and D.R. Shlim. 1995. Prevalence of *Cyclospora* Species and Other Enteric Pathogens Among Children Less than 5 Years of Age in Nepal. *J. Clin. Microbiol.*, 33(11): 3058–3060.

Huang, P., T. Weber, D.M. Sosin, P.M. Griffin, E.G. Long, J.J. Murphy, F. Kocka, C. Peters, and C. Kallick. 1995. The First Reported Outbreak of Diarrheal Illness Associated with *Cyclospora* in the United States. *Annals Intern. Med.*, 123:409–414.

Long, E.G., A. Ebrahimzadeh, E.H. White, B. Swisher, and C.S. Callaway. 1990. Alga Associated With Diarrhea in Patients with Acquired Immunodeficiency Syndrome and in Travelers. *J. Clin. Microbiol.*, 28:1101–1104.

Long, E.G., H. White, W.C. Carmichael, P.M. Quinlisk, R. Rajah, B.L. Swisher, H. Daugharty, and M.T. Cohen. 1991. Morphologic and Staining Characteristics of a Cyanobacterium-Like Organism Associated with Diarrhea. *J. Infect. Dis.*, 164:199–202.

Markus, M.B., and J.A. Frean. 1993. Occurrence of Human *Cyclospora* Infection in Sub-Saharan Africa. *S. African Med. J.,* 83:862–863.

Ortega, Y., C.R. Sterling, R.H. Gilman, V.A. Cama, and F. Diaz. 1993. *Cyclospora* Species—A New Protozoan Pathogen of Humans. *New England J. Med.,* 328:1308–1312.

———. 1994. A New Coccidian Parasite (Apicomplexa: Eimeriidae) from Humans. *J. Parasitol.*, 80:625–629.

Rabold, J.G., C.W. Hoge, D.R. Shlim, C. Kefford, R. Rajah, and P. Echevarria 1994. *Cyclospora* Outbreak Associated with Chlorinated Drinking Water. *Lancet,* 344:1360–1361.

Rijpstra, A.C., and J.J. Laarman. 1993. Repeated Findings of Unidentified Small *Isospora*-Like Coccidia in Fecal Specimens from Travelers Returning to the Netherlands. *Trop. Geograph. Med.*, 45:280–282.

Smith, H.V., C.A. Paton, R.W.A. Girwood, and M.M.A. Mtambo. 1996. *Cyclospora* in Non-Human Primates in Gombe, Tanzania. *Vet. Rec.,* 138:528.

Sun, T., C.F. Ilardi, D. Asnis, A.R. Bresciani, S. Goldenberg, B. Roberts, and S. Teichberg. 1996. Light and Electron Microscopic Identification of *Cyclospora* Species in the Small Intestine. *Clin. Microbiol. Infect. Dis.*, 105(2):216–220.

Wurtz, R. 1994. *Cyclospora*: A Newly Identified Intestinal Pathogen of Humans. *Clin. Infect. Dis.*, 18:620–623.

Chapter 27

Dracunculus medinensis

M. Dale Little

DESCRIPTION OF THE AGENT

Dracunculus medinensis, of the family Dracunculidae, was recognized as a parasite of humans in ancient times by the Egyptians, Persians, Arabs, Hebrews, Greeks, and Romans. It was known as the dragon worm, serpent worm, medina worm, and, more recently, guinea worm. Infections with the worm (dracunculiasis or dracontiasis) were widespread in central and north Africa, the Middle East, India, and Pakistan. At the beginning of the International Drinking Water Supply and Sanitation Decade (1981–1990), a campaign to eradicate this parasite was initiated, and in 1986 was joined by the World Health Assembly. By 1994 dracunculiasis was close to eradication in Pakistan, significantly reduced in India, and new cases reduced by 41 percent in the 16 countries of Africa where it is endemic.

Infection occurs when a small freshwater microcrustacean, *Cyclops*, containing the infective stages of *Dracunculus* in its body cavity, is swallowed by a person drinking contaminated water. Ingested larvae migrate from the intestinal track to the deep somatic connective tissues (such as cartilage) where they develop to maturity and mate. The female later migrates to the subcutaneous and cutaneous tissues of the legs, feet, or other location where it continues to grow to a size of about 70 to 120 cm; the male reaches a length of only 1 to 3 cm and apparently dies soon after mating.

About 12 months after the infected *Cyclops* are ingested, the female worm, now with its uterus completely filled with the first-stage larvae, causes a large blister to be formed where the head end of the worm lies near the surface of the skin. This subsequently ruptures and an ulcer forms. When the lesion comes in contact with water, the worm ruptures and large numbers of minute larvae are released from the uterus into the water. Over the course of several weeks, this process repeats each time the lesion comes into contact with water. The larvae are nearly microscopic in size, less than 1 mm in length, and swim actively in the water. In *Cyclops* the ingested larvae develop to the infectious stage in the body cavity of the copepod in about two weeks. The cycle is repeated when another person drinks water containing infected *Cyclops*. In highly endemic areas, individuals may be reinfected year after year.

DESCRIPTION OF THE DISEASE

Few symptoms are seen before the skin lesion appears. When the initial blister appears, about 12 months after infection occurs, generalized symptoms may develop, including nausea, vomiting, diarrhea, and intense itching at the site of the lesion. Severe inflammation of the tissues surrounding the worm may result from the worm being broken during attempts at extraction. Also, secondary bacterial infection of the lesion is common, especially when the lesion is on the foot. Persons are often incapacitated for several months after the lesion forms in the skin. In some cases, worms may become calcified in a joint, knee, or ankle, and lead to stiffness or a fixed joint.

Definitive diagnosis can be made by observing the worm emerging from the skin. Exposing the lesion to water and observing the discharge of larvae confirms the diagnosis. Roentgenologic examination may be needed to reveal calcified worms.

Traditional treatment consists of removal of the worm by systematically and slowly extracting it, a few centimeters a day. Care must be taken to prevent breaking the worm or increased inflammation will result. Metronidazole is the drug of choice 250 mg is given three times a day over 10 days. The drug reduces inflammation and is said to facilitate the removal of the worm.

RESERVOIRS FOR THE AGENT

Although *D. medinensis* has reportedly been found in dogs and other animals, these reservoir hosts are not likely to transmit this worm to humans. In the United States, a related worm, *D. insignis*, is found in raccoons and mink, but no human infection with this parasite has been reported.

MODE OF TRANSMISSION

Transmission occurs only when a person drinks water containing *Cyclops* infected with *Dracunculus*.

METHODS FOR DETECTING THE AGENT

The infective stage of the parasite occurs only in susceptible species of *Cyclops* and is never free in the environment. Copepods may be collected from standing bodies of water by a plankton sampling net for microcrustaceans. Recovered *Cyclops* are examined under a stereomicroscope for the presence of *Dracunculus* larvae in their body cavity.

OCCURRENCE OF THE AGENT IN PEOPLE, ANIMALS, AND THE ENVIRONMENT

D. medinensis is not known to occur in North America. In endemic areas of Africa, the Middle East, and the Indian subcontinent, infections rarely, if ever, occur from the use of untreated drinking water obtained from running water sources, drilled wells, or draw wells with a circumference of less than 3 metres. In endemic areas, where the main sources of drinking water are ponds and step wells, infection rates may range from below 10 percent to over 80 percent. Animals do not appear to be a source of infection for humans.

The prevalence of dracunculiasis in endemic areas is highest in poor rural areas where drinking water is obtained from unprotected bodies of water, such as seasonal and permanent ponds, and step wells. In a survey carried out in rural settlements in Nigeria in 1988, prevalence rates were generally between 30 and 80 percent.

SURVIVAL OF THE AGENT IN THE ENVIRONMENT

The majority of *Cyclops* infected with *Dracunculus* larvae live for only about three weeks, but some may persist for six weeks or more. The presence of copepod-eating fish in the water may also shorten the time of survival.

INFORMATION SOURCES

American Public Health Association, American Water Works Association, and Water Environment Federation. 1995. *Standard Methods for the Examination of Water and Wastewater.* 19th ed. Eaton, A.D., L.S. Clesceri, and A.E. Greenberg, eds. Washington, D.C.: APHA.

Anon. 1995. Drugs for Parasitic Infections. *Med. Lett.*, 37(961):99–108.

Fabiyi, J.P. 1991. Geographical Distribution of Dracontiasis in Bauchi State, Nigeria. Discovery and Innovation, 3:72–76.

Hoeppli, R. 1959. *Parasites and Parasitic Infections in Early Medicine and Science.* Singapore: University of Malaya Press.

Hopkins, D.R. 1987. Dracunculiasis Eradication: A Mid-Decade Status Report. *Am. J. Trop. Med. Hyg.*, 37:115–118.

———. 1988. Dracunculiasis Eradication: The Tide Has Turned. *Lancet*, July 16:148–150.

Hopkins, D.R., E. Ruiz-Tiben, T. Ruebush II, A.N. Agle, and P.C. Withers, Jr. 1995. Dracunculiasis Eradication: March 1994 Update. *Am. J. Trop. Med. Hyg.*, 52:14–20.

Moorthy, V.N. 1938. Observations on the Development of *Dracunculus Medinensis* Larvae in *Cyclops. Amer. J. Hygiene*, 27:437–460.

Muller, R. 1979. Guinea Worm Disease: Epidemiology, Control, and Treatment. *Bull. World Health Org.,* 57:683–689.

This page intentionally blank.

Chapter 28

Entamoeba histolytica

William Keene

DESCRIPTION OF THE AGENT

Protozoan parasites classified as *Entamoeba histolytica* since 1903 have recently been subdivided into two species. While morphologically indistinguishable, one species, *E. dispar*, is apparently always nonpathogenic, while the other, which retains the name *E. histolytica*, causes human disease. *E. dispar* may be as much as 10 times more common than *E. histolytica*. Despite their similarity, genetic data suggest that these parasites may have diverged millions of years ago. Unless associated with clinical disease, or unless phagocytosed red blood cells can be visualized within trophozoites in fresh stool, infections with *E. histolytica* and *E. dispar* can only be distinguished by isoenzyme typing ("zymodeme" determination) or other sophisticated analyses. In this chapter, *amebiasis* means infection with the pathogenic species. This distinction was never made in the older medical literature. Even today, most clinical laboratory reports do not distinguish between the two species.

E. histolytica has a direct life cycle (i.e., no intermediate hosts) with two stages—trophozoite and cyst. The trophozoite is a "ameboid" blob of changing outline and dimension. Cysts are spheroid (10 to 20 µm in diameter). Humans become infected by swallowing cysts. Trophozoites develop following excystation in the small intestine, and are the form that can cause symptoms. Trophozoites reproduce by fission, and under some conditions develop into cysts. Trophozoites, cysts, or both are shed in feces. Cysts are immediately infective, while trophozoites die rapidly outside the human host, and, because they cannot survive transit through the acidic stomach environment, are not infective.

Although morphologically distinguishable, *E. histolytica* is sometimes confused with other harmless human amoebas, including *E. hartmanni* (formerly called a "small race" of *E. histolytica*, with a cyst diameter less than 10 µm), and *E. coli** (which has up to eight nuclei per cyst). Even human leukocytes found in stool can be

**Entamoeba coli*, not to be confused with the bacterium *Escherichia coli*.

misidentified as amoebas. Pseudo-epidemics resulting from poor laboratory work have been documented.

DESCRIPTION OF THE DISEASE

While most infections with *E. histolytica* are asymptomatic, amebiasis can be a serious and even life-threatening disease. The prevalence of infection worldwide is high enough that amebiasis ranks as the third leading killer among parasitic diseases (far behind malaria and schistosomiasis), causing an estimated 40,000 deaths annually.

Infections begin with parasite excystation in the intestinal lumen, but in some persons, trophozoites burrow into and even penetrate the intestinal wall. If that happens, parasites can spread to adjacent tissues or via the bloodstream to almost any part of the body. The clinical manifestations depend on where the amoebas are localized. Infections are usually categorized as intestinal, extraintestinal, or both.

With symptomatic infections, recurrent diarrhea of varying degrees is common, often with mucus and visible or occult blood, with or without fever, abdominal pain, and tenesmus. In fulminant amebiasis, the onset is abrupt with profuse bloody stools, high fever, and severe abdominal pain. Chronic colitis develops in some patients, with bloody stools and abdominal pain that may persist for months or years without treatment. Liver abscess is the most common form of extraintestinal amebiasis, but the infection can spread to the lungs, brain, perineum, or other sites.

Amebiasis is usually diagnosed by a stool exam for ova and parasites. Trophozoites can be visualized on wet mount of fresh stool or in trichrome-stained material preserved in polyvinyl alcohol (PVA). Cysts can be identified in concentrated and stained stool collected in formalin. Shedding may be intermittent, and three or more samples may be necessary to identify more than 90 percent of cases. Antigen detection tests that can distinguish *E. histolytica* from *E. dispar* in stool specimens have recently been licensed, but they are not yet in widespread use.

Antibodies are usually detectable within 7 to 10 days of invasive infections, and are diagnostic for infection with pathogenic *E. histolytica*. Although titers typically fall with successful treatment, they can remain elevated for years, making serologic results sometimes difficult to interpret.

The incubation period of *E. histolytica* is variable. In one well-studied outbreak of more than 300 cases, incubation periods ranged from several to 120 days, including 25 percent by 11 days, 50 percent by 20 days, and 75 percent by 36 days.

Medical therapy is usually successful for most infections, albeit complicated by side effects of antimicrobials, and, in some areas, drug availability. Noninvasive (intralumenal) infections can be treated with diloxanide furoate, iodoquinol, or paromomycin. Invasive disease (colitis/dysentery, liver abscess, or other extraintestinal infections) is usually treated with metronidazole, followed by a regimen aimed at lumenal parasites.

RESERVOIRS FOR THE AGENT

Infected humans, particularly asymptomatic carriers, are the only reservoirs of significance. Persons with frank diarrhea or dysentery tend to shed predominantly or exclusively trophozoites, hence are unimportant as transmitters of infection. Conversely, asymptomatically infected persons shed most or almost exclusively cysts, up to 15 million a day, according to one estimate. Paradoxically, the sicker the individual may seem, the less likely he or she is to spread the infection. Shedding may be intermittent, and can persist indefinitely in untreated individuals.

MODE OF TRANSMISSION

Transmission is by the fecal–oral route, reflecting direct person-to-person spread or exposure to contaminated food, water, or fomites. Cysts can also be dispersed by flies. Assessing the relative importance of these modes is difficult. Overall, waterborne transmission is probably relatively uncommon, albeit potentially very efficient. The infectious dose is low; inocula of 2,000 to 4,000 cysts produced infections in 100 percent of 42 human volunteers.

METHODS FOR DETECTING THE AGENT

Water samples can be concentrated by filtration and examined microscopically or cultured, but routine testing is not indicated.

OCCURRENCE OF THE AGENT IN PEOPLE, ANIMALS, AND THE ENVIRONMENT

Before *E. histolytica* and *E. dispar* were distinguished, it was estimated that as much as 10 percent of the world's population had amebiasis. In some parts of the world, pathogenic *E. histolytica* are commonly found. In the United States, *E. dispar* is probably much more prevalent than *E. histolytica*, particularly among native-born residents. Amebiasis is most commonly reported among recent immigrants, travelers, gay men, and institutionalized persons, but many of these may be harmless *E. dispar* infections.

Amebiasis was common among homosexual men in the pre-AIDS era, but prevalence has probably declined in recent years. The vast majority of amebic infections in gay men are probably *E. dispar*. In contrast to cryptosporidiosis, amebiasis is not a detectably increased risk for immunocompromised individuals.

In 1989, amebiasis was reportable in 47 of the 50 states. Only a very biased subset of infections are reported; however, surveillance data are difficult to interpret. Surveillance tallies lump *E. dispar* and *E. histolytica* infections, as they are rarely distinguished by clinical laboratories. Many infections are never diagnosed or reported, and even reported cases may get little or no followup by public health agencies. Absent high attack rates, even large, communitywide outbreaks of amebiasis could escape detection.

SURVIVAL OF THE AGENT IN THE ENVIRONMENT

Unlike the fragile trophozoites, amebic cysts are resistant to environmental degradation. Survival is primarily a function of temperature. At temperatures above freezing, *E. histolytica* cysts rarely survive longer than three months. Cysts are rapidly killed by modest heat, with survival times of less than two minutes at 50° C. Cysts are also killed by freezing. *E. histolytica* does not multiply outside the human host.

DOCUMENTED WATERBORNE OUTBREAKS

Waterborne outbreaks of amebiasis are rarely documented because (1) when they occur, they are hard to detect, and (2) they probably do not occur very often. In every case where adequate information is available, local disruptions in distribution systems or consumption of untreated water have been the cause.

According to US Environmental Protection Agency (USEPA) records, only eight waterborne outbreaks have been reported in the United States—the most recent in 1984. These are typically very small clusters (median number of cases, seven). None have involved large community systems.

The largest is the infamous 1933 Chicago World's Fair outbreak, with over 1,400 cases documented, including almost 100 fatalities. This outbreak was traced to cross-connections and contamination of drinking water reservoirs at two hotels with sewage from corroded and leaking waste lines. Chicago was the site of another large waterborne outbreak in 1934 after firefighters and bystanders at a huge stockyard fire drank from watering trough taps, not realizing that they connected to a nonpotable source. The only other sizable US outbreak occurred in 1953 at a large (1,500 employees) factory in South Bend, Ind. That outbreak was traced to a leak in a potable water suction line that ran through a pool of sewage.

Only a handful of outbreaks have been reported in Europe. A British outbreak was attributed to a broken sewer line contaminating a well; a cluster in Sweden was caused by a sewage backup that flooded a drinking water reservoir.

NATIONAL OR INTERNATIONAL GUIDELINES AND MONITORING RECOMMENDATIONS

Amebiasis is a potential problem when unfiltered drinking water is contaminated with human feces. Outbreaks have occurred when chlorinated water supplies became contaminated with sewage. There are no recommendations for specifically monitoring or testing source or effluent drinking water for *E. histolytica*. In the event of a suspected waterborne outbreak, ad hoc protocols would be developed by public health agencies working with water utility engineers.

INFORMATION SOURCES

Adams, E.B., and I.N. MacLeod. 1977a. Invasive Amebiasis. I. Amebic Dysentery and its Complications. *Medicine,* 56:315–323.

———. 1977b. Invasive Amebiasis. II. Amebic Liver Abscess and its Complications. *Medicine*, 56:325–334.

Allason-Jones, E., A. Mindel, et al. 1986. *Entamoeba histolytica* as a Commensal Intestinal Parasite in Homosexual Men. *New England J. Med.*, 315:353–356.

American Public Health Association, American Water Works Association, and Water Environment Federation. 1995. *Standard Methods for the Examination of Water and Wastewater.* Washington, D.C.: APHA.

Andersson, Y., and B. Jong. 1989. An Outbreak of Giardiasis and Amoebiasis at a Ski Resort in Sweden. *Wat. Sci. Tech.,* 21:143–146.

Beaver, P.C., R.C. Jung, et al. 1956. Experimental *Entamoeba histolytica* Infections in Man. *Am. J. Trop. Med. Hyg.,* 5:1000–1009.

Brooke, M.M., D.M. Melvin, et al. 1955. Studies of a Water-Borne Outbreak of Amebiasis, South Bend, Indiana. III. Investigation of Family Contacts. *Amer. J. Hygiene,* 62:214–226.

Bundesen, H.N., J.I. Connolly, et al. 1936. Epidemic Amebic Dysentery: the Chicago Outbreak of 1933. *National Institute of Health Bulletin,* 166:1–187.

Bundesen, H.N., F.O. Tonney, et al. 1934. The Outbreak of Amebiasis in Chicago During 1933. *JAMA,* 102:367–372.

Centers for Disease Control. 1985. Pseudo-Outbreak of Intestinal Amebiasis. California. *MMWR*, 34:125–126.

———. 1990. Mandatory Reporting of Infectious Diseases by Clinicians. *MMWR*, 39(No. RR-9):1–17.

Chang, S.L. 1943. Studies on *Endamoeba histolytica* [sic]. II. Observations Concerning Encystation, Maturation, and Excystation of *E. histolytica,* and on the Longevity of Culture-Induced Cysts in Various Fluids and at Different Temperatures. *J. Infect. Dis.,* 72:232–241.

———. 1950. Kinetics in the Thermodestruction of Cysts of *Endamoeba* [sic] *histolytica* in Water. *Amer. J. Hygiene,* 52:82–90.

———. 1955. Survival of Cysts of *Endamoeba* [sic] *histolytica* in Human Feces Under Low-Temperature Conditions. *Amer. J. Hygiene,* 61:103–120.

Cieslak, P., and S. Stanley. 1992. Advances in Amebiasis; Implications for the Clinician. *Infect. Dis. Clin. Practice,* 1:151–157.

Dritz, S.K. 1980. Medical Aspects of Homosexuality. *New England J. Med.,* 302(8):463–464.

Fassnacht, G.G., and J.H. Fooks. 1954. Engineering Studies on Amebiasis Outbreak at South Bend. *Jour. AWWA,* 46:1129–1140.

Hardy, A.V., and B.K. Spector. 1935. The Occurrence of Infestations with *E. histolytica* Associated with Water-Borne Epidemic Disease. *Public Health Reports,* 50:323–335.

Jones, M.F., and W.L. Newton. 1950. The Survival of Cysts of *Enamoeba histolytica* [sic] in Water at Temperatures Between 45° C and 55° C. *Am. J. Trop. Med. Hyg.,* 30:53–58.

Krogstad, D.J., H.C. Spencer, et al. 1978. Amebiasis: Epidemiological Studies in the United States, 1971–1974. *Ann. Intern. Med.,* 88:89–97.

LeMaistre, C.A., R. Sappenfield, et al. 1956. Studies of a Water-Borne Outbreak of Amebiasis. South Bend, Indiana. I. Epidemiological Aspects. *Amer J. Hygiene,* 64:30–45.

Markell, E.K., R.F. Havens, et al. 1983. Intestinal Parasitic Infections in Homosexual Men at a San Francisco Health Fair. *West. J. Med.,* 139:177–178.

McKerrow, J. 1992. Pathogenesis in Amebiasis: Is it Genetic or Acquired? *Infectious Agents and Disease,* 1:11–14.

Mildvan, D., A. Gelbe, et al. 1977. Venereal Transmission of Enteric Pathogens in Male Homosexuals. *JAMA,* 238(13): 1387–1389.

Morton, T.C., W.P. Stamm, et al. 1952. Indigenous Amoebiasis: A Recent Outbreak in England. *Brit. Med. J.,* 2:114–116.

Muñoz, O. 1986. Epidemiology of Amebiasis. In *Amebiasis.* pp. 213–239. A. Martinez-Palomo, ed. Amsterdam: Elsevier.

Offutt, A.C., B.A. Poole, et al. 1955. A Water-Borne Outbreak of Amebiasis. *Am. J. Public Health,* 45:486–491.

Ravdin, J.I. 1988. Intestinal Disease Caused by *Entamoeba histolytica.* In *Amebiasis: Human Infection by* Entamoeba histolytica. pp. 495–510. New York: John Wiley & Sons.

———. 1995. Amebiasis. *Clin. Infect. Dis.,* 20(6):1453–64.

Reed, S. 1992. Amebiasis: an Update. *Clin. Infect. Dis.,* 14:385–399.

Reed, S.L., and A.I. Braude. 1988. Extraintestinal Disease; Clinical Syndromes, Diagnostic Profile, and Therapy. In *Amebiasis: Human Infection by* Entamoeba histolytica. pp. 511–532. Ravdin, J.I., ed. New York: John Wiley & Sons.

Sawitz, W.G., and E.C. Faust. 1942. The Probability of Detecting Intestinal Protozoa by Successive Stool Examinations. *Am. J. Trop. Med. Hyg.,* 22:131–136.

Sepúlveda, B., and N. Treviño-Garcia. 1986. Clinical Manifestations and Diagnosis of Amebiasis. In *Amebiasis.* pp. 169–188. Martinez-Palomo, A., ed. Amsterdam: Elsevier.

Walsh, J.A. 1986. Problems in Recognition and Diagnosis of Amebiasis: Estimation of the Global Magnitude of Morbidity and Mortality. *Rev. Infect. Dis.,* 8:228–238.

———. 1988. Prevalence of *Entamoeba histolytica* Infection. In *Amebiasis. Human Infection by* Entamoeba histolytica. pp. 93–105. Ravdin, J.I., ed. New York: John Wiley & Sons.

This page intentionally blank.

Chapter 29

Giardia lamblia

Frank W. Schaefer, III

DESCRIPTION OF THE AGENT

Giardia lamblia is a protozoan parasite that infects numerous mammals, including humans, dogs, cats, beavers, and muskrats. Protozoa are unicellular animals that, unlike bacteria and viruses, possess membrane-bound genetic material (nuclei) and other assorted cellular organelles. They move and reproduce in various ways that are used to categorize them into broad groups (phyla); however, the taxonomy of the protozoa is still evolving. Protozoa fall into two broad nontaxonomic groupings depending on whether they are parasitic or free-living.

Parasitic forms live in or on another host organism, and this host–parasite interaction is always detrimental in some fashion to the host. In the case of *Giardia,* the parasite is found within the lumen of the small and large intestine, thus making it an enteric parasite. Most enteric protozoans have two stages in their life cycles, and because *Giardia* is an obligate parasite, it must have a host to complete its life cycle. The *Giardia* cyst is round to oval with dimensions ranging from 8 to 18 µm long by 5 to 15 µm wide. It has up to four nuclei, a claw-hammer-shaped median body (clusters of microtubules), and axonemes (basal portions of flagella within cytoplasm), which give the cyst the appearance of a face. Once inside the host, the cyst is stimulated to excyst and release an undifferentiated trophozoite in the duodenum. The trophozoite is an actively feeding, growing, and reproducing stage with two nuclei, a claw-hammer-shaped median body, and four pairs of bilaterally symmetrical flagella. The trophozoite is shaped like a pear cut in half lengthwise with dimensions ranging from 12 to 15 µm long by 6 to 8 µm wide. Stimuli in the host's intestinal tract induce *Giardia* to produce a resistant, dormant transmission form, which is referred to as a cyst.

Trophozoites generally do not survive outside the host unless they are in a special culture medium. While trophozoites are not thought to be a major mode of transmission, they are capable of initiating infections. Cysts survive for long periods outside the host, especially in cool water.

DESCRIPTION OF THE DISEASE

G. lamblia is known to produce gastrointestinal distress, including diarrhea, weight loss, flatulence, cramps, belching, distention, anorexia, vomiting, fatigue, mucus in the stool, and bloody and foul-smelling stool. The parasite can produce a continuum of pathologies ranging from no symptoms to illness requiring hospitalization. A complete understanding of how pathogenesis is produced is not available; however, the strain of parasite, along with the immune competency and health status of the host, are important factors.

The time from infection until parasites are seen is called the *prepatent period* and depends on the number of parasites in the dose, as well as the health and susceptibility of the host. In a study of human volunteers receiving 10 cysts, the prepatent period averaged 9.1 days. The mean prepatent period of American travelers to the Soviet Union was 12 to 15 days, with a range of 1 to 75 days. Individuals, especially those who are asymptomatic and receive no treatment, may remain infected, pass cysts, and be a source of infection for years.

Diagnosis is based on finding trophozoites or cysts in fecal material, or by demonstrating trophozoites from a duodenojejunal aspirate or biopsy. Because *G. lamblia* produces cysts intermittently in some individuals, finding cysts in fecal material may be difficult. Furthermore, the cyst densities vary depending on how many are being produced by the parasite. For these reasons, collecting three consecutive stools or collecting stool on alternate days for a week has been shown to increase test reliability. In addition to microscopic examination of sample cysts and trophozoites directly in a wet mount of stool, cysts may be concentrated from a stool using either formalethyl acetate sedimentation or zinc sulfate flotation.

Cysts are detected and confirmed using bright field microscopy and Lugol's iodine, which can reveal median bodies, axonemes, and nuclei. Once detected, the cysts are measured using a calibrated ocular micrometer to ensure that they fall within the correct size range. Recently, the use of immunofluorescent antibody stains and epifluorescent microscopy have gained acceptance as reliable diagnostic tools.

G. lamblia infections are susceptible to treatment with quinacrine (Atabrine), metronidazole (Flagyl), furizolidone (Furoxone), and paramomycin (Humatin). The drug of choice depends on the condition of the patient and the experience of the physician.

MODE OF TRANSMISSION

G. lamblia has a simple, direct life cycle, and is transmitted as a fecal contaminant of food or water. Person-to-person transmission has been shown and may take many forms. For example, institutional environments, such as day-care centers and nursing homes with poor hygiene, are well-documented sources of transmission. Sexual activity may also be a source of transmission. Animals, especially pets, may transmit the parasite to humans.

METHODS FOR DETECTING THE AGENT

Immunofluorescence detection is used to detect *Giardia* cysts in environmental water samples. To detect low levels of cysts, large volumes of water are sampled and, currently, *Giardia* cysts are concentrated from water by retention on a yarn-wound filter. Retained particulates and cysts are eluted from the filter and reconcentrated by centrifugation. Pellets of *Giardia* cysts are separated to some extent from other particulate debris by flotation on a Percoll-sucrose solution with a specific gravity of

1.1. A portion of the water/Percoll-sucrose interface is placed on a membrane filter to form a monolayer, stained with an indirect fluorescent antibody, and examined using epifluorescent microscopy. Cysts are classified according to specific criteria, including quality of immunofluorescence, size, shape, and internal morphological characteristics. The results are reported in terms of empty cysts, amorphous cysts with one internal structure, and cysts with more than one internal structure per 100 L. All these cyst categories are added together to calculate the total number of cyst-like objects detected per 100 L. The internal morphological structures that can be detected in some cysts include nuclei, axonenes, and median bodies. Efforts to improve sampling, processing, and detection of enteric parasitic protozoans have been published by the US Environmental Protection Agency (USEPA).

OCCURRENCE OF THE AGENT IN PEOPLE, ANIMALS, AND THE ENVIRONMENT

G. lamblia is cosmopolitan, including the arctic locations. Thirteen percent of adults and up to 50 percent of children may be infected but asymptomatic. *Giardia* is the most frequently identified protozoan parasite in the United States and Britain. Occurrences of clinical symptoms in these countries ranges between 2 and 20 percent, depending on the socioeconomic status and age of the group. A study by the Centers for Disease Control and Prevention (CDC) of stool samples from 55 state and territorial laboratories, found *Giardia* in 3.8 percent of 414,820 specimens examined.

Many mammalian reservoir hosts can carry the parasite. However, the degree to which *Giardia* infections in animals contribute to illness in man remains unclear. Few adequately controlled cross-species transmission studies have been reported. *G. lamblia*-like cysts have been observed in numerous mammals and birds, although isolates from the great blue heron are *G. ardeae* and not *G. lamblia*. Similarly, *G. psittaci* cysts from budgerigars (a small Australian parrot) resemble *Giardia* cysts from humans, but lack the trophozoite ventrolateral flange morphology required for *G. lamblia*. Efforts to infect laboratory mammals with *G. ardeae* and *G. psittaci* have been unsuccessful. Consequently, *Giardia* from birds is not likely to be a threat to humans. *Giardia* cysts isolated from humans have been transmitted to rats, gerbils, guinea pigs, beavers, dogs, cats, raccoons, bighorn sheep, mouflon sheep, and pronghorn sheep. Beavers can be infected with human *Giardia* cysts at doses ranging between 50 and 500 cysts.

SURVIVAL OF THE AGENT IN THE ENVIRONMENT

Temperature affects the viability of *Giardia* cysts. Human source cysts suspended in tap water and stored at –13, 8, 21, 37, and 100° C were evaluated for viability using *in vitro* excystation. Cysts exposed to freezing and thawing, as well as boiling did not survive. Cysts stored at 8, 21, and 37° C remained viable for up to 77, 24, and 4 days, respectively. In a study of storage conditions, *G. muris* cysts were suspended in lake water at 15 feet and at 30 feet as well as in river water. Cysts suspended in tap water and reagent water were stored in a laboratory refrigerator. In the lake water, cysts remained viable for 28 days at 15 feet and 56 days at 30 feet. The cysts exposed to river water remained viable for up to 28 days. Cysts stored in tap water were no longer viable after 14 days. The control cysts, which were stored in reagent water in the laboratory refrigerator, remained viable up to 84 days. The results explain why waterborne outbreaks of giardiasis in the United States have been found clustered in mountainous states, where water temperatures are low but not freezing.

DOCUMENTED WATERBORNE OUTBREAKS

Giardia is the most commonly identified pathogen in waterborne outbreaks in the United States. During the period 1971–1985, it was reported that 92 (18 percent) of the waterborne disease outbreaks were due to giardiasis, resulting in 24,124 cases of illness. By comparison, less than 2 percent of all reported cases of typhoid fever, salmonellosis, shigellosis, or infectious hepatitis have occurred as causes of waterborne outbreaks in the United States since 1951. Some of the more notable giardiasis outbreaks have occurred in Aspen, Colo., in 1965 to 1966; Rome, N.Y., in 1974 to 1975; Camas, Wash., in 1976; Berlin, N.H., in 1977; Vail and Estes Park, Colo., in 1978 and 1979; Bradford, Pa., in 1979; and Pittsfield, Mass., in 1986. For the period 1989 to 1990, *G. lamblia* was identified as the etiological agent for 7 of 12 outbreaks of gastroenteritis for which an agent was identified. Many of these waterborne giardiasis outbreaks involved surface water systems receiving only disinfection. Other outbreaks have occurred in systems using groundwater that were found to have been contaminated with feces. Most of these outbreaks have occurred in systems classified as small community systems, which have a minimum of 15 or more service connections supplying customers year-round. Perhaps less publicized are the outbreaks that have occurred in noncommunity systems, such as those in camps and parks that serve a transient, seasonal population.

EFFECTIVENESS OF WATER TREATMENT PROCESSES

Filtration processes, including diatomaceaous earth filtration, slow sand filtration, and coagulation–filtration, when applied appropriately, can remove *Giardia* cysts at levels of 99 percent or more. Chemical disinfectants, such as free chlorine, chloramine, chlorine dioxide, and ozone are known to inactivate, when appropriate conditions of pH, temperature, disinfectant concentration, and contact time (CT) are used. Disinfectant $C \times T$ (disinfectant concentration multiplied by contact time) required to inactivate 99 percent of *Giardia* cysts range from 9 to 342. Because all surface water is subject to contamination by *Giardia* cysts, a multiple-barrier approach to water treatment is the most prudent policy. In addition to good filtration and disinfection, this multiple-barrier system also must include watershed protection and distribution system maintenance as part of any plan designed to protect the health of the water consumer.

NATIONAL OR INTERNATIONAL GUIDELINES AND MONITORING RECOMMENDATIONS

Currently, there are no numerical US standards (maximum contaminant levels [MCL]) for *Giardia* cysts in water due to the limitations in monitoring methods. US regulations for drinking water are based on the Safe Drinking Water Act (SDWA) of 1974, which was amended in 1986. USEPA proposed filtration of all surface water supplies; however, the US Congress in the SDWA amendment of 1986 required USEPA to establish criteria to be used by the states to decide which water systems must filter. The final regulation was published by USEPA in 1989 and addressed treatment for *Giardia,* viruses, and *Legionella*. In brief, all water systems are required to provide treatment capable of removing or inactivating 99.9 percent of *Giardia* cysts, whether filtration is part of the treatment or not. As part of this rule, $C \times T$ tables for various disinfectants are supplied as well as requirements for effective filter operation.

INFORMATION SOURCES

Bingham, A.K., E.L. Jarroll, E.A. Meyer, and S. Radulescu. 1979. Introduction of *Giardia* Excystation and the Effect of Temperature on Cyst Viability as Compared by Eosin-Exclusion and In Vitro Excystation. In *Waterborne Transmission of Giardiasis*. Jakubowski, W., and J.C. Hoff, eds. USEPA, 600/9-79-001.

Brodsky, R.E., H.C. Spencer, and M.G. Schultz. 1974. Giardiasis in American Travelers to the Soviet Union. *J. Infect. Dis.,* 130:319–323.

Craun, G.F. 1990. Waterborne Giardiasis. In *Giardia and Giardiasis: Biology, Pathogenesis, and Epidemiology*. Erlandsen, S.L., and E.A. Meyer, eds. New York: Plenum Press.

Davidson, R.A. 1990. Treatment of Giardiasis: the North American Perspective. In *Human Parasitic Diseases, Volume 3: Giardiasis*. Meyer, E.A., ed. Amsterdam: Elsevier.

Davies, R.B., and C.B. Hibler. 1979. Animal Reservoirs and Cross-Species Transmission in *Giardia*. In *Waterborne Transmission of Giardiasis*. Jakubowski, W., and J.C. Hoff, eds. USEPA, 600/9-79-001.

deRegnier, D.P., L. Cole, D.G. Schupp, and S.L. Erlandsen. 1989. Viability of *Giardia* Cysts Suspended in Lake, River, and Tap Water. *Appl. Environ. Microbiol.,* 55:1223–1229.

Erlandsen, S.L., and W.J. Bemrick. 1987. SEM Evidence for a New Species, *Giardia psittaci*. *J. Parasitol.*, 73:623–629.

Erlandsen, S.L., W.J. Bemrick, C.L. Wells, D.E. Feely, L. Knudson, S.R. Campbell, H. van Keulen, and E.L. Jarroll. 1990. Axenic Culture and Characterization of *Giardia ardeae* from the Great Blue Heron *(Ardea herodias)*. *J. Parasitol.,* 76:717–724.

Erlandsen, S.L., W.J. Bemrick, and W. Jakubowski. 1991. Cross-species Transmission of Avian and Mammalian *Giardia* spp: Inoculation of Chicks, Ducklings, Budgerigars, Mongolian Gerbils and Neonatal Mice with *Giardia duodenalis (lamblia), Giardia psittaci,* and *Giardia muris*. *Intern. J. Environ. Health Res.,* 1:144–152.

Erlandsen, S.L., L.A. Sherlock, M. Januschka, D.G. Schupp, F.W. Schaefer, III, W. Jakubowski, and W.J. Bemrick. 1988. Cross-Species Transmission of *Giardia* spp: Inoculation of Beavers and Muskrats with Cysts of Human, Beaver, Mouse, and Muskrat Origin. *Appl. Environ. Microbiol.*, 54:2777–2785.

Fout, G.S., F.W. Schaefer, III, J.W. Messer, D.R. Dahling, and R.E. Stetler. 1996. *ICR Microbial Laboratory Manual*. EPA 600/R-95-178. USEPA.

Herwaldt, B.L., G.F. Craun, S.L. Stokes, and D.D. Juranek. 1991. Waterborne-Disease Outbreaks, 1989–1990. *MMWR CDC Surveillance Summary,* 40:1–21

Jarroll, E.L. 1988. Effect of Disinfectants on *Giardia* Cysts. *CRC Critical Reviews in Environmental Control*, 18:1–28.

Jokipii, A.M., M. Hemila, and L. Jokipii. 1985. Prospective Study of Acquisition of *Cryptosporidium, Giardia lamblia,* and Gastrointestinal Illness. *Lancet,* 2:487–489.

Lee, J.J., S.H. Hutner, and E.C. Lee. 1985. *An Illustrated Guide to the Protozoa.* Lawrence, Kan.: Society of Protozoologists.

Logsdon, G.S. 1988. Comparison of Some Filtration Processes Appropriate for *Giardia* Cyst Removal. In *Advances in Giardia Research*. Wallis, P.M., and B.R. Hammond, eds. Calgary, Alta.: University of Calgary Press.

Owen, R.L. 1984. Direct Fecal–Oral Transmission of Giardiasis. In *Giardia and Giardiasis: Biology, Pathogenesis, and Epidemiology*. Erlandsen, S.L., and E.A. Meyer, eds. New York: Plenum Press.

Rendtorff, R.C. 1954. The Experimental Transmission of Human Intestinal Protozoan Parasites. II. *Giardia lamblia* Given in Capsules. *Amer. J. Hygiene,* 59:509–517.

Schaefer, F.W., III. 1990. Methods for Excystation of *Giardia*. In *Human Parasitic Diseases, Volume 3: Giardiasis*. Meyer, E.A., ed. Amsterdam: Elsevier.

USEPA. 1989. National Primary Drinking Water Regulations: Filtration, Disinfection, Turbidity, *Giardia lamblia*, Viruses, *Legionella*, and Heterotrophic Bacteria *Federal Register,* 54:27486–27541.

———. 1998. *Method 1622: Cryptosporidium in Water by Filtration/IMS/FA*. EPA 821-R-98-010. USEPA.

Walzer, P.D., M.S. Wolfe, and M.G. Schultz. 1971. Giardiasis in Travelers. *J. Infect. Dis.,* 124:235–237.

Wolfe, M.S. 1990. Clinical Symptoms and Diagnosis by Traditional Methods. In *Human Parasitic Diseases, Volume 3: Giardiasis.* Meyer, E.A., ed. Amsterdam: Elsevier.

Chapter 30

Gnathostoma spinigerum

M. Dale Little

DESCRIPTION OF THE AGENT

Gnathostoma spinigerum in the family Gnathostomatidae is a robust roundworm that lives in nodules in the stomach walls of wild and domestic cats and dogs in Asia, especially Thailand and Japan. The worms do not develop to the adult stage in the stomach of humans, but immature stages may migrate extensively through somatic and cutaneous tissues causing pain and swelling of the affected parts. While *G. spinigerum* is the species that most commonly infects people, others include *G. doloresi, G. hispidum,* and *G. nipponicum* in Asia, and *G. binucleatum* in Mexico.

The parasite has a complicated life cycle that involves first and second intermediate hosts, paratenic hosts, and hosts that harbor the adult worms. Eggs passed in the feces of the infected mammal develop into embryos in water in about one week. First-stage larvae hatch and swim in the water where they are eaten by microcrustaceans, such as species of *Cyclops* and other genera of copepods. In about two weeks, larvae develop to the third stage in the body cavity of the copepod. When the copepod is ingested by a frog, fish, snake, bird, or mammal, larvae migrate into tissues of the animal and persist there for long periods. In the case of a cat or dog, larvae eventually migrate to the stomach where they mature to the adult stage. Cats and dogs may also become infected by eating infected second intermediate or paratenic hosts, i.e., frogs, fish, snakes, birds, or small mammals.

Persons may become infected by ingesting an infected copepod or by eating the uncooked flesh of an infected paratenic or second intermediate host. Most human infections are acquired by eating raw fish. Other species of *Gnathostoma* known to infect humans have similar life cycles, although the host in which the adult worms live, the definitive host, may be different. *G. doloresi* and *G. hispidum* are natural parasites of pigs, *G. nipponicum* is a parasite of the Japanese weasel, and *G. binucleatum* is a parasite of wild felines.

DESCRIPTION OF THE DISEASE

Immature worms of *Gnathostoma* migrate through the cutaneous tissues in various parts of the body over a few days to many months. Intermittent migratory swellings (creeping eruptions) that are mildly to severely painful are characteristic of this infection. Usually, the swellings are inflamed and an elevated peripheral eosinophilia is present. Infrequently, worms may invade the eye, pulmonary tract, central nervous system, or visceral organs. The disease produced in infections with species other than *G. spinigerum* is essentially the same.

Diagnosis is usually based on the distinct clinical features of the infection and a history of eating raw or inadequately cooked flesh of freshwater fish, chicken, snake, frog, or small mammal, or drinking water from an unprotected source. However, definitive diagnosis can only be made by recovering the worm from the tissues and identifying it as *G. spinigerum* or some other species of *Gnathostoma*.

Gnathostomiasis is endemic throughout Southeast Asia and in Japan, but the prevalence is highest in Thailand. Sporadic cases have been reported in Ecuador and Argentina, and in recent years more than 200 cases have been reported from several states in Mexico.

RESERVOIRS FOR THE AGENT

Cats and dogs are hosts of the adult worms of *G. spinigerum,* and a wide variety of freshwater fish, reptiles, amphibia, birds, and mammals are second intermediate and paratenic hosts of the parasite, i.e., hosts of the third-stage larva that infects humans. The stage developing in the copepod also can infect people.

MODE OF TRANSMISSION

Persons may become infected by drinking water containing infected copepods or by eating the raw or inadequately cooked flesh of an animal, especially fish, containing the third-stage larva of the parasite. Infections in humans cannot be transmitted to another person.

METHODS FOR DETECTING THE AGENT

In water obtained from ponds and other stationary bodies, the larvae stages that infect people only occur in copepods. These microcrustaceans may be collected from standing water by a plankton sampling net. Recovered copepods are examined under a stereomicroscope for the presence of *Gnathostoma* larvae in their body cavity.

OCCURRENCE OF THE AGENT IN PEOPLE, ANIMALS, AND THE ENVIRONMENT

G. spinigerum is common in wild animals in the Far East, and the infection in people is endemic in that area. It is not known to occur in the United States and Canada. A new species causing human infections in Mexico has recently been described, *G. binucleatum*; its definitive host is the ocelot. Three other species have been reported in wild animals in North America, *G. didelphis* in the kidney of opossums (*Didelphis virginia*), *G. procyonis* in the stomach wall of raccoons (*Procyon lotor lotor*), and *G. miyazakii* in the kidney of otters. Autochthonous human cases have not been reported in the United States or Canada.

SURVIVAL OF THE AGENT IN THE ENVIRONMENT

The majority of copepods infected with *Gnathostoma* larvae will live only a few weeks but some have been reported to survive for as long as eight weeks in the laboratory. The life span of the advanced third-stage larvae in the tissues of the second intermediate hosts and paratenic hosts is unknown, but they may remain alive for much of the life span of these host animals.

INFORMATION SOURCES

Almeyda-Artigas, R.J. 1991. Finding of *Gnathostoma binucleatum* n. sp. (Nematoda:Spirurida) in Wild Felids and the Role of Fresh-Water and Oligohaline Fishes as Human Gnathostomiasis Vectors in the Lower Basin of Papaloapan River, Oaxaca-Veracruz, Mexico. *An. Inst. Cienc. del Mar y Limnol. Univ. Nat. Autón. México*, 18:137–155.

American Public Health Association, American Water Works Association, and Water Environment Federation. 1995. *Standard Methods for the Examination of Water and Wastewater.* 19th ed. Eaton, A.D., L.S. Clesceri, and A.E. Greenberg, eds. Washington, D.C.: APHA.

Daengsvang, S. 1980. *A Monograph on the Genus* Gnathostoma *and Gnathostomiasis in Thailand*. Tokyo: Southeast Asian Medical Information Center.

Sunthatasamai, P., M. Rignati, S. Chittamas, and V. Desakorn. 1992. Albendazole Stimulates Outward Migration of *Gnathostoma Spinigerum* to the Dermis in Man. *S.E. Asian J. Trop. Med. Pub. Hlth.*, 23:716–722.

This page intentionally blank.

Chapter 31

Isospora belli

Lynne S. Garcia

DESCRIPTION OF THE AGENT

Isospora belli was first described by Virchow in 1860, and was officially named by Wenyon in 1923. This coccidian is included in the family Eimeriidae and produces oocysts, long and oval, 20 to 33 µm in length by 10 to 19 µm in width (Table 31-1). *I. belli* is the only member of the genus that is parasitic to humans, but many species of *Isospora* are found in wild and domestic animals.

Schizogonic and sporogonic stages in the life cycle of *I. belli* have been described from human intestinal mucosal biopsies. Development in the intestine usually occurs within the epithelial cells of the distal duodenum and proximal jejunum and eventually oocysts are passed with the stool. Usually the oocyst contains only one immature sporont, however, two may also be present. Development continues outside the host where it matures into twin sporocysts, each containing four sporozoites. The sporulated oocyst is the infective stage that excysts in the small intestine, releasing the sporozoites that penetrate the mucosal cells and initiate the life cycle. The life cycle stages are schizonts, merozoites, gametocytes, gametes, and oocysts, and are structurally similar to other coccidia.

DESCRIPTION OF THE DISEASE

Clinical symptoms include foul smelling, foaming diarrhea, which may last for months to years, causing weight loss, abdominal colic, and fever. Patients who are

Table 31-1 Characteristics of *Isospora belli*

Species	Shape and Size	Other Features
Isospora belli	Ellipsoidal oocyst; usual range 20–30 µm long, 10–19 µm wide; sporocysts rarely seen broken out of oocysts, but measure 9–11 µm	Mature cocyst contains two sporocysts with four sporozoites each; usual diagnostic state in feces is immature oocyst containing spherical mass of protoplasm (diarrhea) (intestinal tract)

immunosuppressed, particularly those with acquired immune deficiency syndrome (AIDS), often experience profuse diarrhea associated with weakness, anorexia, and weight loss. The diarrheal and other symptoms may be persistent under immunosuppressive therapy. This infection has been reported in homosexual men, all of whom were immunocompromised and had diarrhea for several months.

Examination of a fecal specimen for the oocysts is recommended. However, wet preparation examination of fresh material either as the direct smear or as concentrated material is preferable to the permanent stained smear. The oocysts are very pale and transparent and can easily be overlooked. They can also be very difficult to see if the concentration sediment is performed from polyvinyl alcohol (PVA)-preserved stool. The light level should be reduced, and additional contrast obtained with the microscope for optimal examination. Oocysts may not be recovered even with a positive biopsy specimen if small numbers of organisms are present. In a patient with diarrhea, the oocyst usually contains only a single sporoblast. These organisms are acid-fast and can also be demonstrated by using auramine-rhodamine stains. Organisms tentatively identified *I. belli* with auramine-rhodamine stains should be confirmed by wet smear examination or acid-fast stains, particularly if the stool contains other cells or excess artifact material as in a stool with more normal consistency. Charcot-Leyden crystals derived from eosinophils are often seen in fecal specimens from infected individuals.

RESERVOIRS FOR THE AGENT

I. belli is thought to be the only species of *Isospora* that infects humans; however, many different species of *Isospora* infect a wide range of carnivores and passeriform birds, as well as amphibians, reptiles, rodents, swine, and primates other than humans.

MODE OF TRANSMISSION

I. belli is transmitted through ingestion of water or food contaminated with mature, sporulated oocysts. The parasite may be transmitted sexually by direct oral contact with the anus or perineum, although this mode of transmission is probably much less common. The oocysts are very resistant to environmental conditions and may remain viable for months if kept cool and moist. Diagnostic methods for laboratory examinations may tend to miss the organisms when they are present. Because transmission is via the infective oocysts, prevention centers on improved personal hygiene measures and sanitary conditions to eliminate possible fecal–oral transmission from contaminated food, water, and environmental surfaces.

METHODS FOR DETECTING THE AGENT

No specific environmental detection methods are available. The same methods for identifying other protozoan parasites (amoebas and flagellates) can be used. Potential problems are the lack of specific monoclonal-based reagents for high specificity and recovery of low organism numbers. The oocysts will stain with auramine-rhodamine and modified acid-fast stains, both of which could be used on environmental isolates. However, oocysts from *I. belli* would have to be differentiated from those found in other animal hosts.

OCCURRENCE OF THE AGENT IN PEOPLE, ANIMALS, AND THE ENVIRONMENT

Although *I. belli* is cosmopolitan, certain tropical areas in the western hemisphere have well-defined locations of endemic infections. These organisms can infect both adults and children, and intestinal involvement and symptoms are generally transient unless the patient is immunocompromised. *I. belli* has also been implicated in traveler's diarrhea.

SURVIVAL OF THE AGENT IN THE ENVIRONMENT

The oocysts of coccidia can withstand exposure to various chemical and physical agents that harm most organisms. The oocyst wall is remarkable in its ability to protect the oocyst contents. Studies indicate that sunlight for as short a time as 4 hours and freezing below about –7° C were lethal for a relative, *Eimeria zuernii,* and survival was directly proportional to relative humidity. Environmental infectivity studies using oocysts from chickens have demonstrated that *E. acervulina* could be recovered from soil plots as long as 86 weeks. *E. tenella* and *E. maxima* oocysts of *I. belli* disappeared from all experimental soil plots in less than a year's time. No severe infection with any of the three species was produced after 34 weeks.

DOCUMENTED WATERBORNE OUTBREAKS

There are no documented waterborne outbreaks of *I. belli.*

EFFECTIVENESS OF WATER TREATMENT PROCESSES

Disinfection studies have not been carried out, but effective coagulation and filtration or slow sand filtration should be effective.

INFORMATION SOURCES

Beaver, P.C., R.C. Jung, and E.W. Cupp. 1984. *Clinical Parasitology.* 9th ed. Philadelphia, Pa.: Lea and Febiger.

Forthal, D.N., and S.S. Guest. 1984. *Isospora belli* Enteritis in Three Homosexual Men. *Am. J. Trop. Med. Hyg.,* 33:1060–1064.

Garcia, L.S., and D.A. Bruckner. 1997. Diagnostic Medical Parasitology. 3rd ed. Washington, D.C.: ASM Press.

Garcia, L.S., S. Bullock-Iacullo, J. Palmer, and R.Y. Shimizu. 1995. Diagnosis of Parasitic Infections: Collection, Processing and Examination of Specimens. In *Manual of Clinical Microbiology*, 6th ed. Murray, P.R., E.J. Baron, M.A. Pfaller, F.C. Tenover, and R.H. Yolken, eds. American Society for Microbiology.

Hammond, D.M. 1973. Life Cycles and Development of Coccidia. In *The Coccidia*. Hammond, D.M., and P.L. Long, eds. Baltimore, Md.: University Park Press.

Godiwala, T., and R. Yaeger. 1987. *Isospora* and Traveler's Diarrhea. *Annals Intern. Med.,* 106:909–910.

National Committee for Clinical Laboratory Standards. 1993. Procedures for the Recovery and Identification of Parasites from the Intestinal Tract, Proposed Guideline, M28-P. Villanova, Pa.: National Committee for Clinical Laboratory Standards.

Ng, E., E.K. Markell, R.I. Fleming, and M. Fried. 1984. Demonstration of *Isospora belli* by Acid-Fast Stain in a Patient with Acquired Immune Deficiency Syndrome. *J. Clin. Microbiol.,* 20:384–386.

This page intentionally blank.

Chapter 32

Microsporidia

Ann Cali

DESCRIPTION OF THE AGENT

Microsporidia is the common name for a group of spore-forming, intracellular, obligate (requiring a host) protozoan parasites of the phylum Microspora. The source of the name for this group is the small, resistant spore, which has a single, long, coiled polar tubule. The tubule everts when ingested and the reproduction portion of its life cycle is intracellular; spores are very resistant to environmental factors and serve as the main source of transmission to other hosts.

Within the order Microsporidia are approximately 20 families, a hundred genera, and hundreds of species. The Microsporidia are ubiquitous, infecting every major group of animals and man Insects, fish, and mammals are the host groups containing the majority of the known Microsporidia. Consequently, their spores are found throughout the environment. In humans, Microsporidia are considered opportunistic, occurring in immune compromised individuals or immune privileged locations, such as the eye. About a dozen different types of Microsporidia are known to infect man.

The microsporidian life cycle is divided into three phases—infective, proliferative, and sporogonic. The infective phase contains the spore stage, from its completed development in a host cell to the stimulus that triggers the eversion of the long polar tubule. This event initiates a new infection and may occur within an infected host with autoinfective spores. This event may also occur in the external environment, when spores are passed out of the body in feces, urine, or other body fluids that may contaminate other individuals or their food. Infective and environmental spores must be properly stimulated by pH or specific ions in order to extrude their polar tubule. The forceful eversion of the polar tubule enables it to pierce a host cell.

The sporoplasm then emerges through the tubule and passes inside a proper host cell, and the proliferative phase begins. Parasite growth and division produce many organisms within the host cell cytoplasm. The sporogonic phase of spore formation is usually indicated by secretions deposited on the parasite plasmalemma, commonly called a *thickened membrane*. These cells (sporonts) may undergo from one to many cell divisions before they become sporoblasts. After the last cell division, the resulting sporoblast cells undergo a metamorphosis into spores.

Because some spores are autoinfective, they evert their polar tubules within the same host in which they were formed, which provides additional sites of infection. The number of spores produced in sporogony, how they are produced, and the host–parasite interface all contribute to genus determination. Three types of host-parasite interfaces are (1) direct contact with the host cells' cytoplasm, (2) indirect contact with the host cells' cytoplasm through an envelope secreted by the parasite called a *sporophorous vesicle* or *pansporoblast*, and (3) indirect contact by production of a parasite-and-host-produced vacuole-like envelope called *aparasitophorous vacuole*.

The transmissible stage of the Microsporidia is the spore. Among the Microsporidia that infect humans, spore sizes range from 1 µm × 0.7 µm to 5 µm × 3 µm. The more common species are in the 1 to 2 µm range. The most distinguishing feature of the spores is the tubule inside the spore. The tubule can sometimes be forced to evert on a microscope slide. The spore's highly refractile coat is visible by phase contrast microscopy of water containing spores or infected cells.

DESCRIPTION OF THE DISEASE

A dozen microsporidian species infect humans. The disease and associated symptoms vary considerably, and depend on the species organism causing the infection. The most commonly reported species are those that infect the intestinal tract (with diarrhea and wasting as the presenting symptoms) and ocular infections causing a keratoconjunctivitis. Among the organisms producing these two clinical syndromes are disseminating species that can cause a myriad of other clinical symptoms. The incubation period is not known. Diagnosis is by microscopic observation of the spore stage collected in fecal samples, biopsies, scrapings, or body fluids. Scattered data on prevalence averages around 25 percent for chronic diarrhea patients.

RESERVOIRS FOR THE AGENT

Encephalitozoon cuniculi, originally described in rabbits and other laboratory animals, is now known to infect two types of birds and over 30 types of mammals, including dogs, cats, rodents, and humans. Most organisms described in humans have not been reported in animals. As Microsporidia are so newly described and so ubiquitous in the environment, other reservoirs are likely.

MODE OF TRANSMISSION

Microsporidia produce a resistant spore stage that survives in the environment and is responsible for infection in new hosts. Those that pass from the body in feces, urine, or other body fluids may contaminate hands, food, clothing, ground, and water. Infection by ingestion is the most common route of infection, but ocular infections could occur by touching the eyes with contaminated fingers. In both instances, water could be a source of infection if the spores are present. Microsporidia are probably as ubiquitous in humans as they are in other organisms, but they may be self-limiting and thus undiagnosed in the immune competent population. Undiagnosed hosts could, however, be responsible for producing great numbers of spores in the environment.

METHODS FOR DETECTING THE AGENT

Detecting environmental spores first requires collection, which may be accomplished in a number of ways. For large quantities of water, a series of progressively smaller sieves should be used to remove other organisms and debris. Microscopic contents can then be concentrated by continuous flow centrifugation at 10,000 rpm into 50-mL tubes. Sediment from these tubes or any other samples may be examined live by phase contrast microscopy. Fresh, unfixed material may be placed on the slide in a small amount of water, cover slipped, and examined on high power. Microsporidian spores are very refractile and many light microscopes equipped for birefringence can be used. Both fresh and fixed spores may be seen in this way.

Other followup procedures should be used on suspected microsporidian spores. Forcing the spore to extrude its polar tubule is positive proof of live material. Seeing the polar tubule in the spore with an electron microscope is the best evidence, although many light microscopic stains can demonstrate the spore's presence. PAS stain (see glossary) reveals a small granule at the anterior end of the spore, which is also diagnostic. For fixed material, Giemsa, Heidenhain iron hematoxylin, Warthin-Starry silver stain, Gomori methenamine silver (GMS) gram stains are the best light microscopy stains for demonstrating spores. General fluorescent stains such as calciflour that combine with the chitinized spore coat or specific fluorescent antibody stains to particular Microsporidia can be used for identification.

OCCURRENCE OF THE AGENT IN PEOPLE, ANIMALS, AND THE ENVIRONMENT

More than 1,000 species of Microsporidia are ubiquitous in nature and infect a wide range of vertebrate and invertebrate hosts. Table 32-1 indicates the incidences of Microsporidia reported in humans.

SURVIVAL OF THE AGENT IN THE ENVIRONMENT

The survival of Microsporidia varies from species to species. Most research has focused on the animal Microsporidia. In insects, some survive a very short time while others survive for years. Some specific studies include the effects of ultraviolet (UV) light and the density of living and dead microsporidian spores. Waller found the viability and infectivity of *E. cuniculi* spores lasted up to four months in the environment, and reported their sensitivity to various temperatures, disinfectants, and drugs.

INFORMATION SOURCES

Ashton, N., and P.A. Wirasinha. 1973. Encephalitozoonosis of the Cornea. *British Journal of Ophthalmology*, 57:669–674.

Avery, S.W., and A.H. Undeen. 1987. The Isolation of *Microsporidia* and Other Pathogens from Concentrated Ditch Water. *J. Am. Mosq. Control Assoc.*, 3(1):54–58.

Bryan, R.T., A. Cali, R.L. Owen, and H.C. Spencer. 1991. *Microsporidia: opportunistic pathogens in patients with AIDS*. Trans. Sun, T. Progress in Clinical Parasitology, 2. New York: Field & Wood Medical Publishers.

Cali, A. 1986. Comparison of the Biology and Pathology of Microsporidia from Different Host Groups. Trans. In *Fundamental and Applied Aspects of Invertebrate Pathology.* pp. 356–359. Samson, R.A., and J.M. Peters, eds. Foundation for the 4th International Colloquium on Invertebrate Pathology. Wageningen, The Netherlands.

Table 32-1 Microsporidia reported in humans

Microsporidian Family	Genus, Species, and Spore Size	Tissues Infected	Manifestations
Enterocytozoonidae	*Enterocytozoon bieneusi*, 1–1.6 × 0.7–1 μm	Intestinal enterocytes Hepatobiliary tract	Diarrhea Hepatitis
Encephalitozoonidae	*Encephalitozoon cuniculi*, 2–2.5 × 1–1.5 μm	Hepatobiliary tract	Hepatitis Peritonitis
	Encephalitozoon-like or sp.,* 2–2.5 × 1–1.5 μm	Ocular conjunctiva	Keratoconjunctivitis
	Encephalitozoon hellem† (Disseminating), 2–2.5 × 1–1.5 μm	Ocular conjunctiva Sinuses, lung, urinary Male genito-urinary tract	Keratoconjunctivitis Sinusitis Renal failure
	Septata intestinalis‡ (Disseminating), 2.0 × 1–1.2 μm	Enterocytes, lamina propria Biliary tree Urinary tract Ocular conjunctiva Sinusitis and respiratory tract	Diarrhea Infected gall bladder Renal failure Keratoconjunctivitis
Pleistophoridae	*Pleistophora* sp., 4 × 2 μm	Skeletal muscle	Myositis
?	*Trachipleistophora hominis*, 4 × 2.4 μm	Skeletal muscle	Myositis
Nosematidae	*Nosema connori*, 4–4.5 × 2–2.5 μm	Intestinal/disseminated	Diarrhea
	Nosema-like,§ 3 × 2 μm	Skeletal muscle	Myositis
?	*Vittaforma corneae* (*Nosema corneum*), 3.7 × 1 μm	Corneal stroma	Blindness
	Nosema ocularum, 5 × 3 μm	Corneal stroma	Blindness
	Brachiola vesicularum 2.9 × 2 μm	Skeletal muscle	Myositis
Unknown affiliation	*Microsporidium africanum*, 4.5–5 × 2.5–3 μm	Corneal stroma	Blindness
	Microsporidium ceylonensis, 3.5 × 1.5 μm	Corneal stroma	Blindness

*These reports were published before *E. hellem* was described and are probably that organism.

†Parasite has been reported to infect many tissues; only primary ones are listed here.

‡Parasite has been reported to infect enterocyte, macrophage, fibroblastic, and endothelial cells, resulting in reports of infection in many tissues. Only some are listed here.

§This report published before *Brachiola vesicularum* described. It is the same organism.

———. 1993. Cytological and Taxonomical Comparison of Two Intestinal Disseminating Microsporidioses. *AIDS*, 7:S12–S16.

Cali, A., and R.L. Owen. 1988. Microsporidiosis. In *The Laboratory Diagnosis of Infectious Diseases: Principles and Practice*, Vol. 1. pp. 929–950. Ballows, A.J., J.W.J. Hausler, M. Ohashi, and A. Turano, eds. New York: Springer-Verlag.

———. 1990. Intracellular Development of *Enterocytozoon*, a Unique Microsporidian Found in the Intestine of AIDS Patients. *J. Protozool.*, 37:145–155.

Cali, A., D.M. Meisler, C.Y. Lowder, R. Lembach, L. Ayers, P.M. Takvorian, I. Rutherford, D.L. Longworth, J. McMahon, and R.T. Bryan. 1991. Corneal Microsporidioses: Characterization and Identification. *J. Protozool.*, 38:2158–2178.

Cali, A., D.P. Kotler, and J.M. Orenstein. 1993. Septata Intestinalis N. G., N. Sp., an Intestinal Microsporidian Associated with Chronic Diarrhea and Dissemination in AIDS Patients. *J. Eukaryotic Micro.*, 40:101–112.

Cali, A., P.M. Takvorain, S. Lewin, M. Rendel, C. Sian, M. Wittner, and L.M. Weiss. 1996. Identification of a New Nosema-Like Microsporidian Associated with Myositis in an AIDS Patient. *J. Eukaryotic Micro.*, 43:108S.

Cali, A., P.M. Takvorian, S. Lewin, M. Rendel, C.S. Sian, M. Wittner, H.B. Tanowitz, E. Keohane, and L.M. Weiss. 1998. Brachioloa Vesicularum, N. G., N. Sp., a New Microsporidium Associated with AIDS and Myositis. *J. Eukaryotic Micro.*, 45:240–151.

Canning, E.U., and J. Lom. 1986. *The Microsporidia of Vertebrates*. London: Academic Press.

Canning, E.U., A. Curry, C.J.N. Laccy, and J.D. Fenwick. 1992. Ultrastructure of Encepluilitozoon sp. Infecting the Conjunctival, Corneal and Nasal Epithelia of a Patient with AIDS. *Europ. J. Protistol.*, 28:226–237.

Chupp, G.L., J. Alroy, L.S. Adelman, J.C. Breen, and P.R. Skolnik. 1993. Myositis Due to Pleistophora (Microsporidia) in a Patient with AIDS. *Clin. Infect. Dis.*, 16:15–21.

Desportes, I., Y. LeCharpentier, A. Galian, F. Bernard, B. Cochand-Priollet, A. Lavergne, F. Ravisse, and R. Modigliani. 1985. Occurrence of a New Microsporidian: *Enterocytozoon bieneusi* N. G., N. Sp. in the Enterocytes of a Human Patient with AIDS. *J. Protozool.*, 32:250–254.

Desser, S.S., H. Hong, and Y.J. Yang. 1992. Ultrastructure of the Development of a Species of Encephalitozoon Cultured from the Eye of an AIDS Patient. *Parasitol. Res.*, 78:677–683.

Didier, E.S., P.J. Didier, D.N. Friedberg, S.M. Stenson, J.M. Orenstein, R.W. Yee, F.O. Tio, R.M. Davis, C. Vossbrinck, N. Millichamp, and J.A. Shadduck. 1991. Isolation and Characterization of a New Human Microsporidian. *Encephalitozoon hellem* (N. Sp.) from Three AIDS Patients with Keratoconjunctivitis. *J. Infect. Dis.*, 163:617–621.

Dore, G.J., D.J. Marriott, M.C. Hing, J.L. Harkness, and A.S. Field. 1995. Disseminated Microsporidiosis Due to Septata Intestinal in Nine Patients Infected with the Human Immunodeficiency Virus: Response to Therapy with Albendazole. *Clin. Infect. Dis.*, 21:70–76.

Hollister, W.S., E.U. Canning, E. Weidner, A.S. Field, J. Kench, and D.J. Marriott. 1996. Development and Ultrastructure of *Trachipleisophora hominis* N.G., N. Sp. After in vitro Isolation from an AIDS Patient with Inoculation into Athymic Mice. *Parasitology*, 112:143–154.

Ledford, D.K., N.D. Overman, A. Gonzalvo, A. Calli, S.W. Mester, and R.F. Lockey. 1985. Microsporidiosis Myositis in a Patient with the Acquired Immunodeficiency Syndrome. *Annals Intern. Med.*, 102:628–630.

Levine, N.D., J.O. Corliss, F.E.G. Cox, G. Deroux, J. Grain, B.M. Honigberg, F. Leedale, A.R. Loeblich, J. Lom, D. Lynn, E.G. Merinfeld, F.C. Page, G. Poljansky, V. Sprague, J. Vavra, and F.G. Wallace. 1980. A Newly Revised Classification of the Protozoa. *J. Protozool.*, 27:37–58.

Lowder, C.Y., J.T. McMahon, D.M. Meisler, E.M. Dodds, L.H. Calabrese, E.S. Didier, and A. Cali. 1996. Microsporidial Keratoconjunctivitis Caused by *Septata intestinalis* in a Patient with Acquired Immunodeficiency Syndrome. *Amer. J. Ophth.*, 121:715–717.

Luna, L.G. 1971. *Manual of Histologic Methods of the Armed Forces Institute of Pathology.* New York: McGraw-Hill.

Margileth, M., A.J. Strano, R. Chandra, and R. Neifie. 1973. Disseminated Nosematosis in an Immunologically Compromised Infant. *Arch. Pathol.,* 95:145–150.

McWhinney, P.H.M., D. Nathwani, S.T. Green, J.F. Boyd, and J.A.H. Forrest. 1991. Microsporidiosis Detected in Associated with AIDS-Related Sclerosing Cholangitis. *AIDS*, 5:1394–1395.

Modigliani, R., C. Bories, Y. LeCharpentier, M. Salmeron, B. Messing, A. Galian, J.C. Rambaud, A. Lavergne, B. Cochand-Priollet, and I. Desportes. 1985. Diarrhoea and Malabsorption in Acquired Immune Deficiency Syndrome: A Study of Four Cases with Special Emphasis on Opportunistic Protozoan Infestations. *Gut*, 26:179–187.

Molina, J.-M., D.T. Dieterich, and D.P. Kotler. 1992. Systemic Dissemination by a Newly Recognized Intestinal Microsporidia Species in AIDS. *AIDS*, 6:1143–1150.

Orenstein, J.M., D.T. Dieterich, and D.P. Kotler. 1992. Systemic Dissemination by a Newly Recognized Intestinal Microsporidia Species in AIDS. *AIDS*, 6:1143–1150.

Orenstein, J. 1992. In *Workshop on Intestinal Microsporidia in HIV Infection*, Paris.

Pinnolis, M., P.R. Egbert, R.L. Font, and F.C. Winter. 1981. Nosematosis of the Cornea Case Report, Including Electron Microscopic Studies. *Arch. Ophth.,* 99:1044–1047.

Pol, S., C. Romana, S. Richard, F. Carnot, J. Dumont, H. Bouche, G. Pialoux, M. Stern, J. Pays, and P. Berthelot. 1992. *Enterocytozoon bieneusi* Infection in Acquired Immunodeficiency Syndrome-Related Sclerosing Cholangitis. *Gasteroentology,* 102:1778–1781.

Schwartz, D.A., A. Cali, G.S. Visvesvara, D. Roseberger, K.O. Hewan-Lowe, and R.T. Bryan. 1993. A Nasal Microsporidian with Unusual Features from a Patient with AIDS. Trans. In International Conference on AIDS, Vol. 1. pp. abstr. PO-1495.

Schwartz, D.A., G.S. Visvesvara, G.J. Leitch, L. Tashjian, M. Pollack, J. Holden, and R.T. Bryan. 1993. Pathology of Symptomatic Microsporidial (*Encephalitozoon hellem*) Bronchiolitis in the Acquired Immunodeficiency Syndrome: A New Respiratory Pathogen Diagnosed from Lung Biopsy, Bronchoalveolar Lavage, Sputum, and Tissue Culture. *Human Pathology,* 24:937–943.

Schwartz, D.A., G.S. Visvesvara, R. Weber, and R.T. Bryan. 1994. Male Genital Tract Microsporidiosis and AIDS: Prostatic Abscess due to *Encephalitozoon Hellem*. *J. Eukaryotic Micro.,* 41:61S

Schwartz, D.A., I. Sobottka, G.J. Leitch, A. Cali, G.S. Visvesvara. 1996. Pathology of Microsporidiosis—Emerging Parasitic Infections in Patients with AIDS. *Arch Pathol. & Lab. Med.,* 120:173–183.

Shadduck, J.A., R.A. Mccoli, R. Davis, and R.L. Font. 1990. Isolation of a Microsporidian from a Human Patient. *J. Infect. Dis.,* 162:773–776.

Silveira, H., and E. Canning. 1995. Vittaforma Corneae N. Comb. for the Human Microsporidiuam Nosema Corneum Shadduck, Meccoli, Davis & Font, 1990, Based on Its Ultrastructure in the Liver of Experimentally Infected Athymic Mice. *J. Eukaryotic Micro.,* 42:158–165.

Sprague, V., J. Becnel, and E. Hazard. 1992. Taxonomy of Phylum Microspora *Crit. Rev. in Microbiol.,* 18(5/6):285–395.

Sprague, V., and J.J. Becnel. 1998. Note on the Name-Author-Date Combination for the Taxon Microsporidies Balbiani, 1882, When Ranked as a Phylum. *J. Invert. Pathol.,* 71:91–94.

Strano, A.J., A. Cali, and R. Neafie. 1976. Microsporidiosis. In *Pathology of Tropical and Extraordinary Diseases*, Vol. 1, pp. 336–339. Binford, C.H., and D.H. Connor, eds. Armed Forces Institute of Pathology Press.

Terada, S., K. Reddy, L.J. Jeffers, A. Cali and E.R. Schiff. 1987. Microsporidian Hepatitis in the Acquired Immunodeficiency Syndrome. *Annals Intern. Med.* 107:61–62.

Undeen, A.H., and S.W. Avery. 1983. Continuous Flow-Density Gradient Centrifugation for Purification of *Microsporidia* Spores. *J. Invert. Pathol.,* 42:405–406.

Undeen, A.H., and R.K. Vander Meer. 1990. The Effect of Ultraviolet Radiation on the Germination of *Nosema algerae* Vavra and Undeen (Microsporidia: Nosematidae) Spores. *J. Protozool.,* 37(3):194–199.

Undeen, A.H., and L.F. Solter. 1996. The Sugar Content and Density of Living and Dead Microsporidian (protozoa: microspora) spores. *J. Invert. Pathol.*, 67:80–91.

Waller, T. 1979. Sensitivity of *Encephalitozoon cuniculi* to Various Temperatures, Disinfectants and Drugs. *Lab Anim.*, 13:227–230.

Weber, R., H. Kuster, G.S. Visvesvara, R.T. Bryan, D.A. Schwart, and R. Luthy. 1993. Disseminated Microsporidosis Due to *Encephalitozoon hellem*: Pulmonary Colonization, Microhematuria, and Mild Conjunctivitis in a Patient with AIDS. *Clin. Infect. Dis.,* 17:415–419.

Weber, R., R.T. Bryan, D.A. Schwartz, and R.L. Owen. 1994. Human Microsporidial Infections. *Clinical Microbiol. Reviews*, 7:426–461.

Zender, H., O. Arrigoni, J. Eckert, and Y. Kapanci. 1989. A Case of *Encephalitozoon cuniculi* peritonitis in a Patient with AIDS. *Am. J. Clin. Pathol.,* 92:352–356.

This page intentionally blank.

Chapter 33

Naegleria fowleri

Govidina S. Visvesvara

DESCRIPTION OF THE AGENT

Small, free-living amoebas belonging to the genus *Naegleria* are commonly found in soil, fresh water, sewage, and sludge. *Naegleria* normally feed on bacteria and multiply in their environmental niche as free-living organisms. They can also cause a fatal disease of the central nervous system (CNS) in humans and feed on human tissue.

Naegleria fowleri and other members of the genus *Naegleria* are also called *ameboflagellates* because of a flagellate stage in addition to the trophozoite and the cyst stages in their life cycle. The trophozoite of *N. fowleri* is a small limax-like amoeba that measures 10 to 35 µm in size and moves with a smooth hemispherical bulge from its body. The uroid or the posterior end is sticky and often has several trailing filaments. The cytoplasm contains a number of dumbbell-shaped mitochondria and abundant ribosomes. All stages of the organism have a single nucleus, although binucleate forms are occasionally seen in the trophic stage. The nucleus has a large, dense, centrally placed nucleolus. The amoebas reproduce by binary division. During the nuclear division, the nucleolus and the nuclear membrane persist and the nucleolus divides to form polar bodies. This type of nuclear division is called *promitosis*.

The pear-shaped biflagellate stage is a transient nonfeeding and nondividing phase formed because of altered environmental conditions. The flagellate usually reverts back to the trophic stage. The cysts measure 7 to 15 µm in size, are smooth-walled, and may have one or two pores flush on the surface of the cyst wall.

DESCRIPTION OF THE DISEASE

N. fowleri causes an acute fulminating (rapidly occurring) disease of the CNS called *primary amebic meningoencephalitis* (PAM). The disease has an abrupt onset and occurs in previously healthy children and young adults who have had contact with fresh water 3 to 10 days before the onset of symptoms. PAM is characterized by severe headache, spiking fever, stiff neck, photophobia, and coma leading to death within 3 to 10 days after the onset of symptoms. The trophozoites of *N. fowleri* enter the nasal passages during water sport activities, make their way into the CNS, and cause an acute hemorrhagic necrosis leading to the destruction of the olfactory bulbs and the cerebral cortex. Patient survival depends on prompt diagnosis and aggressive treatment.

RESERVOIRS FOR THE AGENT

No human or animal reservoir for *N. fowleri* has been identified so far. However, birds such as ducks and geese that have a fairly high body temperature may act as reservoirs for the thermophilic *N. fowleri*. Aquatic mammals (beavers, otters, and muskrats) also may prove to be a source for *N. fowleri*. A comprehensive survey of animals that inhabit aquatic habitats and could be reservoirs needs to be conducted.

MODE OF TRANSMISSION

N. fowleri is transmitted through the nasal passages. The trophozoites and possibly the flagellates enter the nostrils during swimming, diving, splashing while wading, or waterskiing in lakes and other bodies of fresh water. The trophozoites make their way into the olfactory lobes through the cribriform plate and cause an acute hemorrhagic necrosis that destroys the olfactory bulbs and the cerebral cortex.

METHODS FOR DETECTING THE AGENT

Materials suspected of containing *N. fowleri*, such as soil and water, must be collected aseptically in order to detect and isolate the agent. The specimens may be kept at room temperature (24 to 28° C), or at 4° C for short periods of time (but never for more than 24 hours), and should never be frozen. Personnel handling the specimens must take appropriate precautions, such as wearing surgical masks and gloves and working in a biological safety cabinet. Specimens should be sent to the Centers for Disease Control and Prevention (CDC) for identification.

OCCURRENCE OF THE AGENT IN PEOPLE, ANIMALS, AND THE ENVIRONMENT

As of Oct. 1, 1996, more than 175 cases of PAM caused by *N. fowleri* had been reported worldwide, including 81 cases in the United States. *N. fowleri* is found worldwide and has been isolated from fresh water, including tap water, thermal discharges of power plants, heated swimming pools, hydrotherapy and remedial pools, aquaria, sewage, and even from nasal passages and throats of healthy individuals. *N. fowleri* is thermophilic and therefore proliferates when the ambient temperature is raised. PAM cases occur typically in the hot summer months and coincide with the increase in the number of people engaging in aquatic activities in freshwater bodies, such as lakes and ponds, as well as improperly chlorinated swimming pools that may harbor the amoebas. It is estimated that one case of PAM occurs in approximately 2.5 million swimmers.

SURVIVAL OF THE AGENT IN THE ENVIRONMENT

N. fowleri, especially the cyst forms, can likely survive for long periods in moist soil and water. *N. fowleri* cysts held at 4° C for up to 8 months were able to produce PAM in mice. The cysts become nonviable if dried, frozen, or heated above 51° C.

DOCUMENTED WATERBORNE OUTBREAKS

Most cases of PAM have occurred in children and young adults who have had a history of swimming, diving, wading, and waterskiing in swimming pools, lakes, ponds, rivers, thermally polluted water, and hot springs. A series of PAM cases involving 16 young persons in Czechoslovakia between August 1962 and September 1965 was traced to a swimming pool that received heated river water treated with chlorine. Several cases of PAM in the Richmond, Va., area were all traced to one of three lakes in that area. *N. fowleri* has also been isolated from the drinking water in Australia.

INFORMATION SOURCES

Butt, C.G. 1966. Primary Amebic Meningoencephalitis. *New England J. Med.*, 274:1473–1476.

Carter, R.F. 1972. Primary Amoebic Meningo-Encephalitis. An Appraisal of Present Knowledge. *Trans. Royal Soc. Trop. Med. Hyg.*, 66:193–208.

John, D.T. 1993. Opportunistically Pathogenic Free-Living Amebae. In *Parasitic Protozoa*, Vol. 3. pp. 143–246. Kreier, J.P., and J.R. Baker, eds. New York: Academic Press, Inc.

Martinez, A.J. 1985. *Free-Living Amebas: Natural History, Prevention, Diagnosis, Pathology, and Treatment of the Disease.* Boca Raton, Fla.: CRC Press.

Page, F.C. 1985. *A New Key to Fresh Water and Soil Gymnamoebae*. Cumbria, England: Fresh Water Biological Association.

Seidel, J.S., P. Harmatz, G.S. Visvesvara, A. Cohen, J. Edwards, and J. Turner. 1982. Successful Treatment of Primary Amebic Meningoencephalitis. *New England J. Med.*, 306:346–348.

This page intentionally blank.

Chapter 34

Schistosomatidae

Harvey Blankespoor

DESCRIPTION OF THE AGENT

The parasites that cause swimmer's itch (schistosome cercarial dermatitis) belong to a group of flatworms known as digenetic trematodes of the family Schistosomatidae. Although schistosomes found in humans (*Schistosoma*) may be responsible for this condition, the disease is usually associated with nonhuman species, particularly those that use birds as final or definitive hosts. Some common genera that cause swimmer's itch include *Gigantobilharzia, Ornithobilharzia, Schistosomatium,* and *Trichobilharzia*.

The life cycle of nonhuman schistosomes involves an aquatic snail and a warm-blooded vertebrate, usually an aquatic bird. Eggs of the parasite are voided with the host's feces. On contact with water, a free-living, nonfeeding stage (miracidium) hatches from the egg and lies inactive for approximately one day. When the miracidium hatches and contacts an appropriate snail species, it penetrates the tegument or, with some species, is ingested by the snail. It then migrates to a specific region and elongates to form a complex of germinating sacs called *mother sporocysts*. Usually a second generation (daughter sporocysts) are asexually produced and form another life cycle stage known as the *cercaria*. These nonfeeding, free-swimming larvae emerge from the snail and live approximately 24 hours. If they contact a suitable bird species, they enter the host and migrate to the lungs and liver where they enter the mesenteric veins and develop into egg-producing adults. If they enter a human, the cercariae die and sensitive individuals will develop swimmer's itch.

Cercariae are fork-tailed (furcocercous), range in length from 200 to 300 µm, and have a body and tail. The body is elongated and contains four pairs of penetration glands, a ventral sucker, an anterior holdfast organ, and two eye spots. The outer covering, or tegument, is covered with minute spines that make the cercaria difficult to withdraw from vertebrate skin once penetration has begun. The tail is 20 to 40 µm in diameter with a length of 100 to 200 µm. The tail has a main stem and two distal flaps called *furcae* and finfolds may or may not be present. Distinguishing characteristics of the cercaria include the absence of a pharynx, a ventral sucker (protrusible acetabulum), two flame cells near the proximal end of the tail, and four pairs of penetration glands.

DESCRIPTION OF THE DISEASE

Swimmer's itch is a delayed hypersensitivity response to the cercarial stage of the nonhuman schistosomes. Cercariae that are unable to penetrate the dermis layer of the skin of nonsuitable hosts, such as humans, die and within a half hour a small red area may appear at the site of penetration. This spot may continue to increase in size for about 24 to 30 hours. Once it becomes reddened and raised, it is called a *papule* and forms where each cercaria enters the skin. Itching continues for several days. The symptoms vary depending on the age and sensitivity of the individual, type or lack of medication used, amount of irritation from scratching, and the species of schistosome that causes the dermatitis. Diagnosis is based on finding papules only on body areas exposed to water within the past few days. Treatment includes prescription drugs containing antihistamines to minimize itching and topical steroids (cortisone) creams to reduce the swelling. Outbreaks of swimmer's itch in Michigan usually occur from the end of May to early September, but latitude and seasonal fluctuations may affect this timing. Although swimmer's itch has the potential to occur on all lakes, it seems most common on larger recreational lakes with sandy or rocky shorelines. Onshore winds appear to concentrate the cercariae close to the water's edge.

RESERVOIRS FOR THE AGENT

In the Midwest, as many as 20 species of nonhuman schistosomes can cause swimmer's itch. Most of the snail-intermediate hosts belong to families Lymnaeidae or Physidae. A few species of family Planorbidae can harbor dermatitis-causing nonhuman schistosomes. Vertebrates that serve as final or definitive hosts for the dermatitis-producing schistosomes include ducks; geese; swans; gulls; perching birds, such as blackbirds and starlings; and rodents, such as rats, muskrats, and voles.

MODE OF TRANSMISSION

Free-living larval stages of nonhuman schistosomes are only transmitted in water. Hatched, ciliated miracidium must contact the snail intermediate host in the water. Furthermore, cercariae leaving the snail must swim in water to come in contact with the vertebrate host. Transmission is not possible from snail to snail or from bird to bird.

METHODS FOR DETECTING THE AGENT

Cercariae are difficult to detect in natural bodies of water for several reasons. First, the larvae are small and nearly transparent. Second, it is nearly impossible to predict where they will occur. Factors affecting their presence and abundance include the density and location of snail hosts, wave action, water currents, and time of day. If cercariae are subjected to harsh handling techniques, the body and tail separate, leaving the larval flatworm immobile. Finally, they are difficult to distinguish morphologically from cercariae of some other digenetic trematodes (e.g., Strigeidae) that do not cause swimmer's itch. Filtering large volumes of lake or pond water then staining the intact cercariae is not a reliable way to isolate and identify schistosome cercariae.

SURVIVAL OF THE AGENT IN THE ENVIRONMENT

Cercariae of avian schistosomes typically live for one day, depending on the water temperature. The larvae live longer at lower temperatures and die quickly at warmer temperatures. Depending on the species, cercariae emerge at a specific time each day. This emergence coincides with the habits of the vertebrate host involved in the cycle for the maximum contact opportunity.

EFFECTIVENESS OF WATER TREATMENT PROCESSES

Two methods are used to control swimmer's itch. The traditional method is to apply a molluscicide in mid-June to break the life cycle by destroying the snail intermediate host. This type of treatment has met with mixed results and the long-term effects of this toxin on aquatic ecosystems is a concern. A new method of control focuses on capturing and treating the birds with an antihelmitic drug, Praziquantel. Seed-eating birds can be fed treated corn or bread.

INFORMATION SOURCES

Blankespoor, H.D. 1988. Swimmer's Itch: a Preventive Approach. *Lake Line*, 4–5.

Blankespoor, H.D., and R.L. Reimink. 1991. The Control of Swimmer's Itch in Michigan: Past, Present and Future. *Michigan Academician,* 24:7–23.

Brackett, S. 1940. Pathology of Schistosome Dermatitis. *Arch. Derm. and Syphil.,* 42:410–418.

Cort, W.W. 1928. Schistosome Dermatitis in the United States (Michigan). *J. AMAI*, 90:1027–1029.

———. 1950. Studies on Schistosome Dermatitis. *Amer. Jour. Hygiene*, 52:251–307.

Hoeffler, D.F. Swimmer's Itch (Cercarial Dermatitis). *Cutis,* 19:461–465.

———. 1979. Cercarial dermatitis. In *CRC Handbook Series on Zoonoses*, Vol. 3. pp. 7–15. Steele, J.H., ed. Boca Raton, Fla.: CRC Press.

Jarcho, S., and A. Van Burkalow. 1952. A Geographical Study of Swimmer's Itch in the United States and Canada. *Geographical Review,* 42:212–226.

Talbot, S.B. 1936. Studies on Schistosome Dermatitis. *Amer. Jour. Hygiene,* 23:372–384.

This page intentionally blank.

Chapter 35

Spirometra mansonoides

M. Dale Little

DESCRIPTION OF THE AGENT

Spirometra mansonoides, of the family Diphyllobothriidae, is a tapeworm that lives in the intestine of dogs and domestic and wild cats in the United States and other parts of the Western Hemisphere. The worm does not develop to the adult stage in humans, but a larval stage, the sparganum or plerocercoid, can invade the tissues of people and cause sparganosis. Related species in other parts of the world that cause sparganosis include *S. erinacei, S. mansoni,* and *S. ranarum* in Asia.

This group of parasites has a complicated life cycle of first and second intermediate hosts and paratenic hosts in addition to the definitive hosts that harbor adult worms. Undeveloped eggs passed in the feces of the definitive host are deposited into a body of fresh or brackish water, or on damp mud at water's edge, where they develop into embryos in about two to three weeks. A ciliated first larval stage, a coracidium, hatches and swims freely in the water. This larva is eaten by a copepod, a microcrustacean, and in about two to three weeks develops in this host's body cavity to the next larval stage, a procercoid.

Species of *Cyclops* and other genera of copepods may serve as the first intermediate host. When an infected copepod is eaten by a tadpole or is swallowed by another vertebrate animal while drinking water, the procercoid migrates into the tissues and develops to the final larval stage, a sparganum (also called a *plerocercoid*). In dogs and cats, the sparganum then migrates to the intestinal tract and develops to the adult stage. In other vertebrates, frogs, snakes, or mammals (including humans), the sparganum remains in the tissues for a long time. When, for example, an infected frog is eaten by a snake, the sparganum in the frog's tissues will migrate into the tissues of the snake; the snake in this case is a paratenic host. If a dog or a cat ingests a sparganum by eating either an infected second intermediate host or a paratenic host, the larva migrate to the intestine and develop to an adult worm.

DESCRIPTION OF THE DISEASE

Disease in humans, sparganosis, is caused by sparganum migrating through the tissues. The cutaneous tissues in various parts of the body are most frequently involved. The worm produces a nodule or swelling that may or may not be painful. The lesion may disappear at one site and reappear at another days or weeks later. The most serious complications are when the sparganum enters the brain (cerebral sparganosis) or tissues near the eye (ocular sparganosis). The only available treatment is surgical removal of the worm.

Diagnosis is usually made by finding and identifying the sparganum in the affected tissues after surgical removal or at necropsy. About 68 cases of sparganosis have been reported from the United States, mostly from the Southeast, but sporadic cases have occurred throughout the country. Sparganosis occurs worldwide but is most frequently seen in Southeast Asia.

RESERVOIRS FOR THE AGENT

Dogs and wild and domestic cats are the most common hosts of the adult tapeworm. Various species of copepods can serve as hosts for the procercoid stage, and a variety of amphibians, reptiles, and mammals can become infected with the sparganum stage.

MODE OF TRANSMISSION

People may become infected by drinking water containing infected copepods or by eating raw or inadequately cooked flesh of an animal containing the sparganum stage of the worm. A folk remedy of applying a poultice made from the raw flesh of frogs or snakes to an injured eye or another part of the body allows a sparganum to migrate from the raw animal flesh into the orbit or a wound. This transmission method is the usual way ocular sparganosis occurs.

METHODS FOR DETECTING THE AGENT

Water obtained from fresh or brackish ponds, lagoons, and other open bodies of water may contain copepods infected with the procercoid stage. The organisms may be collected from the water with a plankton net for microcrustaceans. Recovered copepods are examined under a stereomicroscope for the presence of *Spirometra* procercoids.

OCCURRENCE OF THE AGENT IN PEOPLE, ANIMALS, AND THE ENVIRONMENT

In the United States, *S. mansonoides* is found primarily in dogs and wild and domestic cats. Where animals are infected, a small percentage of the copepods inhabiting local standing bodies of water are likely to be infected with the procercoid. No free stages are found in the environment. In the United States, various species of water snakes are the most frequently infected second intermediate hosts, and the majority of human cases of sparganosis are in the Southeastern states. The infections in humans cannot be passed on to other people or animals.

SURVIVAL OF THE AGENT IN THE ENVIRONMENT

Copepods infected with *Spirometra* probably live for only a few weeks. The life span of the sparganum in second intermediate and paratenic hosts is unknown but likely they remain alive for much of the life span of these animals.

INFORMATION SOURCES

American Public Health Association, American Water Works Association, and Water Environment Federation. 1998. *Standard Methods for the Examination of Water and Wastewater.* 20th ed. Washington, D.C.: APHA.

Beaver, P.C., R.C. Jung, and E.W. Cupp. *Clinical Parasitology.* Philadelphia, Pa.: Lea and Febiger.

Corkum, K.C. 1966. Sparganosis in Some Vertebrates of Louisiana and Observations on a Human Infection. *J. Parasitol.*, 52:444–448.

Mueller, J.F. 1938. The Life History of *Diphyllobothrium mansonoides* Mueller, 1935, and Some Considerations With Regard to Sparganosis in the United States. *Am. J. Trop. Med.*, 18:41–66.

Sarma, D.P., and T.G. Weilbaecher. 1986. Human Sparganosis. *J. Am. Acad. Dermatol.*, 15:1145–1148.

This page intentionally blank.

Chapter 36

Taenia solium

David W. Fredericksen

DESCRIPTION OF THE AGENT

Taenia solium is a tapeworm of family Taenidae. Taenid cestodes are medically significant, and *T. solium* is the tapeworm potentially most dangerous to humans.

Adults of *T. solium* have a scolex (head) that does not have a rostellum (crown). The scolex supports two rows of hooks and four suckers that allow the worm to attach to the intestinal wall. Adult worms produce ova that can infect through water as well as person to person. Ova hatch into larva that penetrate tissues and form cysticerci (bladderworms). These intermediate stages have a predilection for the connective tissues of the brain, heart, and other vital organs.

DESCRIPTION OF THE DISEASE

Adult worms, which may reach several meters in length, probably cause no symptoms in the majority of patients. The worms may be eradicated by treatment with praziquantel, which cures at a rate approaching 100 percent.

A common larval stage of the worm known as a *bladderworm* or *cysticercus*, may invade the intestinal wall and be carried into the blood stream. They may then lodge in tissue (often muscle), where development is completed. Cysticerci can cause a potentially fatal disease in humans if they invade the central nervous system.

RESERVOIRS FOR THE AGENT

Humans and pigs are the only known reservoirs, and any water contaminated with human or porcine sewage can be a potential threat. Once acquired from water, *T. solium* can spread from person to person throughout entire households.

MODE OF TRANSMISSION

Consuming undercooked infected pork can provide a source of the adult tapeworm, which in turn can spread ova through the fecal–oral route. Drinking water contaminated with human or porcine sewage can contain the ova that develop into cysticerci in the connective tissues of virtually every organ of the body.

METHODS FOR DETECTING THE AGENT

Centrifugation and concentration methods can be used for egg detection. Eggs are infective and precautions should be observed when handling samples.

OCCURRENCE OF THE AGENT IN PEOPLE, ANIMALS, AND THE ENVIRONMENT

Reports of this parasite in the United States are sparse. *T. solium* is cosmopolitan and is most common in underdeveloped regions where personal hygiene is poor and water is contaminated with fecal material. *T. solium* cases are most common in eastern Europe, Africa, Mexico, Central America, Asia, Spain, and Portugal. No published data exist on the length of survival of this particular parasite in the environment. The ova of most taenids can persist for years, depending on weather conditions, and adult worms can reside in the intestinal tract for years.

EFFECTIVENESS OF WATER TREATMENT PROCESSES

Adequate filtration should remove this organism.

INFORMATION SOURCES

Craun, G.F. 1986. *Waterborne Diseases in the United States.* Boca Raton, Fla.: CRC Press, Inc.

Massachusetts General Hospital. 1996. Case Records. *New England J. Med.,* 382–389.

Schmidt, G.D., and L.S. Roberts. 1981. *Foundations of Parasitology.* St. Louis, Mo.: C.V. Mosby.

Sparks, A.K., R.C. Neafie, and D.H. Connor. 1976. *Pathology of Tropical and Extraordinary Diseases,* Vol. II. Binford, C., and D.H. Connor, eds. Washington, D.C.: Department of Defense, Armed Institute of Pathology.

Stunkard, H.C. 1961. Seminar at Tulane University.

White, A.C., Jr., and S.H. Wright. 1992. Host-Parasite Interactions in *Taenia solium* Cystercosis. *Infectious Agents of Disease,* 1(4):185–193.

Chapter 37

Toxoplasma gondii

J.P. Dubey

DESCRIPTION OF THE AGENT

Toxoplasma gondii is an obligate (requiring hosts) intracellular coccidian parasite usually transmitted by ingestion of infective tissues from animals through the placenta, or ingestion of food and water contaminated with infected cat feces. Cats excrete a resistant form of *T. gondii* (oocysts) that are noninfective in their feces. After defecation, the development of infective sporozoites inside the oocyst requires one day or more, depending on environmental conditions. Oocysts are 10 × 12 µm in size, can survive up to 18 months in unfavorable environmental conditions, and are remarkably resistant to most disinfectants.

After a warm-blooded animal ingests fecal-contaminated food or water, the oocyst ruptures in the intestine and releases eight sporozoites. Sporozoites multiply in the intestinal cells and in associated lymph nodes, and tachyzoites (rapidly multiplying forms) are formed. Tachyzoites are banana-shaped and measure 6 × 2 µm. Tachyzoites disperse to the rest of the body through blood and lymph, eventually encysting in the brain, skeletal and cardiac muscles, and liver. Encysted *T. gondii* organisms are called bradyzoites (slowly multiplying forms). Tissue cysts are microscopic (less than 70 µm in diameter) and survive in tissues for the duration of the life of the host. Tachyzoites are found during the acute phase, whereas encysted bradyzoites (tissue cysts) are found predominantly in the latent, chronic phase. Bradyzoites are about 7 × 2 µm in size and a tissue cyst may enclose over 1,000 bradyzoites.

After infected tissues are ingested, enzymes dissolve the wall of the tissue cyst, releasing the bradyzoites that infect intestinal cells of the host. After entering host cells, bradyzoites transform into tachyzoites. These intracellular tachyzoites may undergo repeated intracellular divisions. Ultimately, they are dispersed throughout the body and encyst in tissues. The life cycle of *T. gondii* is completed when tissue cysts are ingested by cats and oocysts are then formed.

DESCRIPTION OF THE DISEASE

T. gondii causes mental retardation, loss of vision, hearing impairment, and mortality in congenitally infected children. Although toxoplasmosis is mostly an asymptomatic infection in adults, it causes serious disease and death in immunosuppressed persons, especially those with acquired immune deficiency syndrome (AIDS). In AIDS patients, latent *T. gondii* infection can be reactivated resulting in an overwhelming disease. Encephalitis is the predominant feature of toxoplasmosis in AIDS patients. *T. gondii* is also a major cause of abortion in sheep and goats and can cause mortality in virtually all warm-blooded animals. It is very pathogenic for marsupials and New World monkeys, especially in zoos.

RESERVOIRS FOR THE AGENT

Cats, including wild Felidae, are the only definitive hosts for this parasite.

MODE OF TRANSMISSION

Human beings and other animals become infected primarily by ingesting food or water contaminated with oocysts or by ingesting infective animal tissues that contain tissue cysts of *T. gondii*. During pregnancy of infected hosts, *T. gondii* can multiply in the placenta and spread to fetal tissues. Although such transplacental infection can occur during any stage of gestation, the fetus is affected most severely when the pregnant female becomes infected during the first half of gestation.

Soil contaminated by feral cats is probably a greater risk than soil contaminated by cats housed indoors. *T. gondii* infection is higher in feral cats than in domestic cats because they hunt birds and small mammals in which a sylvatic cycle of *T. gondii* is found.

METHODS FOR DETECTING THE AGENT

T. gondii oocysts are 10 to 12 μm in diameter and can be seen with a microscope. A bioassay should be performed because other coccidians have similar oocyst morphology. Methods used to concentrate *Cryptosporidium* and *Giardia* oocysts from water by filters can be applied to examine water reservoirs for *T. gondii* oocysts. The final sediment from filters should be inoculated orally into laboratory mice and be examined for *T. gondii* infection.

OCCURRENCE OF THE AGENT IN PEOPLE, ANIMALS, AND THE ENVIRONMENT

T. gondii infects virtually all warm-blooded hosts. It is one of the most widespread infections of human beings.

SURVIVAL OF THE AGENT IN THE ENVIRONMENT

T. gondii oocysts are highly resistant to environmental influences and survive freezing and drying. They are also resistant to ammonia, chlorine, and commonly used disinfectants, including formalin. They are killed by heat (70° C) but will survive for 30 minutes at 56° C. They are killed by 0.30 KgY gamma irradiation. Irradiation may be a practical way of decontaminating fruits and vegetables contaminated with oocysts.

DOCUMENTED WATERBORNE OUTBREAKS

Recently, an outbreak of toxoplasmosis involving many patients was epidemiologically linked to a water reservoir in British Columbia. Another small outbreak occurred in US Army soldiers who drank water from a pond during jungle exercises in Panama. In both of these episodes, persons had persistent symptoms of acquired toxoplasmosis, including chorioretinitis.

INFORMATION SOURCES

Bell, A., J. Isaac-Renton, A. King, L. Martinez, D. Roscoe, D. Werker, S. Eng, T. Johnstone, R. Stanwick, W.R. Bowie, S. Marion, C. Stephen, A. Burnett, J. Cadham, F. Jagdis, P. MacLeod, K. Barnard, J. Millar, S. Peck, J. Hull, et al. 1995. *Canada Communicable Disease Report*, 21(18):161–163.

Benenson, M.V., T.K. Takafuji, S.M. Lemon, R.L. Greenop, and A.J. Sulzer. 1983. Oocyst-Transmitted Toxoplasmosis Associated with Ingestion of Contaminated Water. *New England J. Med.*, 307:666–669.

Dubey, J.P. 1996. Toxoplasmosis. *J. Am. Vet. Med. Assoc.,* 189:166–170.

Dubey, J.P., M.C. Jenkins, D.W. Thayer, O.C.H Kwok, and S.K. Shen. 1996. Killing of *Toxoplasma gondii* Oocysts by Irradiation and Protective Immunity Induced by Vaccination with Irradiated Oocysts. *J. Parasitol.*, 82:724–727.

Dubey, J.P., and C.P. Beattie. 1988. *Toxoplasmosis of Animals and Man*. Boca Raton, Fla.: CRC Press.

Remington, J.S., R. McLeod, and G. Desmonts. 1995. Toxoplasmosis. In *Infectious Diseases of the Fetus and Newborn Infant.* 4th ed. pp. 140–267. Remington, J.S., and J.O. Klein, eds. Philadelphia, Pa.: Saunders Company.

This page intentionally blank.

Chapter 38

Trichuris trichiura

Huw Smith, Tony Grimson, and Celia Holland

DESCRIPTION OF THE AGENT

Trichuris trichiura, superfamily Trichuroidea, is a nematode parasite of man, commonly known as *whipworm* because of the whip-like appearance of the adult stage. The parasite exists in the following three distinct forms: the egg or ovum; the larva, which migrates through various organs of the body; and the adult, which resides in the large intestine of humans. The sexes are separate. Similar species are parasites in other primates, rodents, camels, and some domesticated animals. The genus is also referred to by its former name *Trichocephalus*, especially in Spanish and French medical literature. *Trichuris* is translated as "hairtail," whereas *Trichocephalus* is translated as "hairhead."

Adult males and females are anchored in the caecum. Adult females, fertilized by adult males, can lay up to 20,000 ova daily, and fertilized eggs are excreted in feces. Embryos develop in a moist environment with ambient temperature. The first-stage larva (L1) develop within the eggshell in 14 to 28 days under ideal conditions. At this stage, larva within the eggs are infectious to susceptible human beings if ingested. The infective egg is stimulated to hatch in the intestine. Hatched L1 pass from the small intestine into the large intestine where they develop and molt through the second, third, and fourth larval stages and become adult worms. The cycle from infection to egg-laying adult normally takes about eight weeks.

The transmissive stage of *T. trichiura* infection is the fertilized egg, and the infective stage is the fully embryonated egg that contains the L1 larva. Fertilized eggs that do not contain a fully developed L1 larva are not infective.

The most commonly identified stage is the fertilized egg. Eggs are ovoid (lemon-shaped) and usually brown in color because of the uptake of bile pigments following passage through the intestine. Ova measure 22 to 24 µm by 50 to 55 µm and have a smooth, brown eggshell. At each tip of the ovum is a translucent plug. *T. trichiura* are readily distinguished from the ova of other intestinal parasites of humans. Adult female worms measure 30 to 50 mm in length with a rounded posterior end; adult males measure 30 to 45 mm with a tightly coiled posterior end featuring a single spicule. At the anterior end of adults of both sexes is the mouth, without lips, but with a stylet used to penetrate the mucosal lining of the gut. The posterior end of the female tapers to a point whereas the posterior end of the male is curved or hook-shaped. Both sexes have a narrower anterior portion and a wider posterior portion, the wider posterior portion representing the handle of a whip.

DESCRIPTION OF THE DISEASE

The prepatent period (about two months) is the interval of time between ingesting infectious eggs and the first appearance of ova in the stool. The incubation period is the time between ingesting infectious eggs and the development of recognized symptoms or signs of illness. The interval depends on the number of infectious ova ingested and the susceptibility of the individual. In light infections, individuals are asymptomatic. Symptoms, including abdominal pain, may appear when adult worms number 50 to 150. When several hundred or thousand adult worms are present, chronic pancolitis, known as *Trichuris* dysentery syndrome (TDS) can occur. Principal features of TDS are chronic diarrhea, anemia, and growth retardation. Symptoms include anorexia, pica, lower abdominal pain, mucoid diarrhea, dysentery, and rectal prolapse (especially in intense trichuriasis). As the cycle from infection to egg-laying adult female normally takes about eight weeks, the time between infection and recognition of symptoms, especially systemic symptoms, is often greater.

Trichuris is frequently found concurrently with *Ascaris*, hookworm, and *Entamoeba histolytica*. Significant positive correlations between egg counts for *Ascaris* and *Trichuris* have been demonstrated in individual children.

RESERVOIRS FOR THE AGENT

Humans are the reservoirs of *T. trichiura*. Coprophagous animals, such as pigs, dogs, cats, and chickens that might feed on human feces, can act as transport hosts by dispersing or redistributing fertile ova to other sites associated with human activities. Pigs, lemurs, and monkeys may act as reservoir hosts. *Trichuris* ova have been found in surface water, groundwater, and seawater, but not in treated drinking water. They have also been detected in night soil, sewage (Table 38-1), sludge, soil and on crops and beaches.

Densities of *Trichuris* sp. ova can vary greatly in raw wastewaters, depending on the endemicity of disease within the indigenous animal and human population. Other factors include the size and socioeconomic status of the population, the percentage of the population sewered, shock loadings from the discharge of pit latrine tankers, the provision of separate or combined sewers, and seasonal and sampling factors. *Ascaris* ova occur more frequently and in significantly larger numbers than *Trichuris* ova.

Table 38-1 Occurrence of *Trichuris* spp. ova in raw sewage

Country	*Trichuris*, (*ova/L*)
Russia	—
United States	—
India	1.1–7.3
India	3×10^4–6×10^5
India	6–19
India	—
Nigeria	≤100
Morocco	7

MODE OF TRANSMISSION

T. trichiura is transmitted when infective ova are ingested by a susceptible human host. Because external maturation of ova is necessary in the environment, contact with recently voided feces is not a risk. In endemic areas, major routes of transmission include

- defecation by infected individuals, especially children, in backyards or compounds leading to the contamination of soil, fingers, hands, cooking utensils, and other surfaces
- use of untreated human feces as fertilizer (night soil), especially for crops that receive minimal heating before consumption
- defecation by agricultural workers in or near the fields where they work (defecating in or near flowing water is often believed to be more sanitary than defecating into latrines where water may be unavailable for hand washing)
- use of untreated sewage effluent for irrigating crops that receive minimal heating before consumption
- consumption of contaminated unfiltered drinking water or communal drinking water
- redistribution of fertile ova to other uncontaminated sites associated with human activities by coprophagous animals, such as pigs, dogs, cats, and chickens, which might feed on human feces

METHODS FOR DETECTING THE AGENT

T. trichiura ova are detected in feces or in the environment by morphological and morphometric examination of suspect organisms by bright field microscopy.

OCCURRENCE OF THE AGENT IN PEOPLE, ANIMALS, AND THE ENVIRONMENT

Trichuris ova occur commonly in the environment, with densities depending on the level of infection in the indigenous population. *Trichuris* ova can be found in surface water, groundwater, and seawater, but not in treated drinking water. They can also be present in feces, night soil, sewage, sludge, soil, and on crops and beaches.

The life span of adult female *T. trichiura* is between one and eight years. In endemic areas where reinfection is common, susceptible hosts can excrete fertile ova for extended periods of time. In nonendemic areas, the period of communicability lasts as long as the last fertilized, egg-laying female worm is in the intestine.

Based primarily on cases with positive tests for eggs, the prevalence of *Trichuris* is 902 million (17 percent) worldwide. Prevalence increases rapidly with age in early childhood and attains a plateau in adulthood, remaining high and relatively constant in endemic regions. Socioeconomic and ethnic differences in behavior can influence exposure to infective *Trichuris* eggs. The average worm burden of *Trichuris* peaks in children and shows a marked decline in adulthood. *Trichuris* worm burdens follow an aggregated or overdispersed frequency distribution, with most individuals harboring few or no worms and a few individuals harboring many. Significant correlations between worm burdens before and after anthelmintic treatment can be observed from reinfection studies.

SURVIVAL OF THE AGENT IN THE ENVIRONMENT

Because the embryo develops into the infective larva outside the host, *Trichuris* ova are well-suited to prolonged survival in the environment. Embryo development and survival in the environment depend on aerobic metabolism; however, these ova can also survive in anaerobic conditions. Under conditions of ambient temperature (22 to 35° C), moisture, shade from ultraviolet (UV) light and oxygen, *Trichuris* ova take 11 to 38 days to become infective. At 15° C, *Trichuris* ova may take four to six months to develop to infectivity. Infective ova of *Trichuris* can remain viable for several months, with about 20 percent viable for more than 18 months. However, exposure for short periods of time (hours) to temperatures above 37° C will kill developing embryos.

DOCUMENTED WATERBORNE OUTBREAKS

While associated with foodborne outbreaks of disease, no waterborne outbreak of trichuriasis has been associated with treated public drinking water supplies.

EFFECTIVENESS OF WATER TREATMENT PROCESSES

Effective coagulation and filtration processes remove ova.

INFORMATION SOURCES

Anon. 1989. Health Guidelines for the Use of Wastewater in Agriculture and Aquaculture. *Technical Report Series No. 778*. Geneva: World Health Organization.

Chan, M.-S. 1997. The Global Burden of Intestinal Nematode Infections—50 Years On. *Parasitol. Today,* 13(11): 438–443.

Feacham, R.G., D.J. Bradley, H. Garelick and D.D. Mara. 1982. *Sanitation and Disease. Health Aspects of Excreta and Wastewater Management.* Chapter 35. Chichester, UK: John Wiley & Sons.

Holland, C. 1987. Neglected Infections—Trichuriasis and Strongyloidiasis. In *The Impact of Helminth Infections on Human Nutrition*. pp. 161–201. Stephenson, L.S., ed. London: Taylor and Francis.

Introduction to Viral Pathogenic Agents

Adenoviruses
Astroviruses
Caliciviruses
Enteroviruses
Hepatitis A
Reoviruses
Rotaviruses
Small, Round, Structured Viruses (Human Caliciviruses)

Viruses are the smallest and most basic of known life forms. They consist only of nucleic acid and a protein shell (or capsid), and have no reproductive systems. Their simple genetic system is a single-stranded or double-stranded deoxyribonucleic acid (DNA) or ribonucleic acid (RNA). Because of their inability to autonomously reproduce, they must take over a living cell and use the cell's reproductive mechanism to replicate. After replication, and the subsequent death of the host cell, viral particles are spread to neighboring cells, resulting in the infection of the individual.

VIRUSES IN THE ENVIRONMENT

More than 140 different enteric viruses are known to infect man. Enteric viruses are excreted in the feces of infected individuals and may directly or indirectly contaminate water intended for drinking. These viruses are excreted in high numbers per gram of feces of infected individuals and are commonly isolated in domestic wastewater, even after disinfection. Once in the environment they can survive for long periods of time, even months under the right conditions. The enteric viruses include the enteroviruses, rotaviruses, hepatitis A and E, Norwalk and Norwalk-like viruses, adenoviruses, and reoviruses. These viruses are transmitted by the fecal–oral route, infect the gastrointestinal or respiratory tracts, and are capable of causing a wide range of illness, including diarrhea, fever, hepatitis, paralysis, meningitis, and heart disease. Despite causing a variety of illness in humans, many viral infections are remarkably asymptomatic (with no clinical symptoms). However, viral multiplication in an infected individual occurs, and virus particles are shed in the environment. Virus detection and identification in water supplies has been limited by the difficulties and expense of conventional cell culture assays. However, advances in molecular techniques have provided a simpler and more rapid method for viral monitoring of water samples.

The following chapters discuss the groups of viruses identified as sources of waterborne disease outbreaks or that have the potential to cause outbreaks.

Chapter 39

Adenoviruses

Carlos Enriquez

DESCRIPTION OF THE AGENT

Adenoviruses belong to the Adenoviridae family, which includes human (49 serotypes), simian (27 serotypes), bovine (10 serotypes), equine (1 serotype), porcine (4 serotypes), ovine (1 serotype), and canine (3 serotypes) viruses. These agents are viruses of approximately 70 to 100 nm in diameter.

DESCRIPTION OF THE DISEASE

Human adenoviruses may cause acute respiratory disease, pneumonia, epidemic conjunctivitis, and acute gastroenteritis in children. Most clinical conditions are caused by approximately 30 percent of all types of adenoviruses. Respiratory disease caused by adenovirus is observed mostly among children and characterized by general malaise and fever, nasal congestion, and cough. The most prevalent adenoviruses associated with respiratory infection are types 1, 2, 5, and 6. Waterborne conjunctivitis caused by adenoviruses may occur sporadically or in large groups. The most common adenoviruses causing this type of conjunctivitis are serotypes 3 and 7, but other types have been implicated as well. Swimming pool conjunctivitis is observed mostly among young adults and children during the summer. Conjunctivitis sometimes accompanies respiratory symptoms. Recovery without complications usually follows this condition.

Although many adenoviruses replicate efficiently in the intestine, only the enteric adenoviruses 40 (Ead 40) and 41 (Ead 41) have been recognized as important causes of gastroenteritis in children, second in importance only to rotavirus. Adenoviral gastroenteritis occurs mostly in children under the age of two, particularly during the first year of life. The incubation period is one to three days, and symptoms are watery diarrhea, sometimes with vomiting. Unlike rotaviral infections, enteric adenoviral illness does not vary by season.

RESERVOIRS FOR THE AGENT

Human adenovirus typically is not pathogenic to animals, and animal adenovirus is only pathogenic to the species of origin. However, asymptomatic infections with human adenovirus type 12 has been documented in simian species, and antibodies to bovine, simian, and canine adenoviruses have been found in humans.

MODE OF TRANSMISSION

Adenoviruses can enter a susceptible host by mouth, nose, or eye membranes. Adenoviruses may be shed for months or years, because of low levels of virus replication in tonsils, adenoids, and intestines of infected individuals. Hurst et al. (1988) suggested that enteric adenoviruses could be transmitted through recreational or drinking water. The enteric nature of the adenoviruses 40 and 41, their presence only in the gastrointestinal tract, and their extensive distribution suggest that water may play a role in the transmission of these agents.

METHODS FOR DETECTING THE AGENT

Nonenteric adenoviruses can be grown in Hep-2 cells and both enteric and nonenteric adenoviruses can be grown in human primary liver carcinoma cells (PLC/PRF/5) with the production of cytopathic effect (CPE). Successful growth of enteric adenoviruses 40 and 41 occurs in a cell line derived from a human colon carcinoma (CaCo-2 cells). Polymerase chain reaction (PCR) and gene probe techniques have been used to detect adenoviruses from environmental water.

OCCURRENCE OF THE AGENT IN PEOPLE, ANIMALS, AND THE ENVIRONMENT

A comparative study of disease in cells, immunofluorescence, and *in situ* deoxyribonucleic acid (DNA) hybridization suggested that 80 percent of infectious adenoviruses in raw sewage may be enteric adenoviruses. The number of indigenous adenoviruses detected in primary sewage sludge were 10 times greater than the number of enteroviruses. In addition, a greater number of adenoviruses than enteroviruses have been found consistently in raw sewage around the world.

SURVIVAL OF THE AGENT IN THE ENVIRONMENT

The stability of enterovirus 70 and human adenovirus type 19 were compared under different conditions. Drying these agents at room temperature on ophthalmic instruments resulted in a 99.999 percent (5-log) reduction of enterovirus 70. In contrast, the titer of adenovirus 19 decreased less than 90 percent (1 log) after 11 days under the same conditions. Studies have shown that adenovirus type 2 survived longer than poliovirus 2, vaccinia virus, coxsackievirus B3, and herpes virus. Adenovirus type 5 survived longer than both poliovirus 1 and echovirus 7 in tap water, at either 4 or 18° C. The Ead 40 and Ead 41 survive longer than polio 1 in primary and secondary wastewater and survival of the enteric adenoviruses 40 and 41 was even higher when compared to survival of hepatitis A virus (HAV) and polio 1 in tap and seawater. Evidence shows higher thermal stability of the enteric adenoviruses compared with polio 1 when Ead 40 and polio 1 were held at 50, 65, and 80° C in phosphate buffered saline. The inactivation rate of poliovirus 1 was higher at the three tested temperatures. In addition to thermal stability, Ead 40 shows some resistance at low and high pH levels. An experiment evaluated the stability of this virus at pH values of 3.5, 9.5, 10, and 10.5. No reduction of Ead 40 infectivity was observed after 45 minutes at either pH 3.5, 9.5, or 10. However, after 45 minutes at pH 10.5, Ead 40 suffered a reduction of 2.7 log. Other data have indicated that adenovirus type 5 was sensitive to high pH values, and found that the infectivity of this agent decreased steadily at pH higher than 9.0, with rapid inactivation at pH 10.

DOCUMENTED WATERBORNE OUTBREAKS

Documented waterborne outbreaks of conjunctivitis caused by adenovirus type 3 and type 4 have been reported. The only viral waterborne outbreak from 1991 to 1992 in the United States associated with recreational waters was caused by adenovirus type 3, which affected 595 individuals causing conjunctivitis, pharyngitis, and fever.

EFFECTIVENESS OF WATER TREATMENT PROCESSES

Chlorine disinfection studies of human adenoviruses 3 and 7, and simian adenovirus M2, M3, and M4 have shown that residual chlorine of 0 69 mg/L reduced adenovirus type 3 by 99 percent. A concentration of 0.89 mg/L was needed to achieve the same reduction of adenovirus type 7. Studies of HAV, human rotavirus, poliovirus 1, and adenovirus 5 disinfection in tap water with copper and silver ions and reduced levels of free chlorine have been undertaken. Viruses were exposed to 1.0, 0.5, or 0.2 mg/L of free chlorine, with and without copper and silver ions. They found that adenovirus type 5 was more resistant to all disinfection treatments than poliovirus 1, but less resistant than either HAV or human rotavirus. Depuration of enteric adenovirus 40 from artificially contaminated mussels, in a continuous flow of ozonated marine water, took much longer than the removal of poliovirus 1. However, it was depurated faster than either HAV or human rotaviruses.

Comparative ultraviolet (UV) light inactivation studies showed that enterovirus 70 was more susceptible to inactivation than human adenovirus type 19. It took less than 10 mW/cm^2/min to register a 4.5-log reduction of the enterovirus 70. Ultraviolet doses of 60 mW/cm^2/min were necessary to reach similar levels of inactivation of adenovirus 19. The comparisons of the resistance of enteric adenoviruses to UV light disinfection with poliovirus type 1 and the coliphages MS-2 and PRD-1 have been made. The doses of UV to achieve a 90 percent inactivation of adenovirus 40, adenovirus 41, coliphages MS-2 and PRD-1, and poliovirus type 1 were 30, 23.6, 14, 8.7, and 4.1 mW sec/cm^2, respectively.

INFORMATION SOURCES

Abad, F.X., R.M. Pintó, J.M. Diez, and A. Bosch. 1994. Disinfection of Human Enteric Viruses in Water by Copper and Silver in Combination with Low Levels of Chlorine. *Appl. Environ Microbiol.*, 60:2377–2383.

Albert, M.J. 1986. Enteric Adenoviruses. *Arch. Virol.*, 88:1–17.

Bagdasar, G.A., and R.M. Abieva. 1971 Survival of Enteroviruses and Adenoviruses in Water. *Hyg. Sanitation*, 36:333–337.

Blacklow, N.R, and H.B. Greenberg. 1991. Viral Gastroenteritis. *New England J. Med.*, 325:252–262.

Bosch, A., R.M. Pintó, and F.X. Abad. 1994. Differential Accumulation and Depuration of Human Enteric Mussels by Mussels. In *Proc. Water Quality International. Health-Related Water Microbiology.* IAWQ 17th Biennial International Conference, 24–29 July 1994, Budapest, Hungary.

D'Angelo, L.J., J.C. Hierholzer, R.A. Keenlyside, L.J. Anderson, and W.J. Martone. 1979. Pharyngoconjunctival Fever Caused by Adenovirus Type 4: Report of a Swimming Pool-Related Outbreak with Recovery of Virus from Pool Water. *J. Infect. Dis.*, 140:42–47.

Enriquez, C.E., C.J. Hurst, and C.P. Gerba. 1995a. Survival of the Enteric Adenoviruses 40 and 41 in Tap, Sea, and Waste Water. *Wat. Res.*, 29:2548–2553.

Enriquez, C.E., J. Sandoval-Garzon, and C.P. Gerba. 1995b. Survival, Detection, and Resistance to Disinfection of Enteric Adenoviruses. In *Proc. AWWA Water Quality Technology Conference*. Denver, Colo.: American Water Works Association.

Fields, H.A., and T. Metcalf. 1975. Concentration of Adenovirus from Seawater. *Wat. Res.*, 9:357–364.

Genthe, B., M. Gerike, B. Bateman, R. Kfir, and N. Mjoli. 1994. Detection of Enteric Adenoviruses in South African Waters Using Gene Probes. In *Proc. Water Quality International. Health-Related Water Microbiology.* IAWQ 17th Biennial International Conference, 24–29 July 1994, Budapest, Hungary.

Girones, R., A. Allard, G. Wadell, and J. Jofre. 1993. Application of PCR to the Detection of Adenoviruses in Polluted Waters. *Wat. Sci. Tech.*, 27:235–241.

Grabow, W.O.K., D.L. Putergill, and A. Bosch. 1992. Propagation of Adenovirus Types 40 and 41 in the PLC/PRF5 Primary Liver Carcinoma Cell Line. *J. Virol. Meth.*, 37:201–208.

Hara, J., S. Okamoto, Y. Minekawa, K. Yamazaki, and T. Kase. 1990. Survival and Disinfection of Adenovirus Type 19 and Enterovirus 70 in Ophthalmic Practice. *Jpn. J. Ophthalmol.*, 34:421–427.

Horitz, M.S. 1996. Adenoviruses. In *Fields Virology, 3rd ed.* Fields, B.N., D.M. Knipe, and P.M. Howley, eds. Philadelphia, Pa.: Lippincott-Raven Publishers.

Hurst, C.J., K.A. McClellan, and W.H. Benton. 1988. Comparison of Cytopathogenicity, Immunofluorescence and *In Situ* DNA Hybridization as Methods for the Detection of Adenoviruses. *Wat. Res.*, 22:1547–1552.

Joklik, W.K. 1988. The Structure, Components, and Classification of Viruses. In *Virology.* Englewood, N.J.: Prentice-Hall.

Mahl, M.C., and C. Sadler. 1975. Virus Survival on Inanimate Surfaces. *Can. J. Microbiol.*, 21:819–823.

Martone, W.J., J.C. Hierholzer, R.A. Keenlyside, D.W. Fraser, L.J. D'Angelo, and W.G. Winkler. 1980. An Outbreak of Adenovirus Type 3 Disease at a Private Recreation Center Swimming Pool. *Am. J. Epidemiol.*, 111:229–237.

McMillan, N.S., S.A. Martin, and M.D. Sobsey. 1992. Outbreak of Pharyngoconjunctival Fever at a Summer Camp—North Carolina. *MMWR*, 41:342–344.

Meng, Q.S., and C.P. Gerba. 1996. Comparative Inactivation of Enteric Adenovirus 40 and 41 with Poliovirus 1 and Bacteriophages MS2 and PRD-1 by Ultraviolet Irradiation. *Wat. Res.*, Submitted for publication.

Pinto, R.M., J.M. Diez, R. Gajardo, and A. Bosch. 1994. Detection of Fastidious Viruses by Cell Culture and Molecular Hybridization. In *Proc. Water Quality International Health-Related Water Microbiology.* IAWQ 17th Biennial International Conference, 24–29 July 1994, Budapest, Hungary.

Puig, M., J. Jofre, F. Lucena, A. Allard, G. Wadell, and R. Girones. 1994. Detection of Adenoviruses and Enteroviruses in Polluted Waters by Nested PCR Amplification. *Appl. Env. Microbiol.*, 60:2963–2970.

Straus, S.E. 1984. Adenovirus Infection in Humans. In *The Adenoviruses.* Ginsberg, H.S., ed. New York: Plenum Press.

Uhnoo, I., G. Wadell, L. Svensson and M. Johansson. 1983. Two New Serotypes of Enteric Adenoviruses Causing Infantile Diarrhoea. *Develop. Biol. Standard.*, 53:311–318.

Williams, F.P., and C.J. Hurst. 1988. Detection of Environmental Viruses in Sludge: Enhancement of Enterovirus Plaque Assay Titres with 5-Iodo-2-Deoxyuridine and Comparison to Adenovirus and Coliphage Titres. *Wat. Res.*, 22:847–851.

Chapter 40

Astroviruses

John E. Hermann

DESCRIPTION OF THE AGENT

Astroviruses in the family Astroviridae, are 27 to 32 nm in diameter. They have a characteristic star-shaped surface when viewed by negative-stain electron microscopy. The buoyant density in cesium chloride of the human astroviruses is approximately 1.35 g/mL. They have three structural proteins of M_r 5.5K to 42K. Seven serotypes of human astroviruses have been described, all of which can be cultivated in cell cultures treated with trypsin. Human astroviruses contain single-stranded plus-sense ribonucleic acid (RNA) of 6.8 kilobases with a 3′ poly (A) tail. Astrovirus genomes have been cloned as well and immunoreactive proteins expressed.

Astroviruses from stool samples were originally isolated in trypsin-treated primary human embryo kidney cells. They were subsequently adapted by serial passage to grow in $LLCMK_2$ cells, a continuous line of rhesus monkey kidney cells. CaCo-2 cells have also been used for isolation and cultivation of astroviruses, including two newer types, types 6 and 7.

DESCRIPTION OF THE DISEASE

Astrovirus infections have been studied in natural outbreaks and in volunteers. For example, of eight adult volunteers who ingested astroviruses in a fecal filtrate, only one suffered diarrhea and vomiting and shed astrovirus particles in stools. Nine additional volunteers ingested a fecal filtrate from the volunteer who developed the symptoms. None of these volunteers became ill, but two of them shed astrovirus. A rise in astrovirus-specific antibodies was detected in 13 of 16 volunteers, indicating that infection in adults readily occurs, but that clinical symptoms are uncommon. A seroepidemiological study in England found that over 70 percent of individuals acquired antibodies to astrovirus by 3 to 4 years of age. Several outbreaks of gastroenteritis in children have been reported, with symptoms similar to those caused by rotavirus, including vomiting, diarrhea, and mild dehydration. Data on the incidence of patients requiring hospitalization are not available. Dehydration severe enough to require intravenous fluid replacement therapy would require hospitalization.

In large-scale controlled studies of diarrhea among pediatric outpatients in Thailand, astroviruses were detected in 8.6 percent of ill individuals compared with 2.0 percent of the controls, demonstrating the significance of these viruses in childhood diarrhea. Clinical symptoms were essentially the same as those seen with rotavirus infections.

RESERVOIRS FOR THE AGENT

There have been no reports on infectivity for animals by any of the human astroviruses and there are no known reservoirs for these viruses.

MODE OF TRANSMISSION

Astroviruses are transmitted by the fecal–oral route as with other enteric viruses. Transmission through water and foods has been suspected but not proven.

METHODS FOR DETECTING THE AGENT

Methods for detecting astroviruses have been developed for clinical specimens obtained from patients, primarily stools and serum samples. How well these methods can be adapted to direct detection of astroviruses in water or other environmental samples remains to be determined. One isolation in cell cultures of astroviruses from water has been reported. The incidence of laboratory infections with astroviruses incurred by handling specimens is not known; however, precautions should be taken for other viruses, such as hepatitis A, polioviruses, or coxsackieviruses, or for bacterial pathogens that may be present in the samples being examined. Serum samples obtained from patients with astroviral gastroenteritis present no special hazard, but these samples should be handled with the usual precautions for human serum. Astroviruses are not currently classified by the Centers for Disease Control and Prevention (CDC), but their general characteristics suggest that they should be handled at a Biosafety 2 level.

Electron Microscopy

Before immunoassay or polymerase chain reaction (PCR) methods for astrovirus detection were developed, electron microscopy (EM) or IEM techniques were the major assays used. Although insensitive, these methods are still used to detect astroviruses when other assays are not available. EM may also be important for standardizing new detection methods as they are developed.

Astrovirus serotypes share a common antigen and develop a monoclonal antibody to the antigen that was group-reactive with the five serotypes known at that time. Two new astrovirus serotypes, 6 and 7, also react with this antibody. The enzyme-linked immunosorbent assay (ELISA) most effective for detecting virus in clinical stool samples is an indirect double antibody assay with monoclonal antibody used as the capture antibody and rabbit antiserum as the detector antibody. Presently there are no commercially available antigen detection tests for astroviruses; however, reagents in limited quantities are available from the Viral Gastroenteritis Unit at the CDC.

Nucleic acid probes for astrovirus identification has been used. For routine clinical diagnosis, probes offer no advantage compared with monoclonal antibody assays for astroviruses in gastroenteritis. The sensitivity is similar, but current probe techniques are considerably more complex and require more time to obtain results.

Amplified techniques, such as PCR, offer a more sensitive approach than direct hybridization for astroviruses. The sensitivity in detecting astrovirus infections is improved, but PCR techniques are more time-consuming and cumbersome to perform than ELISA.

Currently no methods for isolating astroviruses in cell cultures are routine. Astroviruses were originally isolated from stools by use of trypsin-treated primary human embryonic kidney (HEK) cells, and CaCo-2 cells can also be used for viral isolation.

Direct detection of astrovirus antigen or nucleic acid in water has not been reported, but astroviruses have been isolated in cell cultures from a natural water source. After three blind passages in CaCo-2 cells of a concentrated river water sample from sites with sewage pollution, astroviruses were detected by nucleic acid hybridization. The findings were confirmed by reverse-transcription PCR.

OCCURRENCE OF THE AGENT IN PEOPLE, ANIMALS, AND THE ENVIRONMENT

Astroviruses have been implicated in diarrhea of lambs and dogs, but no antigenic relationship to the known human astrovirus types has been shown.

SURVIVAL OF THE AGENT IN THE ENVIRONMENT

No studies concerning resistance to chemical or physical agents have been reported for human astroviruses. It can be assumed, based on their biophysical and biochemical properties, that they are similar to other gastroenteritis viruses regarding their stability in the environment. There is one report on isolation of astroviruses from river water.

DOCUMENTED WATERBORNE OUTBREAKS

No reports are available documenting waterborne outbreaks of astrovirus gastroenteritis.

INFORMATION SOURCES

Grohmann, G.S., R.I. Glass, H.G. Pereira, S.S. Monroe, A.W. Hightower, R. Weber, and R.T. Bryan. 1993. Enteric Viruses and Diarrhea in HIV-Infected Patients. *New England J. Med.*, 329:14–20

Herrmann, J.E., R.W. Hudson, D.M. Perron-Henry, J.B. Kurtz, and N.R. Blacklow. 1988. Antigenic Characterization of Cell-Cultivated Astrovirus Serotypes and Development of Astrovirus-Specific Monoclonal Antibodies. *J. Infect. Dis.*, 158:182–185.

Herrmann, J.E., N.A. Nowak, D.M. Perron-Henry, R.W. Hudson, W.D. Cubitt, and N.R. Blacklow. 1990. Diagnosis of Astrovirus Gastroenteritis by Antigen Detection with Monoclonal Antibodies. *J. Infect. Dis.*, 161:226–229.

Herrmann, J.E., D.N. Taylor, P. Echeverria, and N.R. Blacklow. 1991. *Astroviruses* as a Cause of Gastroenteritis in Children. *New England J. Med.*, 324:1757–1760.

Jiang, B., S.S. Monroe, E.V. Koonin, S.E. Stine, and R.I. Glass. 1993. RNA Sequence of Astrovirus: Distinctive Genomic Organization and a Putative Retrovirus-Like Ribosomal Frameshifting Signal that Directs the Viral Replicase Synthesis. *Proc. Nat. Acad. USA*, 90:10539–10543.

Jonassen, T.O., E. Kjeldsberg, and B. Grinde. 1993. Detection of Human Astrovirus Serotype 1 by the Polymerase Chain Reaction. *J. Virol. Meth.*, 44:83–88.

Kurtz, J., and T. Lee. 1978. Astrovirus Gastroenteritis Age Distribution of Antibody. *Med. Microbiol. Immunol.*, 166:227–230.

———. 1987. *Astroviruses:* Human and Animal. In *Novel Diarrhoea Viruses*. CIBA Foundation Symposium 128. pp. 92–101. Chichester, England: John Wiley & Sons.

Kurtz, J.B., T.W. Lee, J.W. Craig, and S.E. Reed. 1979. Astrovirus Infection in Volunteers. *J. Med. Virol.*, 3:221–230.

Lee, T., and J.B. Kurtz. 1981. Serial Propagation of Astrovirus in Tissue Culture with the Aid of Trypsin. *J. Gen. Virol.*, 57:421–424.

———. 1982. Human Astrovirus Serotypes. *J. Hyg. Camb.*, 89:539–540.

———. 1994. Prevalence of Human Astrovirus Serotypes in the Oxford Region 1976–92, with Evidence for Two New Serotypes. *Epidemiol. & Infect.*, 112:187–193.

Lewis, T.L., H.B. Greenberg, J.E. Herrmann, L.S. Smith, and S.M. Matsui. 1994. Analysis of Astrovirus Serotype 1 RNA, Identification of the Viral RNA-Dependent RNA Polymerase Motif, and Expression of a Viral Structural Protein. *J. Virol.*, 68:77–83.

Matsui, S.N., J.P. Kim, H.B. Greenberg, L.M. Young, L.S. Smith, T.L. Lewis, J.E. Herrmann, N.R. Blacklow, L.S. Oshiro, and G.R. Reyes. 1993. Cloning and Characterization of Human Astrovirus Immunoreactive Epitopes. *J. Virol.*, 67:1712–1715.

Moe, C.L., J.R. Allen, S.S. Monroe, H.R. Gary, Jr., C.D. Humphrey, J.E. Herrmann, N.R. Blacklow, C. Carcamo, M. Koch, K.-H. Kim, and R.I. Glass. 1991. Detection of Astrovirus by Immunoassay and RNA Probe in Pediatric Stool Samples. *J. Clin. Microbiol.*, 29:2390–2395.

Monroe, S.S., M.J. Carter, J.E. Herrmann, J.B. Kurtz, and S.M. Matsui. Family Astroviridae. 1995. Taxonomic Structure of the Family. *Arch. Virol.*, Suppl. 10:363–367.

Monroe, S.S., S.E. Stine, L. Gorelkin, J.E. Herrmann, N.R. Blacklow, and R.I. Glass. 1991. Temporal Synthesis of Proteins and RNAs During Human Astrovirus Infection of Cultured Cells. *J. Virol.*, 65:641–648.

Pinto, R.M., F.X. Abad, R. Gajardo, and A. Bosch. 1996. Detection of Astroviruses in Water. *Appl. Microbiol.*, 62:1811–1813.

Willcocks, M.M., and M.J. Carter. 1993. Identification and Sequence Determination of the Capsid Protein Gene of Human Astrovirus Serotype 1. *FEMS Microbiology Letters*, 114:1–7.

———. 1992. The 3' Terminal Sequence of a Human Astrovirus. *Arch. Virol.*, 124:279–289.

Willcocks, M.M., M.J. Carter, F.R. Laidler, and C.R. Madeley. 1990. Growth and Characterization of Human Faecal Astrovirus in a Continuous Cell Line. *Arch. Virol.*, 113:73–81.

Willcocks, M.M., J.G. Silcock, and C.R. Madeley. 1991. A Dot-Blot Hybridization Procedure for the Detection of Astrovirus in Stool Samples. *Epidemiol. & Infect.*, 107:405–410.

Chapter 41

Caliciviruses

Christon J. Hurst

DESCRIPTION OF THE AGENT

Caliciviruses are members of the Caliciviridae family. Two viral species of the Calicivirus are characteristically associated with humans—human caliciviruses and the hepatitis E virus. Included among the human caliciviruses are five recognized strains: Norwalk virus, Hawaii strain, Taunton strain, Snow Mountain strain, and Southampton strain. There are a variety of other strains whose common names are not yet officially recognized. The Norwalk virus and its related strains used to be called small, round, structured viruses based on their morphology as observed using transmission electron microscopy. Other species of caliciviruses infect mammals other than humans. Caliciviruses range in diameter from 27 to 40 nm. The caliciviruses have single-stranded ribonucleic acid (RNA) genomes and an icosahedral capsid structure with an external lattice arrangement. The capsids are not enveloped.

DESCRIPTION OF THE DISEASE

Symptoms of human disease caused by human caliciviruses can be divided into two categories, presumably associated with different viral strains. These categories are classical caliciviral illness and the Norwalk and Norwalk-like illness. Classical caliciviral illness usually strikes infants in the age range of 1 to 24 months, although some geriatric outbreaks have been noted. The principal symptom is diarrhea, with an incubation period of 48 to 72 hours. The ensuing symptoms usually last about 4 days, although symptoms can persist from 1 to 11 days. Illness associated with the Norwalk and Norwalk-like caliciviral strains typically has a shorter course. It incubates in approximately 24 to 48 hours and symptoms typically last from 12 to 48 hours, although they may last up to 60 hours. While this illness typically produces vomiting in children, adults affected by the same viral strains tend to have diarrhea. This illness is common in adults, and in the United States some 40 percent of the outbreaks of gastroenteritis in adults are attributed to the Norwalk and Norwalk-like viruses. Additional symptoms include abdominal pain and cramping, low fever, headache, nausea, malaise, and myalgia.

These diseases may be severe in immunologically debilitated and elderly patients. However, human fatality from either the classical caliciviral illness or Norwalk and Norwalk-like illness is usually rare if the patients are otherwise in good health and proper supportive care is available. Human caliciviruses are present worldwide and most children have been infected with at least one of the strains before leaving primary school.

The illness caused by the hepatitis E virus incubates in two to eight weeks with an average of five to six weeks. Children typically develop subclinical symptoms and jaundice tends to be associated with ages from 15 to 40 years, and can last for many weeks. Bilirubin levels tend to be higher and the jaundice deeper and more prolonged for illness due to the hepatitis E virus compared to the illness caused by the hepatitis A virus, the latter belonging to the *Picornaviridae* family. The hepatitis E virus seems responsible for the majority of cases of hepatitis that occur in Asian countries. The fatality rate for disease caused by the hepatitis E virus generally ranges from 0.1 to 4 percent. However, one notable concern associated with the hepatitis E virus is that in some outbreaks the death rate for pregnant women can be in the 14 to 17 percent range, and can even exceed 20 percent. The greatest risk of death seems to be associated with women who develop illness from hepatitis E virus in their third trimester of pregnancy.

As with most viral infections, the period of infectiousness or transmissibility for caliciviruses can begin before the onset of symptoms and may extend beyond the end of overt symptoms. Even those individuals who develop infections with no symptoms are capable of transmitting their infections. There presently are no known effective antimicrobial therapies for treating human caliciviral diseases.

RESERVOIRS FOR THE AGENT

Some of these viruses can infect other mammals under experimental conditions. However, while humans are considered to be the only natural reservoir for the species human caliciviruses, the hepatitis E virus appears to be zoonotic, with natural reservoirs including swine.

MODE OF TRANSMISSION

Caliciviruses are transmitted by ingestion or other oral contact with feces and fecal-contaminated material. Water is a significant way both the species human caliciviruses and hepatitis E virus are transmitted. Infections have been associated with ingestion of surface water contaminated by fecal material or wastewater, ingestion of groundwater contaminated by septic drainage from sewerage or outhouses, and swimming in sewage-contaminated waters. Infection also occurs by ingesting bivalve molluscan shellfish, including clams, cockles, mussels, and oysters. These shellfish apparently become contaminated during their natural process of filter feeding while growing in sewage-contaminated waters. Use of ice made from contaminated water or by unsanitary handling after the ice was produced has also caused infection.

METHODS FOR DETECTING THE AGENT

Human caliciviruses currently cannot be routinely cultured *in vitro* using animal tissues or animal cell lines. Therefore, detection techniques that do not provide direct evidence of viral infectivity are used. These techniques include visual detection of viruses by transmission electron microscopy and laboratory tests such as ELISA (enzyme-linked immunosorbent assay) and RT–PCR (reverse transcriptase–polymerase chain reaction) that detect the constituent viral proteins and RNA, respectively.

OCCURRENCE OF THE AGENT IN PEOPLE, ANIMALS, AND THE ENVIRONMENT

The caliciviruses that cause infections in humans, producing either classical calciviral illness or Norwalk and Norwalk-like illness, seem to have humans as their only natural reservoir. The calicivirus that causes hepatitis E illness seems to be zoonotic, meaning that animals are its natural reservoir.

SURVIVAL OF THE AGENT IN THE ENVIRONMENT

No information exists about the environmental stability of caliciviruses. This information may become available after the development of *in vitro* infectivity assays for these viruses.

DOCUMENTED WATERBORNE OUTBREAKS

Human caliciviruses and hepatitis E virus have caused numerous waterborne disease outbreaks. Infections and outbreaks of illness can occur year-round with some increased incidence of the classical caliciviral illness during the winter months. Incidence of illness caused by the specie hepatitis E virus tends to peak in autumn in the temperate areas of the world, while in tropical and monsoon areas, it occurs predominantly in flooded areas during the rainy season. Among the largest outbreaks have been those in Kashmir, Somalia, and Delhi. The death rates associated with hepatitis E have varied by a factor of nearly 50, which suggests that the severity of illness caused by this virus may be strongly strain-dependent. For instance, while the Delhi outbreak was estimated to have resulted in 90 deaths among 97,600 cases of illness, the Somalia outbreak reportedly resulted in nearly the same number of deaths while involving only 2,000 cases of illness.

INFORMATION SOURCES

Christensen, M.L., and C. Howard. 1991. Viruses Causing Gastroenteritis. In *Manual of Clinical Microbiology*. 5th ed. pp. 950–958. Balows, A., W.J. Hausler, Jr., K.L. Herrmann, H.D. Isenberg, and H.J. Shadomy, eds. Washington, D.C.: American Society for Microbiology.

Clayson, E.T., B.L. Innis, K.S.A. Myint, S. Narupiti, D.W. Vaughn, S. Giri, P. Ranabhat, and M.P. Shrestha. 1995. Detection of Hepatitis E Virus Infections Among Domestic Swine in the Kathmandu Valley of Nepal. *Am. J. Trop. Med. Hyg.*, 53(3):228–232.

Clayson, E.T., K.S.A. Myint, R. Snitbhan, D.W. Vaughn, B.L. Innis, L. Chan, P. Cheung, and M.P. Shrestha. 1995. Viremia, Fecal Shedding, and IgM and IgG Responses in Patients with Hepatitis E. *J. Infect. Dis.*, 172:927–933.

Cubitt, D., D.W. Bradley, M.J. Carter, S. Chiba, M.K. Estes, L.J. Saif, F.L. Schaffer, A.W. Smith, M.J. Studdert, and H.J. Thiel. 1995. Family Caliciviridae. In *Virus Taxonomy: Classification and Nomenclature of Viruses*. pp. 359–363. Murphy, F.A., C.M. Fauquet, D.H.L. Bishop, S.A. Ghabrial, A.W. Jarvis, G.P. Martelli, M.A. Mayo, and M.D. Summers, eds. Wien: Springer-Verlag.

Dowell, S.F., C. Groves, K.B. Kirkland, H.G. Cicirello, T. Ando, Q. Jin, J.R. Gentsch, S.S. Monroe, C.D. Humphrey, C. Slemp, D.M. Dwyer, R.A. Meriwether, and R.I. Glass. 1995. A Multistate Outbreak of Oyster-Associated Gastroenteritis: Implications for Interstate Tracing of Contaminated Shellfish. *J. Infect. Dis.*, 171:1497–1503.

Fenner, F.J., E.P.J. Gibbs, F.A. Murphy, R. Rott, M.J. Studdert, and D.O. White. 1993. Caliciviridae. In *Veterinary Virology*. 2nd ed. pp. 425–430. San Diego: Academic Press.

Hurst, C.J. 1996. Preventing Foodborne Infectious Disease. In *Modeling Disease Transmission and Its Prevention by Disinfection*. pp. 193–212. Hurst, C.J., ed. Cambridge: Cambridge University Press.

Hurst, C.J., R.M. Clark, and S.E. Regli. 1996. Estimating the Risk of Acquiring Infectious Disease from Ingestion of Water. In *Modeling Disease Transmission and Its Prevention by Disinfection*. pp. 99–139. Hurst, C.J., ed. Cambridge: Cambridge University Press.

Hurst, C.J., and P.A. Murphy. 1996. The Transmission and Prevention of Infectious Disease. In *Modeling Disease Transmission and Its Prevention by Disinfection*. pp. 3–54. Hurst, C.J., ed. Cambridge: Cambridge University Press.

Petric, M. 1995. Caliciviruses, Astroviruses, and Other Diarrheic Viruses. In *Manual of Clinical Microbiology*. 6th ed. pp. 1017–1024. Murray, P.R., E.J. Baron, M.A. Pfaller, F.C. Tenover, and R.H. Yolken, eds. Washington, D.C.: ASM Press, American Society for Microbiology.

Vinjé, J., and P.G. Koopmans. 1996. Molecular Detection and Epidemiology of Small Round-Structured Viruses in Outbreaks of Gastroenteritis in the Netherlands. *J. Infect. Dis.*, 174:610–615.

White, D.O., and F.J. Fenner. 1994. Caliciviridae and Astroviridae. In *Medical Virology*. 4th ed. pp. 407–417. San Diego: Academic Press.

Chapter 42

Enteroviruses

Charles P. Gerba

DESCRIPTION OF THE AGENT

Enteroviruses are a genus of the Picornaviridae family, which are among the smallest ribonucleic acid (RNA) viruses. "Pico" means small RNA virus. Enteroviruses are divided into the following four groups: poliovirus (3 types), coxsackievirus (30 types), echovirus (34 types), and enteroviruses (68 to 71 types). They are all nonenveloped, icosahedral in shape, and 25 to 30 nm in diameter. They contain a genome of single-stranded RNA of the positive sense, which acts like messenger RNA (mRNA). A characteristic of enteroviruses is their resistance to high and low pH. They are stable at pH 3 to 5 for 1 to 3 hours and can tolerate pH 10 to 11 for minutes. They are resistant to all known antibiotics and chemotherapeutic agents. Alcohol (70 percent), Lysol (5 percent), 1 percent quaternary ammonium compounds (Roccal), or similar laboratory disinfectants are not effective. They are also insensitive to ether and detergents that destroy lipid-containing viruses.

DESCRIPTION OF THE DISEASE

Enteroviruses cause a wide variety of illnesses, ranging from paralytic poliomyelitis (polio) to the common cold. Poliomyelitis has been known since ancient times, but became a major concern in the earlier part of the 20th century when epidemics primarily affecting young children became common during the summer and fall. The virus can cause permanent nerve damage that paralyzes arms, legs, or breathing. Most symptomatic infections only cause influenza-like or respiratory illness. Symptoms include aseptic meningitis, fever, rash, and severe headache, followed by stiffness. Only a small percentage of cases (0.1 to 2 percent) develop into paralytic disease. Poliovirus vaccine and large-scale vaccination programs have eradicated paralytic poliomyelitis from the Western Hemisphere. The World Health Organization is hoping to eliminate the disease from the human population in the next few years.

Coxsackie and echoviruses cause a wide range of illnesses in humans (Table 42-1). While most infections result in asymptomatic or mild illnesses, these viruses can cause more serious illness, including myocarditis, diabetes, and acute febrile illness among young children and infants. They are the most common cause of aseptic meningitis in developed countries. Fatalities in more severe illnesses (meningitis, myocarditis, and paralytic disease) can range from 0.01 to 0.9 percent.

The incubation period for enteroviruses varies greatly and may range from 1 to 35 days. Shorter incubation periods (two to three days) are typical for respiratory-tract infections. Laboratory diagnosis has usually been by isolation of the virus from stool, rectal swabs, throat swabs, or spinal fluid in primate cell culture. Serological typing with antisera pools is used to identify the specific enterovirus. Persons with enterovirus infections usually excrete the virus several days before clinical symptoms, during the acute illness, and often for several weeks afterwards. The period of communicability is potentially long. Enteroviruses are also excreted by persons who have asymptomatic infections.

Table 42-1 Clinical syndromes associated with enteroviruses

Enterovirus	Clinical Syndrome
Poliovirus types 1–3	Paralysis (complete to slight muscle weakness) Aseptic meningitis Febrile illness
Coxsackie, group A, types 1–24	Aseptic meningitis Herpingina Paralysis (infrequently) Exanthema Hand, foot, and mouth disease "Common cold" Hepatitis Infantile diarrhea Acute hemorrhagic conjunctivitis
Coxsackie, group B, types 1–6	Aseptic meningitis Pleurodynia Paralysis (infrequently) Severe systemic infection in infants, meningoencephalitis, and myocarditis Myocarditis Rash Febrile illness Upper respiratory illness and pneumonia Hepatitis Postviral fatigue syndrome Diabetes
Echoviruses, types 1–34	Aseptic meningitis Paralysis Encephalitis Exanthema Respiratory disease Diarrhea Pericarditis Myocarditis
Enterovirus, types 68–71	Pneumonia and bronchiolitis Acute hemorrhagic conjunctivitis Paralysis Meningoencephalitis Hand, foot, and mouth disease

In temperate climates, enterovirus infections peak in the late summer and fall. Enterovirus infections are greater in lower socioeconomic groups and are very common in young children. The incidence of children excreting enteroviruses has been observed to range from 2 percent in late fall to 22.2 percent in the summer. Peterson (1974) observed that 10 percent of all fecal-soiled diapers contained enteroviruses.

RESERVOIRS FOR THE AGENT

Humans are the only known natural host for enteroviruses. Although serologically distinct enteroviruses have been found in many animals, humans do not usually have recognizable infections with "animal" enteroviruses. Some laboratory animals, however, are susceptible to infection with human enteroviruses, including primates and neonatal mice for the coxsackieviruses.

MODE OF TRANSMISSION

Enteroviruses may be transmitted by the fecal–oral route or the respiratory route. One route may be more predominant than another, depending on the serotype. All enteroviruses are believed to be capable of transmission by the fecal–oral route, with the possible exception of enterovirus type 70. This type, which causes acute hemorrhagic conjunctivitis, may be transmitted only by direct contact with contaminated hands and fomites. Most transmission is believed to be person-to-person. Outbreaks of coxsackie and echoviruses from water and food have been documented.

METHODS FOR DETECTING THE AGENT

Enteroviruses can be grown in primate or human animal cell cultures with the production of cytopathogenic effects (CPE), although they may not all grow in the same cell line. Enteroviruses in water or other environmental samples are usually isolated by the production of CPE in the buffalo green monkey kidney (BGMK) cell line. Many of the enteroviruses also can be isolated by the plaque-forming unit (PFU) method.

OCCURRENCE OF THE AGENT IN PEOPLE, ANIMALS, AND THE ENVIRONMENT

Because enteroviruses grow easily in cell culture, they have been the human virus most commonly isolated from the environment. The concentration of enteroviruses in raw sewage has been reported to vary from a few hundred per litre to more than 100,000 per litre in some parts of the world. The concentration of enteroviruses in sewage is greater during the late summer and fall, and depends on the incidence rates in the community and the sanitation condition within the population. The average concentration of enteroviruses in raw sewage in the United States is estimated to be approximately 7,000 per litre.

With the exception of poliovirus, coxsackieviruses are the enteric viruses most often isolated from water, including treated drinking water. Enteroviruses are not completely removed by domestic sewage treatment, including standard disinfection, and can usually be isolated. Enteroviruses have been isolated in almost any source exposed to human fecal contamination, including groundwater, marine waters and sediments, shellfish, crabs, crops irrigated with sewage, domestic solid waste, soil, aerosols, and where spray irrigation of sewage is practiced.

The incidence of the virus in human fecal material depends on the same factors that influence its occurrence in sewage. The incidence in young children, which is higher than adults, may range from 10 to 40 percent during the summer months in some age groups.

Although animals are not the normal hosts of enteroviruses, they have been isolated from the stools of dogs, cats, and other domestic animals. They are not known to cause disease in these animals. Their occurrence is thought to be related to the often close association with these animals in developing world households.

SURVIVAL OF THE AGENT IN THE ENVIRONMENT

The survival of enteroviruses in the environment has been shown to depend on many factors, e.g., temperature, sewage pollution, bacteria, and adsorption to solids (clays and sediments). Typically, the lower the temperature, the longer the survival time. Enteroviruses may survive for years below 5° C in the environment.

DOCUMENTED WATERBORNE OUTBREAKS

Before the advent of the poliovirus vaccine, several published reports attributed outbreaks in part to contaminated drinking water. The studies, however, were not adequate to be conclusive. Coxsackieviruses have been associated with two recreational outbreaks and an epidemiological study of bathers in surface waters found a significant increased risk of enteroviral infection in children. Echovirus 30 was associated with an outbreak of gastroenteritis among bathers in a swimming pool. Although enteroviruses have been isolated during waterborne disease outbreaks associated with drinking water, epidemiological investigations have been lacking.

EFFECTIVENESS OF WATER TREATMENT PROCESSES

Enteroviruses have been the most studied of all enteric viruses for their ability to be removed by water treatment processes. Enteroviruses appear to be capable of being removed easily by conventional water treatment involving disinfection (99.99 percent or greater). Coxsackieviruses appear to be more resistant to ultraviolet (UV) light disinfection than the other enteroviruses.

NATIONAL OR INTERNATIONAL GUIDELINES AND MONITORING RECOMMENDATIONS

The European Economic Community (EEC) has had an enterovirus standard for bathing waters of 0 PFU per 10 litres since at least 1985. The EEC has also recommended that enteroviruses be absent in 10-litre volumes of drinking water. The state of Arizona, under its wastewater reuse standards, has had an allowable limit of 1 enteric virus per 40 litres of full-body contact water.

INFORMATION SOURCES

Arizona Administrative Code. 1991. Title 18, chapter 18, Article 7. *Regulations for the Reuse of Wastewater Suppl.,* 91-1:15–20.

Dagan, R., and M.A. Menegus. 1995 Non-polio Enteroviruses and the Febrile Infant. In *Human Enterovirus Infections.* pp. 239–254. Rotbart, H.A., ed. Washington, D.C.: ASM Press.

D'Alessio, D.J., T.E. Minor, D.B. Nelson, C.I. Allen, and A.A. Tsiatis. 1980. *Epidemiologic Studies on Virus Transmission in Swimming Waters.* EPA-600/1-80-006. Cincinnati, Ohio: US Environmental Protection Agency.

Denis, F.A., E. Blanchovin, F. Poitiers, and P. Flamen. 1974. Coxsackie A16 Infection from Lake Water. *J. Am. Med. Assoc.,* 226:1370–1371.

Grew, N., R.S. Gohd, J. Arguedas, and J.I. Kato. 1970. Enteroviruses in Rural Families and Their Domestic Animals. *Am. J. Epidemiol.,* 91:518–526.

Kee, F., G. McElroy, D. Stewart, P. Coyle, and J. Watson. 1994. A Community Outbreak of Echovirus Infection with an Outdoor Swimming Pool. *J. Pub. Health Med.*, 16:145–148.

Lundgren, D.L., A. Sanchez, M.G. Magnuson, and W.E. Clapper. 1968. Isolation of Human Enteroviruses from Beagle Dogs. *Proc. Soc. Exp. Biol. Med.,* 128:463–466.

Hawley, H.B., D.P. Morin, M.E. Geraghty, J. Tomkow, and A. Phillips. 1973. Coxsackievirus B Epidemic at a Boys' Summer Camp. *JAMA,* 226:33–36.

Mosley, J.W. 1966. Transmission of Viral Diseases by Drinking Water. In *Transmission of Viruses by the Water Route.* pp. 5–23. New York: Interscience.

Payment, P. 1991. Antibody Levels to Selected Enteric Viruses in a French-Canadian Population in the Province of Quebec (Canada). *Immunol. Infect. Dis.*, 1:317–322.

Peterson, M.L. 1974. Soiled Disposable Diapers: A Potential Source of Viruses. *Amer. J. Public Health,* 64:912–914.

Saliba, L. 1993. Legal and Economic Implications in Developing Criteria and Standards. In *Recreational Water Quality Management, Volume 2: Fresh Waters.* pp. 57–73. Kay, D., and R. Hanbury, eds. Chichester, UK: Ellis Horwood.

This page intentionally blank.

Chapter 43

Hepatitis A

Mark Sobsey

DESCRIPTION OF THE AGENT

Hepatitis A virus (HAV), the main cause of infectious hepatitis in the United States, is a member of the Picornaviridae family. For a time, HAV was classified as enterovirus 72 in the *Enterovirus* genus, but based on the extent of genetic (nucleic acid sequence homology) and phenotypic (temperature and pH resistance) differences, it is now classified as a hepatovirus. One species or antigenic type of HAV exists. However, there are several groups or genotypes of HAV, including at least two primarily human groups (genotypes I and III) and two nonhuman primates groups (genotypes II and IV). The human and nonhuman strain distinctions are not absolute, as a strain from *Aotus* monkeys is similar to human genotype III viruses.

HAV is a nonenveloped or "naked," icosahedral virion of about 27 nm in diameter. Virions consist of single-stranded, plus-sense ribonucleic acid (RNA) about 7,500 nucleotides long.

HAV is one of the most resistant viruses to a variety of physical, chemical, and biological agents. Compared to most other viruses, it is quite stable in water up to a temperature of 60° C, or even 80° C if stabilized with high concentrations of divalent cations. It is very stable to pH extremes, tolerating pH levels as low as 1 and as high as 10 for hours. It can be inactivated by strong oxidizing agents, such as free chlorine and ozone, and by powerful alkylating agents, such a gluteraldehyde. Compared to other enteric viruses, HAV is quite resistant to a variety of proteolytic enzymes, including those produced by naturally occurring microbes in water and soil.

DESCRIPTION OF THE DISEASE

HAV causes the disease known as "infectious hepatitis," which is an acute inflammation of the liver. Hepatitis E virus (HEV), a member of the Caliciviridae family described in chapter 41, also causes infectious hepatitis that is nearly indistinguishable from HAV and can also be waterborne. HEV is rare in the human population of the United States, although widespread in some other parts of the world, such as the Indian subcontinent, North Africa, parts of Eastern Europe, and Asia.

Infectious hepatitis is caused by ingesting fecal matter containing the virus. Infection is thought to begin in the epithelial cells of the intestinal tract, although the initial site has not been identified. The virus apparently spreads in the bloodstream to the liver where it destroys parenchymal cells. The incubation period averages about four weeks, ranging from two to six weeks, and symptoms typically last four weeks with a range of two weeks up to six months.

The mortality rate of hepatitis A is low, less than 0.3 percent in the United States, but can be higher in more susceptible members of the population and in other countries where additional factors contribute to poor health. The ratio of symptomatic to asymptomatic (subclinical or inapparent) infection varies with age. More than 90 percent of infections in infants and young children are asymptomatic. The rate of symptomatic infection increases with age and reaches 70 percent by adulthood. The severity of illness also increases with age, with most adults experiencing jaundice.

Hepatitis A has an abrupt onset with clinical symptoms of malaise, loss of appetite, dark urine, nausea, and vomiting. Scleral icterus (yellowing of the whites of the eyes) often occurs, as does jaundice (yellowing of the skin), and a tender liver. Shedding of the virus in feces, which can reach a billion virions per gram, begins during the incubation period and as early as two weeks before the onset of symptoms. Fecal shedding of viruses declines during the acute phase of illness, but can continue for weeks. Fecal material from HAV cases is infectious for weeks and highest in infection risk before clinical illness occurs. Virus is present in blood, serum, and saliva, but at much lower levels than in feces. Liver damage results not only in jaundice, but also increased levels of certain serum enzymes indicative of liver damage, primarily alanine and aspartate aminotransferase (ALT and AST). Liver damage is reversible, and the virus disappears from the body and recovery is complete.

Serum antibodies indicative of an immune response begin to appear about four weeks after infection. Initially, the levels of immunoglobulin M (IgM) are higher than the levels of immunoglobulin G (IgG), and this is diagnostic for current or recent infection. Over several months, levels of IgM wane and levels of IgG rise, which indicates past or historical infection. Immunity is considered to be lifelong. Studies indicate that HAV is less common in the United States, and other developed countries seroprevalence is less than 10 percent in young children and rises with age to about 50 percent in young adults. In developing countries with poor sanitation and hygiene, HAV infection is acquired early in life and seroprevalence approaches 100 percent in young adults.

RESERVOIRS FOR THE AGENT

Humans are the main reservoir for HAV. Nonhuman primates can be experimentally infected with human isolates of HAV and they also harbor their own unique genotypes or strains of HAV. Natural infection of humans with nonhuman primate strains of HAV may be possible.

MODE OF TRANSMISSION

Hepatitis A is transmitted primarily by ingesting feces containing HAV. In addition to direct and indirect personal contact, the virus is transmitted in fecally contaminated water, foods, fomites, and other objects. Less commonly, HAV is parenterally transmitted by infectious blood, serum, and therapeutic factors from blood, such as clotting factors. HAV transmission by exposure to respiratory exudates or urine is not likely. Water is an important vehicle of HAV transmission, but the other routes (especially food) account for the majority of reported cases of illness.

METHODS FOR DETECTING THE AGENT

Detecting HAV in water and other environmental samples is difficult and requires special techniques. In feces and other clinical samples containing high virus concentrations, HAV antigens can be detected by immunoassays, but laboratory diagnosis of suspected cases of HAV is primarily by detection of IgM antibodies in serum. HAV can be recovered and concentrated from water and other environmental samples by methods developed and used for other enteric viruses. HAV from clinical and environmental samples grows poorly and without cytopathogenic effects (CPE) in known cell cultures, so cell culture isolation is unreliable and often difficult, even when samples are known to be contaminated. The best cell cultures for HAV isolation are primary monkey kidney and FRhK4 (fetal rhesus monkey kidney derived) cells, but typically, several weeks or even months are required to achieve and confirm virus isolation. Confirmation of HAV isolation requires additional analytical methods, such as immunofluorescence assay, nucleic acid hybridization, or nucleic acid amplification by reverse transcription–PCR (RT–PCR). HAV in water can be detected directly by RT–PCR and nucleic acid hybridization of specially processed sample concentrates.

OCCURRENCE OF THE AGENT IN PEOPLE, ANIMALS, AND THE ENVIRONMENT

Persons actively infected or ill with HAV are major reservoirs and shed the virus in feces. Infected nonhuman primates also may be sources of HAV exposure. Once a person recovers from HAV infection or illness, virus shedding ceases. There is no evidence of chronic carriage, but long-term virus shedding occurs for some immunocompromised persons and some infants. Children experiencing asymptomatic infection can transmit HAV to others, especially in group settings like day-care centers. Other important settings for HAV transmission are overcrowded communities with poor sanitation and hygiene, such as those found in underdeveloped countries and underserved areas of the United States (e.g., Native American reservations in the Southwest); male homosexual and intravenous drug-use communities; institutions such as mental-health facilities, prisons, and jails; and facilities for nonhuman primates, such as zoos and animal research facilities. There is some evidence for increased risk of occupational exposure to HAV among sewer workers.

Besides direct and indirect person-to-person contact, major sources of HAV exposure are fecally contaminated water and food, especially in areas highly endemic for HAV. Water and fresh produce contaminated with sewage or other sources of human fecal waste, and foods, such as salads and sandwiches, prepared by infected persons are significant sources of HAV exposure. Of particular risk are bivalve molluscan shellfish (e.g., oysters, clams, and mussels) harvested from fecally contaminated waters and eaten raw or only partially cooked. Another risk is bathing in waters contaminated with sewage. As indicated in the next section, fecally contaminated drinking, bathing, and molluscan shellfishing waters and their associated sediments, molluscan shellfish, and other foods, and inadequately treated feces, sewage, or sludge can serve as reservoirs and potential transmission vehicles for HAV.

In the United States, 20,000 to 30,000 cases of HAV are reported annually, which is considered a substantial underestimate (perhaps by a factor of 10) of the true annual incidence. There is a minor seasonal peak of HAV in the fall and winter and annual peaks occur every decade (except in the 1980s). HAV vaccines have been licensed recently but are not universally required. These are expensive, killed-virus vaccines. Vaccination is recommended for persons in high-risk groups, including health-care and sewage workers, travelers to hyperendemic regions, military personnel, day-care workers, primate handlers, commercial food handlers, and sexually active homosexual men.

SURVIVAL OF THE AGENT IN THE ENVIRONMENT

HAV is one of the more persistent enteric viruses in the environment. Inactivation rates in feces, sewage, water, soil, and sediments are so slow that infectious viruses may persist for months to years, especially at lower temperatures. Fresh, frozen, and partially cooked shellfish have been vehicles of HAV because the viruses are highly protected and persistent in shellfish tissues and are not readily degraded or eliminated by live shellfish. HAV is relatively resistant to high temperatures and survives some pasteurization conditions. It is resistant to drying and desiccation and survives on fomites and other surfaces. It is also resistant to proteolytic enzymes and persists in microbially active water, soil, and sediments. HAV adsorption to soils is between the most highly and poorly adsorbed enteric viruses, but it survives longer than many other enteric viruses in soils and thus can contaminate groundwater sources of drinking water. Like other enteric viruses, HAV is not completely removed by sewage treatment processes, including disinfection. It is relatively resistant to combined chlorine, with $C \times T$-99.99 (disinfectant concentration by contact time for 99.99 percent inactivation) values in the hundreds to thousands of mg-min/L.

DOCUMENTED WATERBORNE OUTBREAKS

Waterborne outbreaks of hepatitis A continue to be reported in the United States and other countries. There were no waterborne outbreaks of HAV in 1993–94, two well water outbreaks in 1991–92, and two well water outbreaks in 1989–90. One outbreak was due to a community well water system with deficient treatment. The other three were due to untreated groundwater wells, of which two were individual systems serving homes and the other served a school and church. The report for 1989–90 also reported a previously undocumented 1988 outbreak due to an untreated community well water system serving a trailer park. These outbreaks are typical of most waterborne HAV outbreaks since the 1970s. From 1971 to 1988, 23 drinking waterborne outbreaks of HAV involving 737 cases were reported. Most outbreaks are due to untreated or inadequately treated groundwater that becomes contaminated from deficient on-site sewage treatment and disposal systems, usually septic tank–soil absorption systems.

EFFECTIVENESS OF WATER TREATMENT PROCESSES

Removal of HAV by conventional physicochemical water treatment processes of coagulation–flocculation and filtration is similar to that of other enteric viruses, with reductions up to 99 percent. Disinfection of water with free chlorine, chlorine dioxide, ozone, and ultraviolet (UV) light radiation can achieve up to 99.99 percent inactivation of HAV under optimum conditions. $C \times T$-99.99 values for the chemical disinfectants are less than 20 mg-min/L. If HAV is protected within organic matter or other particles, however, rates of inactivation can be dramatically reduced and $C \times T$ values can be more than 10-fold higher than for dispersed virions. UV radiation inactivates HAV better than some other enteric viruses, with 99.99 percent reduction at a dose of less than 20 mW-sec/cm^2. Like other enteric viruses, HAV is relatively resistant to combined chlorine. For monochloramine, HAV $C \times T$-99.99 values are in the thousands of mg-min/L. A small fraction of hepatitis A virions are highly resistant to monochloramine, probably because they are aggregated. Overall, complete conventional treatment of surface water should reduce HAV by 99.99 percent, as required by the Surface Water Treatment Rule (SWTR). Under optimum conditions, it should be possible to achieve substantial inactivation of HAV in groundwater by disinfection processes. However, the numerous groundwater outbreaks of HAV reported in the United States and elsewhere suggest that current groundwater supplies and their treatment practices (typically disinfection only) are not always adequate.

NATIONAL OR INTERNATIONAL GUIDELINES AND MONITORING RECOMMENDATIONS

International drinking water guidelines, such as those of the World Health Organization, recognize the importance of HAV as a waterborne viral pathogen, but it is not singled out for special treatment. Instead, HAV and other enteric viruses are expected to be essentially absent from drinking water and to pose a negligible risk to consumers. Alternative treatment options are recommended for different sources of groundwater and surface water to achieve essentially virus-free drinking water.

Currently, national guidelines or standards for drinking water quality in the United States do not specify requirements to monitor or treat for HAV. The Information Collection Rule (ICR) in support of the Enhanced Surface Water Treatment Rule (ESWTR) requires monitoring for enteric viruses in drinking water supplies from surface sources serving 100,000 people or more. But, the methods used in the ICR would not detect HAV. The current SWTR set many of the $C \times T$ requirements for enteric virus disinfection on the basis of HAV inactivation, although inactivation of *Giardia* cysts is usually the more stringent and therefore controlling basis for the $C \times T$ requirements of this rule.

INFORMATION SOURCES

Battigelli, D., D. Lobe, and M.D. Sobsey. 1993. Inactivation of Hepatitis A Virus and Other Enteric Viruses in Water by Ultraviolet Light. *Wat. Sci. Tech.*, 27(3–4):339–342.

Callahan, K.M., D.J. Taylor, and M.D. Sobsey. 1995. Comparative Survival of Hepatitis A Virus, Poliovirus and Indicator Viruses in Geographically Diverse Seawaters. *Wat. Sci. Tech.*, 31(5–6):189–193.

Craun, G.F. 1991. Causes of Waterborne Outbreaks in the United States. *Wat. Sci. Tech.*, 24(2):17–20.

Hall, R.M., and M.D. Sobsey. 1993. Inactivation of Hepatitis A Virus (HAV) and MS-2 by Ozone and Ozone-Hydrogen Peroxide in Buffered Water. *Wat. Sci. Tech.*, 27(3–4):371–378.

Herwaldt, B.L., G.F. Craun, S.L. Stokes, and D.D. Juranek. 1992. Outbreaks of Waterborne Disease in the United States: 1989–90. *Jour. AWWA*, 84(4):129–135.

Hollinger, F.B., and J.R. Ticehurst. 1996. Hepatitis A Virus. In *Fields Virology*. 3rd ed. pp. 735–782. Fields, B.N., D.M. Knipe, P.M. Howley, R.M. Chanock, J.L. Melnick, T.P. Monath, B. Roizman, and S.E. Strauss, eds. Philadelphia, Pa.: Lippincott-Raven Publishers.

Kramer, M.H., B.L. Herwaldt, G.F. Craun, R.L. Calderon, and D.D. Juranek. 1996. Waterborne Disease: 1993–1994. *Jour. AWWA*, 88(3):66–80.

Moore, A.C., B.L. Herwaldt, G.F. Craun, R.L. Calderon, A.K. Highsmith, and D.D. Juranek. 1994. Waterborne Disease in the United States, 1991 and 1992. *Jour. AWWA,* 86(2):87–99.

Rao, V.C., J.M. Symons, A. Ling, T.G. Metcalf, and J.L. Melnick. 1988. Removal of Hepatitis A Virus by Drinking Water Treatment. *Jour. AWWA,* 80(2):59–67.

Sobsey, M.D., S.E. Oglesbee, and D.A. Wait. 1985. Evaluation of Methods for Concentrating Hepatitis A Virus from Drinking Water. *Appl. Environ. Microbiol.,* 50(6):1457–1463.

Sobsey, M.D., P.A. Shields, F.S. Hauchman, A.L. Davis., V.A. Rullman, and A. Bosch. 1988. Survival and Persistence of Hepatitis A Virus in Environmental Samples. In *Viral Hepatitis and Liver Disease.* pp. 121–124. Zuckerman, A.J., ed. New York: Alan R. Liss, Inc.

Sobsey, M.D., T. Fuji, and P.A. Shields. 1989. Inactivation of Hepatitis A Virus and Model Viruses in Water by Free Chlorine and Monochloramine. *Wat. Sci. Tech.,* 20(11/12):385–391.

Sobsey, M.D., T. Fuji, D. Battigelli, and R.M. Hall. 1990. Inactivation of Cell-Associated and Dispersed Hepatitis A Virus by Free and Combined Chlorine and Chlorine Dioxide. In *Proc. 1989 AWWA Water Quality Technology Conference.* pp. 167–179. Denver, Colo.: American Water Works Association.

Sobsey, M.D., T. Fuji, and R.M. Hall. 1991. Inactivation of Cell-Associated and Dispersed Hepatitis A Virus in Water. *Jour. AWWA,* 83(11):64–67.

Sobsey, M.D., R.M. Hall, and R.L. Hazard. 1995. Comparative Reductions of Hepatitis A Virus, Enteroviruses and Coliphage MS2 in Miniature Soil Columns. *Wat. Sci. Tech.,* 31(5–6):203–20[illegible].

Sobsey, M.D., D.A. Battigelli, T.R. Handzel, and K.J. Schwab. 1995. *Male-specific Coliphages as Indicators of Viral Contamination of Drinking Water.* Denver, Colo.: American Water Works Association Research Foundation and American Water Works Association.

Sobsey, M.D., K.J. Schwab, R. De Leon, and Y.-S.C. Shieh. 1996. *Enteric Virus Detection in Water by Nucleic Acid Methods.* Denver, Colo.: American Water Works Association Research Foundation and American Water Works Association.

USEPA. 1989. *Guidance Manual for Compliance with the Surface Water Treatment Requirements for Public Water Systems.* Washington, D.C.: Criteria and Standards Division, USEPA, Office of Drinking Water.

Venczel, L.V., M.D. Sobsey, and D. Crawford-Brown. 1992. The Inactivation Kinetics of Monochloramine on Monodispersed Hepatitis A Virus and MS2. In *Proc. 1991 AWWA Water Quality Technology Conference.* pp. 531–550. Denver, Colo.: American Water Works Association.

World Health Organization. 1993. *Guidelines for Drinking-water Quality.* 2nd ed. Vol. 1. Geneva: World Health Organization.

Chapter 44

Reoviruses

Syed A. Sattar and V. Susan Springthorpe

INTRODUCTION

Reoviruses are very widely distributed in nature and are commonly found in sewage and fecal-polluted waters; they are perhaps the most commonly isolated viruses from water. They belong to the genus *Orthoreovirus* in the family Reoviridae. Reoviruses have been found in mammals, including humans, and in birds, reptiles, fish, invertebrates, and plants. Basic characteristics of mammalian reoviruses are summarized in Table 44-1.

ASSOCIATION OF REOVIRUSES WITH DISEASE IN HUMANS AND ANIMALS

Reoviruses were first isolated in 1951 from the respiratory and gastrointestinal tracts of humans. Reovirus infections in humans occur early in life and most cases are subclinical or very mild. Unconfirmed reports associate reoviruses with biliary atresia, juvenile onset diabetes, fever, exanthema (rash), respiratory disease, diarrhea, hepatitis, pneumonia, eye infections, encephalitis, meningitis, myocarditis, and other symptoms. The name *reo* was derived from the fact that these viruses are found in the respiratory and enteric tracts and are orphans because of a lack of association with a human disease.

Human reoviruses are pathogenic in newborn mice. The three serotypes of reoviruses of humans and other mammals are indistinguishable. Avian reoviruses are antigenically distinct from mammalian types. In poultry, reoviruses can cause arthritis and other symptoms. Avian reoviruses can also induce immunosuppression in chickens by destroying B cells. It is not yet known if reoviruses can cross species barriers.

BASIC CHARACTERISTICS AND PROPAGATION

Virions are icosahedral in shape with a double protein shell. They are 75 to 82 nm across and lack an envelope. The genome is double-stranded ribonucleic acid (RNA) with 10 segments. Reoviruses can grow in animals or cell cultures, but not in embryonated eggs. The virus replicates exclusively in the cytoplasm. Complete particles can be assembled as soon as six to eight hours after infection.

Mammalian reoviruses can be grown in kidney cells from a variety of animals. L cells, derived from mice, are often used for this purpose. For virus isolation from human clinical specimens, bovine kidney cells (MDBK) are the most sensitive. Monkey kidney cells (LLC-MK_2, MA104, Vero, or BGM) are commonly used to isolate reovirus from environmental samples.

Reoviruses produce a highly distinctive and characteristic cytopathology. The large cytoplasmic inclusions initially appear as cytoplasmic granules and develop

Table 44-1 Basic characteristics of mammalian reoviruses

Characteristic	Description
Shape, size, and structure	Round, icosahedral symmetry; nonenveloped; double-shelled protein capsid; virions 75 to 82 nm in diameter, two stable subvirion forms (infectious subviral particles and cores) can be derived by treating virions with proteolytic enzymes; molecular weight of intact virions 129.5×10^6 Dalton.
Genome	Linear, double-stranded RNA with 10 segments; virions contain 15–20% nucleic acid; total genome 23,700 nucleotides long.
Proteins and antigens	Contain at least 12 types of proteins including a hemagglutinin, an RNA polymerase, and other enzymes for virus replication; 80–85% of virion is protein; the 3 serotypes share a group-specific antigen; can be distinguished based on neutralization and hemagglutination-inhibition tests; isolates from humans and other mammals hard to separate based on such tests.
Resistance to physicochemical agents	Resistant to lipid solvents and 1% phenol; inactivated by 70% ethanol and 800 ppm sod. hypochlorite; stable at pH 3.5; proteases and sod. thiocyanate can disrupt outer capsid.
Host range	Can infect humans, chimpanzees, monkeys, dogs, horses, cats, cattle, sheep, swine, mice, bats, etc.
Diseases caused	Antibodies to reoviruses common in humans and virus only occasionally found in mild cases of respiratory and enteric infections; not considered important human pathogens; in other mammals known to cause many clinical conditions, including jaundice, meningitis, encephalitis, pneumonia, myocarditis, gastroenteritis, biliary atresia; mice experimental animals of choice and, depending on the route of inoculation, develop diarrhea, runting syndrome, oily hair, encephalitis, etc.
Isolation in the laboratory	Cell cultures of human, monkey, and mouse origin hosts of choice; infection of cells lytic with characteristic cytopathology and formation of large, perinuclear cytoplasmic inclusions. Do not grow in embryonated eggs.
Epidemiology	Ubiquitous in nature; antibody to all 3 types acquired in early life; not known if animal reoviruses can infect humans; frequently found in sewage and fecally polluted waters; spread mainly by fecal–oral route and airborne spread suspected; no water-, food-, or airborne outbreaks documented.
Survival in water and wastewater	Survives in experimentally contaminated water from months to years; survives in wastewater and can also be isolated from sewage treatment train.
Reduction during water and wastewater treatment	No reliable figures available for water treatment but probably reovirus removals were comparable to other human viruses. Relative stability to wastewater treatment processes, although varying decay observed.

into large, irregular-shaped masses in the perinuclear region. They are readily recognized before cell destruction occurs, and are diagnostic of reoviruses even if the numbers are too low to be readily confirmed with electron microscopy.

Infected mice, the most common experimental animals, show diarrhea with high fat content in the stools, pneumonia, myocarditis, runting, oily hair, jaundice, and involvement of the central nervous system. Infection of the bile duct in mice can lead to chronic biliary atresia and jaundice. Injury to the pancreas, pituitary gland, and thyroids also occurs in mice. Intracerebral injection of reovirus type 3 into newborn mice leads to fatal encephalitis; intramuscular injection can cause myositis.

SURVIVAL AND RESISTANCE TO PHYSICAL AND CHEMICAL AGENTS

Reoviruses are relatively long-lived in water. In surface waters, with an input dose of 10^4 infective units, more than 200 days were required for infectious reovirus to become undetectable. *In situ* survival studies in cellophane tubes indicated survival in excess of six months. When samples of river water were filtered or centrifuged to remove bacteria, then experimentally contaminated with reovirus and held at approximately 5° C, the viruses remained infective for longer than three years. All of these systems are to some extent artificial and may overestimate actual survival in the water column. On the other hand, viruses in natural systems can be protected by adsorption to particulate matter. Reovirus survival may vary with the type of organic and mineral material contacted and heterogeneity exists within the reovirus population.

Reoviruses are stable over a wide range of pH, even at pH 3.5. Aerosol stability of reoviruses appears favored by relative humidities above 75 percent or below 40 percent. Recreational water users could be exposed without water ingestion. Reovirus may also survive aerosolization during spray irrigation of crops. The virus is relatively resistant to the levels of disinfectants normally used for water and wastewater disinfection.

REOVIRUS OCCURRENCE IN WATER AND WASTEWATER

Many studies have reported reoviruses in natural waters. These studies typically report a spectrum of other virus isolations and frequently reoviruses are the most numerous viruses isolated. When few or no reoviruses are reported, it may be the result of a failure to look for them, use of a cell line not highly sensitive to reoviruses, or use of concentration and isolation methods that inactivate or fail to recover small numbers of reoviruses. Reoviruses have also been found in piped spring water and potable supplies.

Reoviruses occur in relatively high numbers in sewage, comprising 26 to 57 percent of the isolated organisms, and in slaughterhouse wastes. In Ottawa, Ont., reoviruses accounted for 57, 43, and 59 percent of virus isolates identified from samples of raw sewage, and primary effluent before and after chlorination, respectively. At a smaller plant, the number of samples positive for reovirus dropped from 43.5 percent in the raw sewage to 21.7 percent in the chlorinated primary effluent (Table 44-2). Although the total virus numbers dropped by approximately 60 percent, mixed infections made it difficult to account for the exact reductions in reovirus. Some studies did not detect seasonal patterns of reovirus recovery. Other studies, however, have suggested that reovirus isolations are seasonal, occurring with the greatest frequency in late summer, fall, and early winter. Sample size and reduced water flow at that time of year should also be considered when evaluating possible seasonal variations in reovirus recovery.

ISOLATION OF REOVIRUSES FROM WATER AND WASTEWATER

Isolation of reoviruses from surface water will almost certainly require sample concentration. Samples of 20 to 100 L are often used. Reoviruses can be concentrated by adsorption–elution on a variety of electronegative or electropositive matrices, by precipitation with flocculating agents, or by tangential ultrafiltration. The best method for concentration of reoviruses from natural waters has not been determined. Most isolation methods, including a tentative standard method for virus isolation, were developed primarily for enteroviruses rather than reoviruses. Any method that uses pH values above 10 for elution from the adsorption matrix may not be suitable for optimal recovery of reoviruses.

Cell lines are often used for recovering infectious reovirus from sample concentrates. MA-104 cells appear to be more sensitive than BGM cells or BSC-1 cells. Several cell lines for reovirus isolation have been determined and indicate the superiority of primary RhMK cells. Primary HEK cells were found to be very sensitive for reovirus isolation. The difficulties and costs of working with and obtaining primary cells, however, will almost certainly be outweighed by the relative ease and consistency obtained from an established cell line. Recently CaCo-2 cells

Table 44-2 Reovirus isolation from the Ottawa River, Canada*

Collection sites, in upstream to downstream progression	Samples positive for virus(es), *percent*	Samples positive for reovirus, *percent*
1. Raw sewage from small upstream sewage treatment plant	100 (23/23)	43.5 (10/23)
2. Chlorinated effluent from small upstream sewage plant. Plant discharged into lagoon with long (>6 months) retention	56.5 (13/23)	21.7 (5/23)
3. Bay water downstream from sewage plant lagoon	43.8 (7/16)	25 (4/16)
4. Beach water, year 1	55.0 (11/20)	30.0 (6/20)
5. Beach water, year 2	77.3 (17/22)	50.0 (11/22)
6. Raw water intake for upstream treatment plant (located midstream)	43.5 (10/23)	26.1 (6/23)
7. Treated water—plant 1	0.00 (0/25)	0.00 (0/25)
8. Raw water intake (located midstream) for second treatment plant. This intake is upstream from the major sewage plant on one river bank but may be influenced by discharges from the other river bank.	82.9 (29/35)	65.7 (23/35)
9. Treated water—plant 2	0.00 (0/38)	0.00 (0/38)
10. Just below discharge of large downstream sewage treatment plant with primary treatment only	100.0 (25/25)	76.0 (19/25)
11. Downstream site 1†	100.0 (24/24)	75.0 (18/24)
12. Downstream site 2†	100.0 (15/15)	66.7 (10/15)
13. Downstream site 3†	100.0 (12/12)	100.0 (12/12)

*Adapted from Sattar et al. (1978/1979).

†These sites receive sewage discharge from both river banks and from significant tributaries.

have been proposed as a universal cell line for virus isolation because of their sensitivity to fastidious viruses; however, more work is needed to validate this suggestion. Ultimately, cell line selection will be governed by both the desired targets for isolation as well as individual experience. This is because it is well recognized that the same cell line can behave quite differently between laboratories. Sera used for cell culture isolation of reovirus must be free from reovirus antibodies.

SOURCES OF REOVIRUSES IN WATER

The source of reoviruses in surface waters is mainly fecal material discharged directly or through incomplete treatment of wastes. Studies in Japan and Germany on reoviruses in water indicate their main source to be human excreta. While such studies are important in understanding the primary sources of reoviral pollution of surface waters, any reoviruses recovered from water cannot be assumed necessarily to be of human origin. Therefore, risk assessment for contact with these viruses is difficult until more is known about their ability to cross species boundaries.

REOVIRUS ELIMINATION DURING WATER AND WASTEWATER TREATMENT

No studies that specifically examined reovirus removal during conventional water treatment have been found. However, no reoviruses were found in the 500- to 1,000-L samples of treated drinking water when levels of reoviruses were detected in 26 or 66 percent of the raw water samples (100-L) studied. Reovirus removal by slow sand filtration demonstrated that such treatment can remove up to 99.99 percent (4 $\log_{10}$ units) depending on water quality, flow rate, and bed construction. Adsorbed reovirus was detected throughout the bed, but concentrations decreased with increasing bed depth. Some work on inactivation of viruses by 0.5 ppm chlorine suggests that 4 $\log_{10}$ reduction in reovirus titer can be achieved after 2 to 4 minutes. The degree of reovirus clumping may have an impact on disinfection rates.

Most studies of virus removal from wastewater during treatment do not specifically examine reductions for reoviruses. However, a treatment plant handling domestic sewage removed reoviruses less efficiently than enteroviruses. Studies isolated reoviruses from chlorinated primary effluent at approximately 50 percent of that isolated from raw sewage. Dewatering of sludge led to only a small drop in reovirus recovery until sludge solids were greater than 90 percent.

CONCLUDING REMARKS

Information on reoviruses is limited because they are not regarded as major human pathogens. Because they are ubiquitous and easily recognized, they could play a role as indicators of other pathogenic viruses. More work is needed to optimize methods for reovirus recovery from natural waters and wastewaters, to determine whether they are seasonal or year-round contaminants, and to determine if they can cross species boundaries.

INFORMATION SOURCES

Aulicini, F.A., A. Mastrantonio, P. Orsini, et al. 1996. Enteric Viruses in a Wastewater Treatment Plant in Rome. *Water, Air & Soil Pollu.*, 91:327–334.

Gilbert, R.G., R.C. Rice, H. Bouwer, et al. 1976. Wastewater Renovation and Reuse: Virus Removal by Soil Filtration. *Science,* 192:1004–1005.

Goyal, S.M., and C.P. Gerba. 1982. Concentration of Viruses from Water by Membrane Filters. In *Methods in Environmental Virology.* pp. 59–116. Gerba, C.P., and S.M. Goyal, eds. New York: Marcel Dekker, Inc.

Grandien, M., M. Forsgren, and A. Ehrnst. 1995. Reoviruses. In *Diagnostic Procedures for Viral, Rickettsial, and Chlamydial Infections.* Lennette, E.H., D.A. Lennette, and E.T. Lennette, eds. Washington, D.C.: American Public Health Association.

Lipson, S.M., and G. Stotsky. 1984. Effect of Proteins on Reovirus Adsorption to Clay Minerals. *Appl. Environ. Microbiol.,* 48:525–530.

Mahnel, H., K. Ottis, and M. Herlyn. 1977. Stabilitaet von Neun Viruatren Unterschiedlisher Genera in Trink- und Oberflaechenwasser. *Zbl. Bakt. Hyg. I. Abt. Orig. B,* 164:64–84.

Matsuura, K., M. Ishikura, T. Nakayama, et al. 1988. Ecological Studies on Reovirus Pollution of Rivers in Toyama Prefecture. *Microbiol. & Immunol.,* 32:1221–1234.

———. 1993. Ecological Studies on Reovirus Pollution of Rivers in Toyama Prefecture II. Molecular Epidemiological Studies of Reoviruses Isolated from River Water. *Microbiol. & Immunol.*, 37:305–310.

McConnell, L.K., R.C. Sims, and B.B. Barnett. 1984. Reovirus Removal and Inactivation by Slow Sand Filtration. *Appl. Environ. Microbiol.,* 48:818–825.

Milde, N., D. Tougianidou, and K. Botzenhart. 1995. Occurrence of Reoviruses in Environmental Water Samples. *Water Sci. Tech.,* 31:363–366.

Nibert, M.L., L.A. Schiff, and B.N. Fields. 1996. Reoviruses and Their Replication. In *Fundamental Virology.* 3rd ed. pp. 691–730. Fields, B.N., D.M. Knipe, and P.M. Howley, eds. New York: Lippincott-Raven.

Palfi, A.B. 1971. Virus Content of Sewage in Different Seasons in Hungary. *Acta Microbiol Acad. Sci. Hung.,* 18:231–237.

Patti, A.M., F.A. Aulicini, A.L. Santi, et al. 1996. Enteric Virus Pollution of Tyrrhenian Areas. *Water, Air & Soil Pollu.,* 88:261–267.

Pinto, R.M., R. Gajardo, F.X. Abad, and A. Bosch. 1995. Detection of Fastidious Infectious Enteric Viruses in Water. *Envir. Sci. and Tech.,* 29:2636–2638.

Sattar, S.A. 1978. *Viral Pollution of the Ottawa River and Its Possible Impact on the Quality of Potable and Recreational Waters in the Ottawa Area—Phase I.* May 1978. Ontario Ministry of the Environment Research Study—Contract #77-004-11.

———. 1979. *Viral Pollution of the Ottawa River and Its Impact on the Quality of Potable and Recreational Waters in the Ottawa Area—Phase II.* May 1979. Ontario Ministry of the Environment Research.

Sattar, S.A., and J.C.N. Westwood. 1978. Viral Pollution of Surface Waters Due to Chlorinated Primary Effluents. *Appl. Environ. Microbiol.,* 36:427–431.

Sattar, S.A., V.S. Springthorpe, and S. Ramia. 1978–79. Sewage Disposal and Viral Pollution of the Ottawa River. *Water Poll. Res. Canada*, 14:45–62

Schwartzbrod, L., C. Finance, M. Aymard, et al. 1985. Recovery of Reoviruses from Tap Water. *Z. Bakt. Mikrobiol. Hyg. 1-Abt. Orig B, Hygiene,* 181:383–389.

Sharma, J.M., K. Karaca, and T. Pertile. 1994. Virus-Induced Immunosuppression in Chickens. *Poultry Sci.,* 73:1082–1086.

Smith, E.M., and C.P. Gerba. 1982. Laboratory Methods for the Growth and Detection of Animal Viruses. In *Methods in Environmental Virology.* pp. 15–47. Gerb, C.P., and S.M. Goyal, eds. New York: Marcel Dekker, Inc.

Spendlove, J.C., and K.F. Fannin. 1982. Methods for Characterization of Virus Aerosols. In *Methods in Environmental Virology.* pp. 261–329. Gerba, C.P., and S.M. Goyal, eds. New York: Marcel Dekker, Inc.

Sproul, O.J. 1973. Effectiveness of Water and Wastewater Treatment Processes in Virus Removal and Inactivation. In *Proc. Symp. Viruses in the Environment and their Potential Hazards Nov. 1973.* Mahdy, M.S., and B.J. Dutka, eds. Ontario: Canada Centre for Inland Waters.

Tani, N., Y. Dohi, N. Kurumatani, and K. Yonemasu. 1995. Seasonal Distribution of Adenoviruses, Enteroviruses and Reoviruses in Urban River Water. *Microbiol. & Immunol.,* 39:577–80.

Ward, R.L. 1983. Destruction of Viruses in Sludges by Treatment Processes. In *Viral Pollution of the Environment.* pp. 95–114. Berg, G., ed. Boca Raton, Fla.: CRC Press, Inc.

Chapter 45

Rotaviruses

Morteza Abbaszadegan

DESCRIPTION OF THE AGENT

The rotaviruses belong to a family of viruses known as Reoviridae. There are six known rotavirus groups (A–F). Groups A, B, and C rotaviruses are found in humans and animals, and groups D, E, and F have been only reported in animals to date. Group A, which contains nine serotypes is the most studied. They are nonenveloped, icosahedral viruses with a double-layer protein capsid. They have both an outer and inner layer and a core, and are 65 to 75 nm in diameter. The genome is composed of 11 segments of double-stranded ribonucleic acid (RNA). Rotaviruses are capable of genetic reassortment and replicate in the cytoplasm of host cells.

DESCRIPTION OF THE DISEASE

Rotaviral infections are the cause of many serious diarrheal illnesses, mostly in infants and children under age two. Rotavirus infections are responsible for 3.5 million cases of diarrhea and 125 deaths in infants and young children in the United States and more than 500,000 deaths worldwide per year. There are an estimated 500,000 physician visits and 50,000 hospitalizations yearly related to rotavirus. In addition, rotavirus accounts for 30 to 50 percent of US hospitalizations for diarrhea in children younger than five years.

Rotaviruses also infect adults and are thought to be the primary cause of traveler's diarrhea. The incubation period of rotavirus infection is less than 48 hours, with a duration of illness for typically 5 to 8 days. The clinical symptoms usually include vomiting, abdominal distress, diarrhea, and dehydration. Fever and respiratory involvement are often associated with the illness in children, and adults usually have more asymptomatic infections than children. The virus is excreted in large numbers in the feces of infected individuals, with concentrations as high as 10^{10} rotavirus per gram of fecal materials.

Rotaviruses are the leading cause of acute infantile gastroenteritis and diarrhea-related infantile death. The virus has also been associated with diarrhea outbreaks among the elderly and among immunocompromised patients.

RESERVOIRS FOR THE AGENT

Humans and animals are the primary reservoirs for rotaviruses. The virus has been isolated from humans, monkeys, cattle, sheep, mice, cats, dogs, and other mammals, and from chickens and turkeys. Although the various strains of rotavirus are usually associated with a specific species, reports have documented infections through interspecies transmission, including a human infection by a bovine strain of rotavirus. Additionally, recent work has shown that an isolated rotavirus surface protein alone can produce diarrhea in mice.

MODE OF TRANSMISSION

Rotaviruses are transmitted via the fecal–oral route. They may also be transmitted via the respiratory route, but that is not yet proven. In a significant number of cases, the viruses were isolated from the nasopharyngeal area. Most rotavirus infections and illness occur in the winter in temperate climate. This seasonal pattern is apparent worldwide, except in the tropics where it occurs year-round.

METHODS FOR DETECTING THE AGENT

Rotavirus detection in water samples can be accomplished by cell culture assays or polymerase chain reaction (PCR). In addition, group A rotavirus can be detected using enzyme-linked immunosorbent assay (ELISA), latex agglutination, and counter-immunoelectric-osmophoresis. Non-group A rotaviruses are difficult to grow in cell culture, only one has been successfully cultivated. Both group A and non-group A rotavirus can be detected by electron microscopy.

OCCURRENCE OF THE AGENT IN PEOPLE, ANIMALS, AND THE ENVIRONMENT

Rotaviruses have been isolated from humans and the environment. The virus is stable in feces at room temperature, with infectivity persisting for a minimum of a week. The virus has been detected on contaminated surfaces in day-care centers. Rotaviruses have been detected in wastewater, with concentrations as high as 90,700 per litre. Based on a limited number of studies on the occurrence of rotavirus in raw sewage in the United States, the average concentration was reported to range from 10 to 218 per litre. Rotaviruses have been detected in surface, ground, and recreational waters in the United States. The virus has also been detected in marine waters, including both bathing and shellfish harvesting waters.

SURVIVAL OF THE AGENT IN THE ENVIRONMENT

Rotaviruses, like most enteric viruses, are resistant to inactivation at both low (3.5) and high (10.0) pH. Rotaviruses can survive secondary sewage treatment, including disinfection. They also can survive in water for days to weeks, depending on water quality and temperature. Although true evidence of waterborne outbreaks has proven scarce, rotavirus group A has been documented as a cause of such outbreaks in humans.

DOCUMENTED WATERBORNE OUTBREAKS

Rotaviruses have been studied in conjunction with other enteric viruses as possible sources of waterborne illness and are thought to be the cause of gastrointestinal waterborne illnesses.

The organism has been detected in fresh water and sewage. There have been at least nine documented waterborne outbreaks. The outbreaks were associated with direct fecal contamination of a water supply or improper treatment. Rotaviruses are known to have high attack rates in adults. In an outbreak of rotaviral gastroenteritis in a community water system in Vail, Colo., the attack rate among adults was 43.8 percent.

EFFECTIVENESS OF WATER TREATMENT PROCESSES

Currently, the understanding for removal of rotaviruses by conventional water treatment processes is similar to other enteric viruses. They are effectively removed during the processes, especially through disinfection. Rotaviruses are susceptible to disinfection in water with free chlorine, ozone, and ultraviolet (UV) radiation. They are more resistant to inactivation by UV light than enteroviruses, probably because they contain double-stranded RNA.

Most viruses are known to be substantially inactivated by free chlorine, but are more resistant to free chlorine than most enteric bacteria. Viruses in feces, wastewater, tapwater, and associated with solids are much more resistant to inactivation.

NATIONAL OR INTERNATIONAL GUIDELINES AND MONITORING RECOMMENDATIONS

In the United States, rotavirus infections are monitored by the National Respiratory and Enteric Virus Surveillance System (NREVSS). National guidelines for drinking water quality do not specify requirements to monitor or treat for rotavirus.

INFORMATION SOURCES

Abbaszadegan, M., P. Stewart, C.P. Gerba, and M.W. LeChevallier. 1998. *Application of PCR Technologies for Virus Detection in Groundwater.* Denver, Colo.: American Water Works Association Research Foundation and American Water Works Association.

Ball, J.M., P. Tian, C. Zeng, A.P. Morris, and M.K. Estes. 1996. Age-Dependent Diarrhea Induced by a Rotaviral Nonstructural Glycoprotein. *Science*, 272:101–104.

CDC. 1997. Laboratory-Based Surveillance for Rotavirus—United States, July 1996–June 1997. *MMWR*, 46:1092–1094.

Estes, M.K., Palmer, E.L., and J.F. Obijeski. 1983. Rotaviruses: A Review. *Current Topics in Microbio. Immun.*, 105:123–184.

Estes, M.K. 1990. Rotaviruses and Their Replication. *Virology*, 48:1329–1347.

Gerba, C.P., J.B. Rose, and S.N. Singh. 1985. Waterborne Gastroenteritis and Viral Hepatitis. *CRC Crit. Rev. Environ. Contr.*, 15:213–236.

Gerba, C.P., and J.B. Rose. 1990. Viruses in Source and Drinking Water. In *Drinking Water Microbiology.* McFeters, G.A., ed. New York: Springer-Verlag.

Glass, R.I., P.E. Kilgore, R.C. Holman, et al. 1996. The Epidemiology of Rotavirus Diarrhea in the United States: Surveillance and Estimates of Disease Burden. *J. Infect. Dis.*, 174(suppl.):S5–S11.

Gouvea, V., R.I. Glass, P. Woods, K. Taniguchi, H.F. Clark, B. Forrester, and Z.-Y. Fang. 1990. Polymerase Chain Reaction and Amplification and Typing of Rotavirus Nucleic Acid for Stool Specimens. *J. Clin. Microbiol.*, 28:276–282.

Hopkins, R.S., G.B. Gaspard, F.P. Williams, R.J. Karlin, G. Cukor, and N.R. Blacklow. 1984. A Community Waterborne Gastroenteritis Outbreak: Evidence for Rotavirus as the Agent. *Amer. J. Public Hlth.*, 74:263–265.

Hrdy, D.B. 1987. Epidemiology of Rotaviral Infection in Adults. *Rev. Infect. Dis.*, 9:461–469.

Kapikian, R.Z., and R.M. Chanock. 1990. Rotaviruses. *Virology*, 49:1353–1387.

Keswick, B.H., L.K. Pickering, H.L. DuPont, and W.E. Woodward. 1983. Survival and Detection of Rotaviruses and Environmental Surfaces in Day-Care Centers. *Appl. Environ. Microbiol.*, 46:813–816.

Matson, D.O., and M.K. Estes. 1990. Impact of Rotavirus Infection at a Large Pediatric Hospital. *J. Infect. Dis.*, 162:598–604.

Moe, K., and J.A. Shirley. 1982. The Effects of Relative Humidity and Temperature on Survival of Human Rotavirus in Feces. *Arch. Virol.*, 72:179–186.

Nakagomi, O., Y. Isegawa, R.L. Ward D.L. Knowlton, E. Kaga, T. Nakagomi, and S. Ueda. 1994. Naturally Occurring Dual Infection with Human and Bovine Rotaviruses as Suggested by the Recovery of G1P8 and G1P5 Rotaviruses from a Single Patient. *Arch. Virol.*, 137:381–388.

Rao, V.C., T.G. Metcalf, and J.L. Melnick. 1986. Development of a Method for Concentration of Rotavirus and its Application to Recovery of Rotaviruses from Estuarine Waters. *Appl. Environ. Microbiol.*, 52:484–488.

Sobsey, M.D. 1989. Inactivation of Health-Related Microorganisms in Water by Disinfection Process. *Wat. Sci. Tech.*, 21:179–195.

Chapter 46

Small, Round, Structured Viruses (Human Caliciviruses)

Kellogg Schwab

DESCRIPTION OF THE AGENT

Electron microscopy (EM) used for examining fecal specimens from persons with nonbacterial gastroenteritis revealed a group of viruses generically described as small, round, structured viruses (SRSVs). These viruses have been difficult to characterize because researchers cannot grow them in cell culture and they lack a suitable animal infectivity model. SRSVs range in size from 20 to 40 nm, and are nonenveloped icosahedral particles. Many of the SRSVs recently analyzed by their nucleic acid have been shown to be human caliciviruses (HuCVs), suggesting that most, if not all, SRSVs are HuCVs. The viral genome of the characterized SRSVs consists of single-stranded, positive-sense ribonucleic acid (RNA), 7,000 to 8,000 nucleotides in length. Originally, other viruses, such as parvovirus, were classified as SRSVs based on morphological characteristics.

DESCRIPTION OF THE DISEASE

Outbreaks due to SRSVs are characterized by median incubation periods of 24 to 48 hours, median durations of 12 to 48 hours, and a high percentage of patients with diarrhea, nausea, abdominal cramps, and vomiting. Symptoms are typically self-limiting and not life-threatening, with adequate fluid replacement to prevent dehydration, which is the only treatment needed. Strains of SRSVs can be highly infectious with rapid spread of infection. In volunteer studies, attack rates are greater than 50 percent and sometimes as high as 90 percent. Patients suffered a rapid onset of explosive diarrhea, vomiting, or both.

RESERVOIRS FOR THE AGENT

For SRSVs associated with human disease, the only reservoir appears to be humans.

MODE OF TRANSMISSION

SRSV is predominantly transmitted via the fecal–oral route. Viruses have been transmitted through contamination of private wells, small water systems, community water systems, and recreational waters. Cold food contaminated by food handlers and consumption of raw and cooked shellfish (predominantly bivalve mollusks) has been documented.

METHODS FOR DETECTING THE AGENT

Norwalk virus (NV), the prototype SRSV, was first isolated from an outbreak of epidemic gastroenteritis in an elementary school in Norwalk, Ohio. The virus was observed using immuno-electron microscopy (IEM) in specimens from volunteers fed stool filtrates from the school outbreak. IEM uses sera from convalescent patients as a source of specific antibodies to agglutinate the virions and make them easier to recognize. Solid-phase, immuno-electron microscopy (SPIEM) fixes the antibodies onto the EM grid, providing a platform to capture virus particles for subsequent IEM detection. These methods have serious limitations because specific hyperimmune animal sera are not available for many of the viruses and human sera contain a wide spectrum of antibodies. In addition, the surface morphology of the virus may be obscured by antibodies. As a result, unrelated viruses might be classified with other morphologically distinct viruses merely on the basis of similar size and buoyant density. Detection of viruses by IEM requires approximately 10^5 virus particles per mL; the concentration of SRSVs present in environmental samples often are below this detection level, limiting the diagnostic value of IEM.

Immunologic assays, such as the radioimmunoassay (RIA) and enzyme-linked immunoassays (ELISA) were developed using human volunteer reagents to detect both antibody and virus. When stable virus-like particles (VLPs) were produced, sensitive and specific ELISAs using hyperimmune antisera were developed. ELISAs using these new reagents have significantly improved the sensitivity of detecting these viruses over older methods using human reagents.

Reverse transcription–polymerase chain reaction (RT–PCR) assays are the most sensitive diagnostic methods currently available for the detection of SRSVs. Primer pairs that amplify a number of different regions in the viral genome have been used diagnostically. Unfortunately, the genetic diversity of SRSVs has prevented the development of a universal primer pair that can amplify all such viruses. Techniques to overcome the diversity of SRSVs are being developed.

A confirmation test should be performed following the RT–PCR reaction. Hybridization assays (dot/slot or Southern blot hybridization) are the most common confirmatory assays used. They also increase the sensitivity of virus detection by 10- to 100-fold over that obtained with agarose gel electrophoresis alone. However, the genetic diversity of SRSVs limits the usefulness of hybridization assays. The use of as many as 10 different oligoprobes was not sufficient to confirm all PCR results obtained using a panel of different HuCV strains.

Direct sequencing of PCR products is an alternate, although more labor-intensive, technique to confirm PCR results. Stool and environmental samples contain a variety of substances that may inhibit reverse transcription or PCRs. When working with stool and environmental samples, the use of appropriate controls is essential to detect any inhibition. The addition of low concentrations of an internal standard RNA control allows the detection of inhibitory substances without compromising the sensitivity of the RT–PCR assay. False positive results due to carryover contamination may occur due to the sensitivity of RT–PCR assays. Physical separation of pre- and post-PCR working areas, dedicated reagents and equipment for pre-PCR sample processing, and appropriate controls for each PCR reaction to prevent such occurrences should be followed.

OCCURRENCE OF THE AGENT IN PEOPLE, ANIMALS, AND THE ENVIRONMENT

SRSVs that infect humans appear to have humans as their only reservoir.

SURVIVAL OF THE AGENT IN THE ENVIRONMENT

Because SRSVs cannot be grown in cell culture, nothing is known about survival of intact and potentially infectious SRSVs in the environment. Although SRSVs are unique because their capsid is composed of only one protein, SRSV resistance to environmental degradation might be similar to other nonenveloped, single-stranded RNA viruses, such as hepatitis A virus. Human volunteer studies have shown that NV retained infectivity for volunteers following exposure to pH 2.7 for 3 hours at room temperature, treatment with 20 percent ether at 4° C for 18 hours, or incubation at 60° C for 30 minutes. Research indicates that NV may be as resistant as poliovirus type 3 and bacteriophage MS2 to inactivation by chlorine dioxide (ClO_2).

DOCUMENTED WATERBORNE OUTBREAKS

SRSVs cause outbreaks of waterborne and foodborne gastroenteritis, and studies have estimated that at least 42 percent of outbreaks of nonbacterial gastroenteritis in the United States are caused by such infections. Outbreaks of waterborne viral gastroenteritis have been associated with private wells, small water systems, community water systems, and groundwater contamination. Several outbreaks have been associated with recreational waters and outbreaks have also occurred when food such as celery was washed with contaminated water. One such outbreak involved over 1,500 cadets and staff at the US Air Force Academy. Celery had been soaked for one hour in water from a hose used earlier in the day to clear clogged drains in the kitchen after sewage had backed up.

EFFECTIVENESS OF WATER TREATMENT PROCESSES

Very little information has been reported on the survival characteristics of SRSVs during standard water treatment processes. In one study, human volunteers were given NV treated with chlorine. A dose of 3.75 mg/L, resulting in no free residual Cl, failed to inactivate NV. A dose of 10 mg/L, with a free residual Cl level of 5–6 mg/L, apparently did inactivate the virus. The study concluded that NV was very resistant to Cl as compared to other indicator viruses. Because an infectivity model has not been developed for SRSVs, the effectiveness of water treatment procedures in eliminating or inactivating these important human pathogens is difficult to determine. Researchers are attempting to identify specific human intestinal cells that will support the growth of SRSVs to establish such an infectivity model. However, recent studies using Norwalk virus VLPs in filtration experiments show great promise as model systems for enteric virus transport through treatment processes.

NATIONAL OR INTERNATIONAL GUIDELINES AND MONITORING RECOMMENDATIONS

There are no guidelines for monitoring SRSVs in water at this time.

INFORMATION SOURCES

Ando, T., S.S. Monroe, J.R. Gentsch, Q. Jin, D.C. Lewis, and R.I. Glass. 1995. Detection and Differentiation of Antigenically Distinct Small Round-Structured Viruses (Norwalk-like Viruses) by Reverse Transcription–PCR and Southern Hybridization. *J. Clin. Microbiol.,* 33:64–71.

Baron, R.C., F.D. Murphy, H.B. Greenberg, C.E. Davis, D.J. Bregman, G.W. Gary, J.M. Hughes, and L.B. Schonberger. 1982. Norwalk Gastrointestinal Illness: An Outbreak Associated with Swimming in a Recreational Lake and Secondary Person-To-Person Transmission. *Am. J. Epidemiol.,* 115:163–172.

Beller, M., A. Ellis, S.H. Lee, M.A. Drebot, S.A. Jenkerson, E. Funk, M.D. Sobsey, O.D. Simmons, S.S. Monroe, T. Ando, J. Noel, M. Petric, J.P. Middaugh, and J.S. Spika. 1997. Outbreak of Viral Gastroenteritis Due to a Contaminated Well. International Consequences. *JAMA,* 278:563–568.

Dolin, R., N.R. Blacklow, H. DuPont, R.F. Buscho, R.G. Wyatt, J.A. Kasel, R. Hornick, and R.M. Chanock. 1972. Biological Properties of Norwalk Agent of Acute Infectious Nonbacterial Gastroenteritis. *Proc. Soc. Exp. Biol. Med.,* 140:578–583.

Estes, M.K., R.L. Atmar, and M.E. Hardy. 1997. Norwalk and Related Diarrhea Viruses. In *Clinical Virology.* pp. 1073–1095. Richman, D.D., R.J. Whitley, and F.G. Hayden, eds. New York: Churchill and Livingstone.

Graham, D.Y., X. Jiang, T. Tanaka, A.R. Opekun, H.P. Madore, and M.K. Estes. 1994. Norwalk Virus Infection of Volunteers: New Insights Based on Improved Assays. *J. Infect. Dis.,* 170:34–43.

Gray J.J., J. Green, C. Cunliffe, C.I. Gallimore, J.V. Lee, K. Neal, and D.W. Brown. 1997. Mixed Genogroup SRSV Infections Among a Party of Canoeists Exposed to Contaminated Recreational Water. *J. Med. Virol.,* 52:425–429.

Hedberg, C.W., and M.T. Osterholm. 1993. Outbreaks of Food-borne and Waterborne Viral Gastroenteritis. *Clin. Microbiol. Reviews,* 6:199–210.

Jiang, X., M. Wang, D.Y. Graham, and M.E. Estes. 1992. Expression, Self-assembly, and Antigenicity of the Norwalk Virus Capsid Protein. *J. Virol.,* 66:6527–6532.

Kapikian, A.Z., R.G. Wyatt, R. Dolin, T.S. Thornhill, A.R. Kalica, and R.M. Chanock. 1972. Visualization by Immune Electron Microscopy of a 27 nm Particle Associated with Acute Infectious Nonbacterial Gastorenteritis. *J. Virol.,* 10:1075–1081.

Kaplan, J.E., G.W. Gary, R.C. Baron, N. Singh, L.B. Schonberger, R. Feldman, and H.B. Greenberg. 1982a. Epidemiology of Norwalk Gastroenteritis and the Role of Norwalk Virus in Outbreaks of Acute Nonbacterial Gastroenteritis. *Annals Intern. Med.,* 96:756–761.

Kaplan, J.E., R.A. Goodman, L.B. Schonberger, E.C. Lippy, and G.W. Gary. 1982b. Gastroenteritis Due to Norwalk Virus: An Outbreak Associated with a Municipal Water System. *J. Infect. Dis.,* 146:190–197.

Keswick, B.H., T.K. Satterwhite, P.C. Johnson, H.L. DuPont, S.L. Secor, J.A. Bitsura, G.W. Gary, and J.C. Hoff. 1985. Inactivation of Norwalk Virus in Drinking Water by Chlorine. *Appl. Environ. Microbiol.,* 50:261–264.

Lawson, H.W., M.M. Braun, R.I. Glass, S.E. Stine, S.S. Monroe, H.K. Atrash, L.E. Lee, and S.J. Englender. 1991. Waterborne Outbreak of Norwalk Virus Gastroenteritis at a Southwest US Resort: Role of Geological Formations in Contamination of Well Water. *Lancet,* 337:1200–1204.

Le Guyader, F., M.K. Estes, M.E. Hardy, F.H. Neill, J. Green, D. Brown, and R.L. Atmar. 1996. Evaluation of a Degenerate Primer for the PCR Detection of Human Caliciviruses. *Arch. Virol.,* 141:2225–2235.

Redman, J.A., S.B. Grant, T.M. Olson, M.E. Hardy, and M.K. Estes. 1997. Filtration of Recombinant Norwalk Virus Particles and Bacteriophage MS2 in Quartz Sand: Importance of Electrostatic Interactions. *Envir. Sci. & Tech.,* 31:3378–3383.

Schwab, K.J., M.K. Estes, F.H. Neill, and R.L. Atmar. 1997. Use of Heat Release and an Internal RNA Standard Control in Reverse Transcription–PCR Detection of Norwalk Virus from Stool Samples. *J. Clin. Microbiol.,* 35:511–514.

Shin, G., and M.D. Sobsey. 1997. Norwalk Virus Reduction by Chlorine Dioxide as Determined by Alternative PCR Assays. New Orleans: ASM Proceedings.

Taylor, J.W., G.W. Gary, Jr., and H.B. Greenberg. 1981. Norwalk-Related Viral Gastroenteritis Due to Contaminated Drinking Water. *Am. J. Epidemiol.,* 114:584–592.

Warner, R.D., R.W. Carr, F.K. McCleskey, P.C. Johnson, L.M. Elmer, and V.E. Davison. 1991. A Large Nontypical Outbreak of Norwalk Virus. Gastroenteritis Associated with Exposing Celery to Nonpotable Water and with *Citrobacter freundii. Arch. Intern. Med.,* 151:2419–2424.

Appendix A

Introduction to Web Sites

Many web sites are dedicated to pathogenic microorganisms reviewed in this manual. These sites may be useful for updating information and to access current information. Web sites can provide a wealth of information; however, the information is not regulated or peer-reviewed. Anyone can place information on a web page. As supplements to the information presented in this manual, it is suggested that the following web sites be used as initial searches for further information:

http://www.cdc.gov/ncidod/nica.htm of the National Center for Infectious Diseases, Centers for Disease Control and Prevention.

http://vm.cfsan.fda.gov/~mow/intto.html US Food and Drug Administration Center for Food Safety and Applied Nutrition Foodborne Pathogenic Microorganisms and Natural Toxins Handbook.

http://www.ksu.edu/parasitology/topics is a web site maintained by Dr. Steve Upton of Kansas State University, which gives a bibliographic list of select articles dealing with *Cryptosporidium*.

http://www.epa.gov/nerlcwww provides access to microbiology-related information developed or managed by USEPA. From this site, you can access an on-line publication, an image gallery, and a directory of publications.

This page intentionally blank.

Glossary

aerobic Living or occurring only in the presence of oxygen.

aerosolization To be in water vapor.

agar A gelatinous material prepared from certain marine algae and used as a solidification agent for bacterial culture media.

agglutination Adhesion of distinct parts

aggregation To clump or grow together.

alveolar A small cavity or pit, such as a honey comb cell.

ambient temperature 22 to 35° C.

amebic Caused by an amoeba, as in amebic dysentery.

ameboflagellate Amoeba that has a flagellate stage in addition to the trophozoite and cyst stages.

ameboid Shapeless or shape-changing.

amino acid An organic compound containing both an amino group (NH_2) and a carboxylic acid group (COOH).

amphotericin B Antibiotic.

anaerobic Living or occurring without the presence of oxygen.

anoxic Absence of oxygen.

antihelminthic Acting to expel or destroy intestinal worms.

antigen A substance that when introduced into the body stimulates the production of an antibody.

antimicrobial Capable of destroying or suppressing the growth of microorganisms.

AOC Assimilable organic carbon.

artifacts Unknown material, other than that being tested for.

ascariasis Infestation with nematode worms of the species *Ascaris lumbricoides*.

asymptomatic Neither causing nor exhibiting symptoms.

autochthonous Native to a particular place; indigenous.

axillae The armpit or an analogous part.

axoneme Basal portions of flagella within cytoplasm.

backsiphon Water flow in a backward direction caused by the siphon effect.

bacteria Any of numerous unicellular microorganisms of the class schizomycetes, occurring in a wide variety of forms, existing either as free-living organisms or as parasites, and having a wide range of biochemical, often pathogenic, properties.

bacteriophage A submicroscopic, usually viral organism that destroys bacteria.

bacteriostatic agent Inhibits growth or multiplication of bacteria.

Baird-Parker agar Growth medium that permits the detection, enumeration, and isolation of coagulase-positive staphylococci after 24 hours of incubation.

barrier A method or obstacle preventing passage.

biliary atresia Closure of bile ducts.

biofilm A build-up of agents.

birefringence The resolution or splitting of a light wave into two waves with mutually perpendicular vibration directions by an optically anisotropic medium, such as calcite or quartz.

BOD Biochemical oxygen demand.

boil Painful, localized, pus-filled swelling of the skin and subcutaneous tissue caused by bacterial infection.

bradyzoite Slowly multiplying forms of parasites.

CaCo-2 cell Cell line derived from cells; colon carcinoma.

caecum A cavity with only one opening; the large blind pouch forming the beginning of the large intestine.

capsule A mucopolysaccharide layer enveloping certain bacteria.

carbol fuchsin technique, modified Used for examination of fecal specimens.

carbuncle A painful, localized, pus-producing infection of the skin and subcutaneous tissue.

casein A white, tasteless, odorless milk and cheese protein used to make plastics, adhesives, paints, and foods.

catalase An enzyme in the blood and tissues that catalyzes the decomposition of hydrogen peroxide into water and oxygen.

cellulitis Inflammation of subcutaneous tissue.

cercariae Free-swimming larvae of schistosomes.

cestode A flatworm of the class Cestoda, which includes the tapeworms.

cfu Colony-forming units.

Charcot-Leyden crystal Minute crystals occurring in the sputum of patients with asthma and bronchitis.

chemorganotrophic Chemical affinity of substances for certain organs or tissues of the body.

chitinized spore coat A hard, white, horny polysaccharide that is the principal constituent of the spore coating.

chloramine Any of several compounds containing nitrogen and chlorine.

chorioretinitis Inflammation of the choroid and retina.

chromogenic colony Colony producing a pigment or coloring matter.

citrate A salt or ester of citric acid.

clearwell A reservoir of treated water.

coagulation The transformation of a liquid or solid into a soft, semisolid, or solid mass.

coccal bodies Spherical in shape.

coccobacilli Bacilli that are short and oval in shape.

coliform Of, pertaining to, or resembling the colon bacillus.

colony A group of the same kind of animals, plants, or one-celled organisms living or growing together; visible growths of microorganisms in a nutrient medium.

commensal organism Close association of two organisms in which one or both may derive some benefit but neither harms or is parasitic on the other.

community water system Water systems serving at least 25 residents year-round.

conjugation A process of sexual reproduction in which ciliate protozoans of the same species temporarily couple and exchange genetic material.

conjunctivitis Inflammation of the conjunctiva (the mucous membrane that lines the inner surface of the eyelid and the exposed surface of the eyeball).

connective tissue Tissue such as tendons and muscles.

contact time (CT) The period of disinfection in water treatment.

cribiform plate A plate that is perforated like a sieve.

cross-connection Potable and nonpotable water supplies that become connected.

cutaneous Of, pertaining to, or affecting the skin.

cyst A resting stage formed by some bacteria and protozoa in which the whole cell is surrounded by a protective layer.

cysticerci Bladderworms.

cytopathic effect The effect of pathological/morphological change.

cytoplasm The protoplasm outside a cell nucleus.

cytostome The mouth aperture (opening) of certain protozoa.

depuration Cleansing or purifying, or becoming cleansed or purified.

desiccation The process of drying out completely.

diatomaceous earth (DE) A white or cream-colored siliceous earth composed of the shells of diatoms.

diplopia A disorder of vision that causes objects to appear double.

direct plating Taking a sample aliquot from specimen and applying directly to a culture plate.

disinfection Destruction of harmful microorganisms, usually by the use of bactericidal chemical compounds.

disinfection by-products Compounds created by the reaction of a disinfectant with organic compounds in water.

DNA Deoxyribonucleic acid; a polymeric chromosomal constituent of living cell nuclei, consisting of two long chains of alternating phosphate and deoxyribose units twisted into a double helix and joined by hydrogen bonds between the complementary bases adenine and thymine or cytosine and guanine, each of which projects toward the axis of the helix from one of the strands where it is bonded in a sequence that determines individual hereditary characteristics.

DNA–DNA homology group Genomic species.

duodenojejunal aspirate Aspirate from the area containing duodenum and jejunum (the first portion of the small intestine).

dyspepsia Functional disturbance of the intestine, which can result in malnutrition.

ectocyst Outside the cyst.

elevated eosinophilia High counts of eosinophils.

eluted One material extracted from another, usually by means of a solvent.

embryonation To develop into the embryo stage.

empyema Pus in a body cavity, such as the pleural cavity or gall bladder.

encapsulated Enclosed by a protective coating or membrane, as in certain bacteria.

endemic Prevalent in or peculiar to a particular locality or people.

endocarditis Inflammation of the endocardium (the thin, endothelial, serous membrane that lines the interior of the heart).

endocyst Within the cyst.

endotoxin A toxin produced within a microorganism and released on destruction of the cell in which it is produced.

enteric Of or within the intestine.

enterotoxin A toxin produced by bacteria that is specific for intestinal cells and causes the symptoms of food poisoning.

enzyme-linked immunosorbent assay (ELISA) The basic system consists of antibodies bonded to enzymes that remain able to catalyze a reaction yielding a visually discernible end product while attached to the antibody. The antibody-binding sites remain free to react with their specific antigen.

eosinophilia An increase in the number of eosinophils (any microorganism, cell, or histological element easily stained by eosin dye) in the blood.

epidemiology The study of wide-spread, infectious diseases.

epifluorescent microscopy A microscope designed to observe organisms that have been treated with fluorescent stains or dyes.

epithelial Membranous tissue, usually in a single layer, composed of closely arranged cells separated by very little intercellular substance and forming the covering of most internal surfaces, organs, and the outer surface of an animal body.

erythema edema A redness of the skin and swelling as caused by chemical poisoning or sunburn.

erythermatous nodule A nodule that has redness associated with it.

estuary The part of the wide lower course of a river where its current is met by the tides.

etiological agent Something that causes a disease.

eugonic media Media that encourages luxuriant growth.

eukaryotic protozoa Organism with a nucleus.

eutrophic Designating a body of water in which the increase of mineral and organic nutrients has reduced the dissolved oxygen, producing an environment that favors plant over animal life.

excystation When a cyst ruptures or opens.

extraintestinal Outside the intestine.

family A taxonomic category ranking below an order and above a genus.

febrile Of, pertaining to, or characterized by fever; feverish.

fermentative Causing chemical reactions induced by living or nonliving ferments that split complex organic compounds into relatively simple substances.

filtration The process of passing a liquid or a gas through a porous substance to remove constituents such as suspended matter.

fimbriae A fringe-like part or structure.

flagellate Having a flagellum or flagella.

flagellum A long filamentous process; whiplike extensions of certain cells or unicellular organisms, usually functioning locomotion.

flocculation To form lumpy or fluffy masses.

flora Plants collectively; the plants of a particular region or time.

fluorescent antibody test (FA) A technique to identify an organism using a fluorescently labeled antibody specific to the organism.

folliculitis Inflammation of a follicle (an approximately spherical group of cells containing a cavity).

fomite An inanimate object or substance that serves to transfer infectious organisms from one individual to another.

formalin A 37 percent by weight aqueous solution of formaldehyde with some methanol.

GAC Granulated activated carbon.

GAE Granulomatous amoebic encephalitis.

gas chromatography Chromatography in which the substance to be analyzed is vaporized and diffused along with a carrier gas through a liquid or solid adsorbent for differential adsorption.

gastroenteritis Inflammation of the mucous membrane of the stomach and intestine.

genera (pl.), genus (sing.) Taxonomic categories ranking below a family and above a species.

genome A complete haploid set of chromosomes.

GN A broth used as a selective medium for cultivation of gram-negative bacteria.

gram-negative Loses the stain or becomes decolorized by alcohol in Gram's method of staining. This is a primary identifying characteristic of certain microorganisms.

granulomatous amoebic encephalitis (GAE) A meningoencephalitis caused by freshwater amoebas; may occur as a subacute or chronic disease with focal granulomatous lesions in the brain; the skin or lungs are primary sites of invasion; causative organism is an *Acanthamoeba* spp.

Guillane-Barre syndrome A syndrome described in encephalitis of virus origin consisting of absence of fever, pain or tenderness in the muscles, motor weakness, abolition of tendon reflexes, great increase in the protein in the cerebrospinal fluid without corresponding increase in cells.

HAV Hepatitis A virus.

helminth ova Eggs of the helminth (intestinal parasite).

hematogenous Containing red blood cells.

hemiparesis Muscular weakness affecting one side.

hemodialysis Dialysis of the blood.

hemolysin An agent or substance that initiates lysis of red blood cells, thereby liberating hemoglobin (a constituent of blood).

hemolytic reaction The lysis of red blood cells releasing hemoglobin. Usually a reaction due to parasitism or immunopathogenic mechanisms.

Hep-2 cells Cell line that can be used to grow certain organisms.

hepatotoxin A substance causing hepatotoxicity (the quality or condition of being toxic to the liver).

homologous antisera Serum containing an antibody or antibodies that is derived from a consistent source.

homology The quality or condition of corresponding in structure and evolutionary origin; having the same linear sequence of genes as another chromosome.

HPC Heterotrophic plate count.

hypochlorite A salt or ester of hypochlorous acid.

icosahedral A polyhedron having 20 faces.

IEM Immuno-electron microscopy.

IFA Immunofluorescent antibody.

immunosuppressed A reduced immune response of an organism to pathogens, also immunocompromised.

impetigo A contagious skin disease characterized by superficial pustules that burst and form characteristic thick yellow crusts.

indole A white crystalline compound, C_8H_7N, obtained from coal tar and used in perfumery, medicine, and as a flavoring.

infantile methemoglobinemia The presence of methemoglobin (a modified form of oxyhemoglobin) in the blood. Methemoglobin contains ferric iron with normal hemoglobin (an oxidized heme). Oxygen is held firmly so it cannot be pumped off, therefore it does not function in respiration, resulting in anemia.

infectious Capable of causing invasion by pathogenic microorganisms of a bodily part in which conditions are favorable for growth, production of toxins, and subsequent injury to tissue.

inositol Any of nine isomeric alcohols $C_6H_6(OH)_6$; especially one of these substances found in plant and animal tissue and classified as a member of the vitamin B complex.

isolate Something isolated from another substance.

jejunum The section of the small intestine that lies between the duodenum and the ileum.

labile Likely to undergo chemical change; unstable.

lactose A white crystalline disaccharide, $C_{12}H_{22}O_{11}$, made from whey and used in pharmaceuticals, infant foods, bakery products, and confections.

latent Present or potential but not evident or active.

leukocyte Any of the white or colorless nucleated cells occurring in blood.

lipid Fatty or waxy material.

lipolytic Has the power to produce lipolysis, which is the decomposition or splitting up of fat.

lysed blood Blood that has gone through the lysis process. Lysis is the dissolution; a loosing, setting free, releasing of. Usually the destruction/decomposition of the blood cell.

M-Endo Liquid growth medium used for detection of bacteria.

MacConkey agar Selective growth medium used for growth of many enteric bacteria.

Macroinvertebrate Visible invertebrate organism.

maximum contaminant level (MCL) USEPA-established standard.

megacolon Abnormally large colon; usually due to dilatation and hypertrophy. Usually seen in children.

meningitis Inflammation of any or all of the meninges of the brain and the spinal cord, usually caused by bacterial or viral infection.

mesenteric lymph glands Lymph glands that are found in and around the mesentery. This a membrane that connects portions of the intestines to the abdominal wall.

mesenteric veins Veins found in the peritoneal folds that connect the intestines to the dorsal abdominal wall.

mesophilic An organism whose optimal growth temperature is between 30° and 45° C.

metabolite Any of various organic compounds produced by metabolism.

methyl-red test A qualitative test for acid production. It is based on the use of a pH indicator, methyl red, to determine the hydrogen ion concentration present when an organism ferments glucose or other fermentable sugar.

MF Membrane filtration, a technique used to determine the number of coliforms in raw and treated water.

microbiology The science that deals with microorganisms (protists).

microvilli A microscopic projection from the surface of a cell.

MIO Media used for identification on the basis of motility, ornithine decarboxylase activity, and indole production.

mitochondria-bearing Organisms that carry mitochondria within the cytoplasm of their cells.

mitosis The sequential differentiation and segregation of replicated chromosomes in a cell nucleus that precedes complete cell division.

monoclonal antibodies Produced by cells that are cloned from a single hybrid cell and produce only one molecular species of antibody.

monotrichous Having one flagellum at only one pole or end, as certain bacteria.

morbidity Of, relating to, or caused by disease.

morphology The biological study of the form and structure of living organisms; the structure and form of an organism, excluding its functions.

mortality Frequency of number of deaths in proportion to a population.

motility Moving or having the power to move spontaneously.

MTF Multiple tube fermentation, a technique that requires water samples to be placed in a set of fermentation tubes that contain lactose or lauryl tryptose broth. Tubes are incubated at 35° C for 24 to 48 hours.

mucoid Any of a group of organic compounds similar to the mucins or mucoproteins, descriptive of a bacterial colony that is very sticky or stringy.

mucosal Mucous membrane.

myositis Inflammation of a voluntary muscle; seen in trichinosis or Sarcocystis infections.

necrotizing fasciitis Inflammation and necrosis of the fascia.

nematode A worm of the phylum Nematoda, having unsegmented, thread-like bodies, many of which, as the hookworm, are parasitic.

neonate A newborn.

neurocysticercosis The brain is infested with cysticerci (a form of larval tapeworm resembling Cysticercus), but having the cyst small and almost devoid of fluid.

neurotoxin A substance that can damage nerve cells.

noncommunity water system Water systems providing service to primarily transient populations, such as camps, hotels, and industries.

nonsporulating Does not produce spores.

nosocomial Disease acquired in a hospital.

obligate Must have a host to complete its life cycle.

oncogenic Tending to cause the formation of tumors.

ONPG O-nitrophenyl-B-D-galactopyranoside; tests for B-D-galactosidase produced by some coliforms.

oocyst The encysted form of some sporozoan zygotes.

operculum A lid or flap covering an aperture, such as the gill cover in some fishes or the horny shell cover in snails or other mollusks.

ornithine decarboxylase Biochemical test used in differentiating coliform types.

osteomyelitis Inflammation of the bone marrow.

otitis Inflammation of the ear.

ova The female reproductive cells of animals (eggs); ovum (egg) is singular.

ovoid Lemon-shaped.

oxidase Any of various plant or animal enzymes that act as oxidants.

pandemic Widespread; general; epidemic over an especially wide geographic area.

parasite An organism that grows, feeds, and is sheltered on or in a different organism while contributing nothing to the survival of its host.

paratenic host Host of third-stage larvae that infect humans.

parenchyma The tissue characteristic of an organ, as distinguished from connective tissue.

parenchymal cell Found in the liver.

PAS Periodic acid-Schiff, a staining procedure used to distinguish Microsporidia spores.

passeriform birds Perching birds and songbirds, such as jays, blackbirds, finches, warblers, and sparrows.

pathogen An agent that causes disease, especially a microorganism.

pathogenesis The development of a diseased or morbid condition.

pathogenicity Capable of causing disease.

PCR Polymerase chain reaction.

peptide Any of various natural or synthetic compounds containing two or more amino acids linked by the carboxyl group of one amino acid and the amino group of another.

perineum The portion of the body in the pelvis occupied by urogenital passages and the rectum, bounded in front by the pubic arch, in the back by the coccyx, and laterally by part of the hipbone.

peritoneal-dialysis effluent Fluid from the flushing of the peritoneal cavity.

peritonitis Inflammation of the membrane lining the walls of the abdominal cavity and enclosing the viscera.

PFU Plaque forming unit.

phenospecies Species that look alike.

phototaxis The movement of an organism in response to a source of light.

pica Abnormal craving for clay, paint, chalk, or other substances not fit for food.

pico- A combining form meaning one trillionth; 10^{-12}.

plasmid A genetic element occurring outside of the nucleus that is found in the cytoplasm of some bacterial cells.

polymerase Any of various enzymes that aid in the linkage of nucleotides in the formation of DNA or RNA, with an existing strand of DNA or RNA acting as a template.

polymyxin B Antibiotic; cyclic polypeptide; causes direct membrane damage by a detergent-like action.

pour plate A bacterial culture method in which an aliquot of sample is placed in a petri dish and melted; tempered agar growth medium poured in, mixed, and allowed to solidify; and the plate then incubated at an appropriate temperature.

prepatent period The time from infection to when parasites are seen in diagnosis.

prodromal Showing the symptom of the onset of a disease.

proteolytic Able to break down proteins into simpler, soluble substances, as in digestion.

protozoa Any of the single-celled, usually microscopic organisms of the phylum or subkingdom Protozoa, which includes the most primitive forms of animal life.

pseudopod Projections of cell membranes that move a cell.

psychrophilic Thriving at relatively low temperatures, usually at or below 15° C.

pustule A slight, inflamed elevation of the skin filled with pus.

PVA Polyvinyl alcohol.

quality control A system for ensuring the maintenance of proper standards in manufactured goods, especially by periodic inspection of the product.

R2A An agar; a low-nutrient medium used in heterotrophic plate counts.

reactive arthritis Inflammation of the joints; a result of injury, toxin exposure, etc.

rectal prolapse Protrusion of the rectal mucous membrane through the anus.

refractive hyaline cell wall A cell wall that has semitransparent properties and refracts light.

reverse osmosis A water filtration process using pressure to force water through a membrane.

RFLP Restriction fragment length polymorphism analysis.

ribosome A spherical cytoplasmic RNA-containing particle active in the synthesis of protein.

rifampicin An antibiotic that has both antibacterial and antiviral action.

rostellum Crown.

saccharolytic Has the capability of chemically splitting up sugar.

salt flotation A method by which one can concentrate parasites either through sedimentation or by flotation. Concentration is specifically designed to allow recovery of protozoan cysts, coccidian oocysts, microsporidian spores, and helminth eggs and larvae.

sanitary survey An investigation of the sanitary conditions of an area.

saprophytic A plant that derives its nourishment from dead or decaying organic matter.

schizogonic stage Asexual multiplication (merogony); multiple intracellular nuclear division precedes cytoplasmic division; reproductive stage that results in many merozoites.

schmutzdecke The carpet-like layer of bacteria, algae, and other microorganisms and inorganic and organic matter that forms on the surface of a slow sand filter and that aids in purifying the water.

scolex Head.

sedimentation The act or process of depositing sediment (material that settles to the bottom of a liquid).

selenite broth A selective enrichment medium used for the growth–isolation of *Salmonella*. Very inhibitory for most Enterobacteriaceae.

self-limiting Limiting itself, as in a disease that clears without treatment.

sepsis The presence of pathogenic organisms or their toxins in the blood or tissues.

septicemia A systemic disease caused by pathogenic organisms or their toxins in the blood stream.

seroepidemiology Study of disease outbreak–spread using serological responses.

serological group Related organisms distinguished by their antigenic properties.

serology The medical science that deals with serums (clear yellowish fluids obtained by separating whole blood into its solid and liquid components; the fluid from the tissues of immunized animals, used especially as an antitoxin; watery fluid from animal tissue, such as that found in edema).

serotyping A test to determine a group of related microorganisms distinguished by its antigenic composition.

sp. and spp. Abbreviations for species (singular and plural, respectively).

speciation The evolutionary process by which new species are formed.

species A fundamental category of taxonomic classification, ranking after genus and consisting of organisms capable of interbreeding.

spicule A small needle-like structure or part, such as one of the silicate or calcium carbonate processes supporting the soft tissue of certain invertebrates.

spore An asexual, usually single-celled reproductive organ; a microorganism, as a bacterium, in a dormant or resting state.

sporocyst A resting cell that produces asexual plant spores; a protective case containing spores of certain protozoans; a sac-like larval stage in many trematode worms.

sporogonic state, sporogony The production of spores resulting from sexual fusion of gametes prior to multiple fission, characteristic of certain protozoans.

sporont Parasitic cells with thickened membranes seen prior to becoming sporoblasts.

sporozoite A sporozoan that has been released from a spore and is ready to penetrate a new host cell.

sporulation Producing or releasing spores.

spp. (See sp.)

stylet A slender, pointed instrument; a surgical probe.

subacute Somewhat acute (reaching a crisis rapidly).

subcutaneous Located or found just beneath the skin.

substrate The material or substance on which an enzyme acts; a surface on which a plant or animal grows or is attached.

suppurative infection An infection associated with the formation or discharge of pus.

symptomatology The medical science of disease symptoms.

tachyzoite Rapidly multiplying forms of parasites.

taxonomy The science, laws, or principles of classification; the theory, principles, and process of classifying organisms in established categories.

tegument Outer covering of an organism.

tenesmus A painfully urgent but ineffectual attempt to urinate or defecate.

tetrathionate broth A peptone-based selective broth; used for the culture of *Salmonella* and *Shigella*.

thermophilic Pertaining to organisms whose optimal temperature for growth is above 50° C.

thiosulfate-citrate-bile salts-sucrose agar Has a color indicator—bromthymol blue; a selective medium used for culture of vibrios.

titer The concentration of a substance in solution or the strength of such a substance determined by titration (the process or method of determining the concentration of a substance in solution by adding to it a standard reagent of known concentration in carefully measured amounts until a reaction of definite and known proportion is completed); the minimum volume needed to cause a particular result in titration.

TOC Total organic carbon.

toxic Of or pertaining to a toxin (a poisonous substance having a protein structure secreted by certain organisms and capable of causing toxicosis when introduced into the body tissues, but also capable of inducing a counteragent or an antitoxin); harmful, destructive, or deadly.

transient Passing through from one place to another.

trimethoprim An antibiotic.

trophozoite A vegetative stage of amoeba.

trypsin One of the proteolytic enzymes of the pancreatic juice, important in the digestive processes.

tryptophane An amino acid, $C_{11}H_{12}N_2O_2$, produced in the digestive process and essential in human nutrition.

urea broth Hydrolysis of urea by urease releases ammonia. This causes a change in alkalinity and the color indicator (phenol red) will change from yellow to red. Urease-positive organisms produce a pink color while urease-negative organisms cause no change in the broth color.

vacuole A small cavity in the protoplasm of a cell.

vasculature The arrangement of blood vessels in the body or in an organ or part of the body.

vibrio Any of various S-shaped or comma-shaped microorganisms of the genus *Vibrio*, especially *V. cholerae*, which causes cholera.

virion Infective form of a virus.

virulent Extremely poisonous or pathogenic.

virus Any of various submicroscopic pathogens consisting essentially of a core of a single nucleic acid surrounded by a protein coat, having the ability to replicate only inside a living cell.

Voges-Proskauer test Used to assist in differentiating between different Enterobacteriociae.

waterborne Found in water or transmitted through water supplies.

zoonosis, zoonotic A disease such as rabies or malaria that can be transmitted from animals to man.

zygote The cell formed by the union of two gametes.

This page intentionally blank.

Index

NOTE: *f.* indicates a figure; *t.* indicates a table.

This page intentionally blank.

AWWA Manuals

M1, *Water Rates*, Fourth Edition, 1991, #30001PA

M2, *Automation and Instrumentation*, Second Edition, 1983, #30002PA

M3, *Safety Practices for Water Utilities*, Fifth Edition, 1990, #30003PA

M4, *Water Fluoridation Principles and Practices*, Fourth Edition, 1995, #30004PA

M5, *Water Utility Management Practices*, First Edition, 1980, #30005PA

M6, *Water Meters—Selection, Installation, Testing, and Maintenance*, Second Edition, 1999, #30006PA

M7, *Problem Organisms in Water: Identification and Treatment*, Second Edition, 1995, #30007PA

M9, *Concrete Pressure Pipe*, Second Edition, 1995, #30009PA

M11, *Steel Pipe—A Guide for Design and Installation*, Fourth Edition, 1989, #30011PA

M12, *Simplified Procedures for Water Examination*, Second Edition, 1997, #30012PA

M14, *Recommended Practice for Backflow Prevention and Cross-Connection Control*, Second Edition, 1990, #30014PA

M17, *Installation, Field Testing, and Maintenance of Fire Hydrants*, Third Edition, 1989, #30017PA

M19, *Emergency Planning for Water Utility Management*, Third Edition, 1994, #30019PA

M20, *Water Chlorination Principles and Practices*, First Edition, 1973, #30020PA

M21, *Groundwater*, Second Edition, 1989, #30021PA

M22, *Sizing Water Service Lines and Meters*, First Edition, 1975, #30022PA

M23, *PVC Pipe—Design and Installation*, First Edition, 1980, #30023PA

M24, *Dual Water Systems*, Second Edition, 1994, #30024PA

M25, *Flexible-Membrane Covers and Linings for Potable-Water Reservoirs*, Second Edition, 1996, #30025PA

M26, *Water Rates and Related Charges*, Second Edition, 1996, #30026PA

M27, *External Corrosion—Introduction to Chemistry and Control*, First Edition, 1987, #30027PA

M28, *Cleaning and Lining Water Mains*, First Edition, 1987, #30028PA

M29, *Water Utility Capital Financing*, Second Edition, 1998, #30029PA

M30, *Precoat Filtration*, Second Edition, 1995, #30030PA

M31, *Distribution System Requirements for Fire Protection*, Second Edition, 1992, #30031PA

M32, *Distribution Network Analysis for Water Utilities*, First Edition, 1989, #30032PA

M33, *Flowmeters in Water Supply*, Second Edition, 1997, #30033PA

M34, *Alternative Rates*, Second Edition, 1999, #30034PA

M35, *Revenue Requirements*, First Edition, 1990, #30035PA

M36, *Water Audits and Leak Detection*, Second Edition, 1999, #30036PA

M37, *Operational Control of Coagulation and Filtration Processes*, First Edition, 1992, #30037PA

M38, *Electrodialysis and Electrodialysis Reversal*, First Edition, 1995, #30038PA

M41, *Ductile-Iron Pipe and Fittings*, First Edition, 1996, #30041PA

M42, *Steel Water-Storage Tanks,* First Edition, 1998, 30042PA

M44, *Valve Installation and Maintenance*, First Edition, 1996, #30044PA

M45, *Fiberglass Pipe Design*, First Edition, 1996, #30045PA

M46, *Reverse Osmosis and Nanofiltration*, First Edition, 1999, #30046PA

M47, *Construction Contract Administration*, First Edition, 1996, #30047PA

To order any of these manuals or other AWWA publications, call the Bookstore toll-free at 1-(800)-926-7337.